AWAKEN THE
WELLNESS WITHIN

#1 Best-Selling author, Dr. Kaplan, is one of the most highly endorsed authors—ever! Dr. Kaplan and his books have been highly acclaimed and endorsed by such people as Donald Trump, Former Congressman Tom McMillen, Brian Tracy, Marla Maples, Kathy Coover, Norman Vincent Peale, Mark Victor Hansen, Duane Clemmons, Ken Blanchard, Patch Adams, Les Brown, Jack Canfield, Wally "Famous" Amos, Rudy Ruettiger, and many, many more.

Praise for *Awaken the Wellness Within*

Awaken the Wellness Within will change the way you think about healthcare and wellness. Finally, a practical book full with solutions for what is making us sick. Thank you, Dr. Kaplan.

—Dr. Fabrizio Mancini
BE FABulous, Dr. Fab
International Best-Selling Author, Speaker, and Media Personality
America's #1 "Healthy Living" Media Expert, World-Renowned Chiropractor,
and President Emeritus of Parker University.

Awaken the Wellness Within is an insightful resource for how we become ill and how we can awaken our inner natural power to become well.

—Dr. John Demartini
International Best-Selling Author of *Count Your Blessings: The Healing Power of Gratitude and Love*

According to World Health Organization stress-related diseases will be the number two cause of death in our generation. Don't be part of this statistic! Dr. Kaplan's new book *Awaken the Wellness Within* will help you deal with the ever-abundant social, environmental, and work-related stress we all face. So it's simple—read it, absorb it, live it, and share it!

—Dr. Peter Kash Ed.D./MBA
Biotech Venture Capitalist, Former Adjunct Professor Wharton School of Business, Visiting Professor Nihon University Japan and Hebrew University Jerusalem, Best-Selling Author of *Freedom from Disease, Make Your Own Luck*, and *Take Two Tablets: Medicine from the Bible*

In his new book, *Awaken the Wellness Within*, author Dr. Kaplan says, "There is only one disease, cytopathology, and two causes of disease, deficiency and toxicity." As a long-time medical intuitive healer, I could not agree more. Many people want to look good, and this is relatively easy up until the age of 30. At that point, deficiencies and toxicities become outwardly apparent. Most of us want to feel good and to have the vitality we search for, we must follow the principles Dr. Kaplan outlines here so simply and clearly, including positive mental attitude, exercise, proper diet, motivation, and taking responsibility. Few of us are aware how quickly our body regenerates. Follow the guidelines Dr. Kaplan blesses you within this book and you will not only feel good, you'll also end up looking good.

—Catherine Carrigan
Amazon #1 Best-Selling Author of *Unlimited Energy Now*

Game Over! *Awaken the Wellness Within* has peeled back all the layers and allows both doctors and patients to understand the root cause of disease. Dr. Kaplan has created the "plug & play" return-to-health game plan that empowers both doctors and patients alike with the tools necessary to reach the highest levels of heath and wellness possible.

The real "magic" is how Dr. Kaplan communicates concisely, congruently, completely and chiropractically the cellular message of health, (The 6 C's). Then again that is Dr. Kaplan's genius. His ability to deliver a message that resonates through every cell in your body. *Awaken the Wellness Within* is Dr. Kaplan's crowning achievement and a gift beyond measure for the readers fortunate enough to get their hands on this book that unlocks the door to one's own health and life potential!

—Dr. Perry Bard, DC
CEO Concierge Coaches

Awaken the Wellness Within is a revolutionary approach to healthcare. Exposing ObamaCare and providing a personal solution is the essence of this powerful book. This book is not only a must-read, it is a must for every person's personal health library. I will share this model with my patients so they can take a practical approach to health. Thank you, Dr. Kaplan.

—**Dr. Glenn Zuck**
Orthopedic Surgeon
Former Sports Fellow
Philadelphia Eagles/Flyers

As a pioneer in the natural healing movement, Dr. Eric Kaplan expounds upon an alternative paradigm for both the health professional and the lay person. Having healed himself from a so-called incurable condition, he fully embraces the mind-body connection to wellness. He points out that while lost in "a glut of complex and confusing health information" many do not understand their own power to heal, and thus become powerless and dependent. Seeking natural solutions to health rather than just prescribing a pill or a surgery, he says, "No doctor and no drug have ever truly healed anyone. They can only assist if they act in harmony with the laws of nature." There are many components to health, the combination of which results in either health or dis-ease. By breaking down the components, Kaplan educates the reader to become his own best healing advocate. This is a valuable book that paves the way for advancing the natural healing movement in the Western world of medicine.

—**Wendy E. Slater**
Quantum Healer
#1 Best-Selling Author of *Into the Hearth: Poems—Volume 14*

Thank you, Dr. Kaplan for having the inspiration to bring forth a new paradigm in health care. Our entire health care culture will evolve to the next level when they embrace your words of wisdom. Finally, someone has the insight and courage to reveal the truth about sickness and disease!

—**Dr. James Cronin, DC**

Dr. Kaplan's new book is destined to be a best seller as he clearly illustrates the innate power of every individual. *Awaken the Wellness*

Within is one of the few books I have ever read that clearly shows the reader that we have the power within us to live a healthy and abundant life, a life free of sickness and disease. Step by step, chapter by chapter, Dr. Kaplan proves that we are as strong and powerful as we want to be. That our body and mind can not only survive and eliminate illness but thrive no matter what obstacles or toxins are thrown at us on a daily basis. This book teaches us that it is never too late to apply these principals of health and longevity into our lives. As a nurse, a doctor, on behalf of myself and my patients, we want to thank you for all your passionate work. This book is a Life Changer.

—Dr. Ginny Steiner, DC, RN, BSN

Awaken the Wellness Within is another fine example of the easy-to-implement, new, and contemporary concepts for understanding wellness and healthcare shared by best-selling author Dr. Kaplan. A must-read for anyone who is looking to polish their communication abilities in this new era!

—Dr. Rob Jackson
Co-Author of *You Can Expect a Miracle: With Chiropractic*
CEO Back Talk Systems Inc.

Dr. Kaplan picks up where Dr. Deepak Chopra left off.

—Dr. Leo R. Boisvert, DC

The often neglected and forgotten definition of doctor is that it means to teach. Dr. Kaplan exemplifies that responsibility with his book *Awaken the Wellness Within*. Step by step he guides and educates his readers to understand the effects that deficiencies and toxicity have on our cells and how that reflects their ability to create wellness. Understanding the how to and why we need to maintain the integrity of our temple within is clearly defined throughout the book. His readers will come to understand a time-honored truth in a new paradigm. Essential knowledge for maintaining wellness in this challenging society.

—Dr. Pat Gibson
Amazon #1 Best-Selling Author

WOW. This is 21st century medical wisdom shared by an internationally renowned physician to his readers, just as a wise teacher would speak lovingly and personally to his students. Dr. Kaplan is a pioneer in a new paradigm of medicine that all physicians of all specialties will see as revolutionary now but as "why didn't I accept that" within a decade. Unlike other books in its category, *Awaken the Wellness Within* is not trendy, it is scientific truth. Cytopathology, or simply put, the health or illness of our cells, as Dr. Kaplan teaches us, is the root of health or disease. Do you want to live a life of vitality, wellness, mental acuity, passion, and longevity? Of course you do. The good news is that you have what you need right in your hands. AND, most importantly, share this gift with those you love the most. Like yourself, give them a present that brings years to their lives and life to their years.

—Steven M. Rosman, DC, PhD, Rabbi, MS
Dipl. Ac.(NCCAOM), LMHC (New York), Author, Director of Rosman Whole Person Healthcare, Wellness Clinic, in Sarasota, Florida

Dr. Kaplan has done it again: his book is easy to read and understand, teaches us the basics of health and wellness in a comprehensive new paradigm that exposes medical myths as well as getting to the cause of disease, while providing a pathway to health. This book is a must-read. I highly recommend it.

—Bob Mangat
#1 Best-Selling Author of *The Automated Entrepreneur*

Dr. Kaplan's new book *Awaken the Wellness Within* is a modern approach to healthcare. If your goal is to be healthy and you want to find the secrets to being healthy, Dr. Kaplan has exposed the truth about "inner Healing" and has template a modern, natural way to health and well being.

—Salvatore D. LaRusso DC, F.I.C.A.(Hon.)
Chair, I.B.C.E.
Director, N.B.C.E.

As Dr. Eric Kaplan so brilliantly points out, our bodies will heal themselves. We become vulnerable to attacks to our health due to our mental suggestions. If we recognize this is true, our diseases disappear. Dr. Kaplan's research is important, clear, and contemporary. His topic is very important in this day and age. His book, *Awaken the Wellness Within*, gives us a special gift of aha moments that can bring you health and joy.

–Dr. Anna Maria Prezio
Best-Selling Author of *Confessions of a Feng Shui Ghostbuster*

Our brains are wired to find things we're looking for; our spinal nerves are the pathways through our souls—if you're always cynical or waiting for things to go wrong, then your life will reflect that. On the other hand, having a positive outlook on life will bring you joy and provide you with inspiration when you least expect it. Dr. Kaplan from day one has always been a positive influence. He has not given up on me meeting my potential even when I have been cynical. His books are clearly genius.

—Dr. Tammy Costello
Myrtle Beach, SC

Too often people search for the answers to their health problems in the wrong places. *Awaken the Wellness Within* is the right place and is a valuable resource for discovering health solutions that begin at the very core of all our health issues. Dr. Kaplan's newest best-selling book teaches us to assume responsibility for our own well-being, to understand that the answers we hunger for lie within ourselves and he explains how we can...*Awaken the Wellness Within*. A book not to be missed!

—Dr. Michael Axelrod, DDS

Oral Health has a wide-ranging impact on our overall health and well-being. Dr. Kaplan's book will change the way we all look at the process of health and healthcare. His simple approach is a must read for all people concerned with their health and well-being. Bravo, Dr. Kaplan.

—Dr. Roy Hart, DDS
Developer of Power Flosser

In his book *Awaken the Wellness Within*, Dr. Eric Kaplan shares the underlying mechanisms of health and disease in easy-to-understand layman's terms for readers. I know first-handedly from my own healing experience from Crohn's Disease Colitis that what he shares in this book makes total sense and will assist people who are looking to take control of their health and lives to find their way back to wellness.

—Barbara Steingas
Author #1 Bestseller *Solving The Crohn's & Colitis Struggle*

Awaken the Wellness Within is surely destined to be a blockbuster that revolutionizes the health game. Dr. Kaplan finally puts into perspective precisely why health is not a game of chance, but rather a choice. From this day forward you no longer need to be confused about health. Through Dr. Kaplan's stories and useful techniques, you'll know how to unlock your innate healing potential. You've taken the first step. Now read and apply the wisdom, just like I am doing to improve my understanding of cellular health and take control of my health.

—Patrick K. Porter, PhD
Best-Selling Author and Inventor of BrainTap Technology

Awaken the Wellness Within is the missing book in health. If every doctor and patient would apply the information in it, their approach to health would change. Dr. Kaplan's message is one to be shared by the masses, which explains why wellness is your best health insurance! Thank you, Dr. Kaplan, for a most dynamic read!

—Dr. John N. Zilliox, DC CDN, DACBN
Positive Health and Wellness

Thank you! Thank you! Thank you! For years I've looked for different and better ways to help my clients reach their full health potential. I love the way *Awaken the Wellness Within* weaves together stories that are practical and inspiring. The bottom line every reader will walk away with is: The body will heal itself. It is our basic nature. The body is inherently healthy and self-healing and always strives to maintain or reestablish optimal healthy conditions. This is a book I can recommend to all my clients, family and friends. Dr. Kaplan has done it again!

—Dr. Cynthia J. Porter, PhD
Best-Selling Author/Speaker/Coach

Dr. Eric Kaplan has done it again! With *Awaken the Wellness Within*, he has done a masterful job of demonstrating the healing power of the human body, as well as how you can take control of your health and well-being. A must-read for anyone that is truly interested in learning and enjoying the benefits of a natural approach to health.

—Dr. Daniel T. Drubin
Best-Selling Author of *Busting Your Rut* and *Letting Go of Your Bananas*

Practicing for over 25 years, I believed I new everything on how to treat my patients naturally with optimizing their health. *Awaken the Wellness Within* just Awoke me to amazing new potentials I hadn't dreamed about! This is taking health care to a whole new level, and the ones who benefit are all our patients. Though it's been only a few months, I'm honored and privileged to call Dr. Eric Kaplan my Friend.

—Dr. Michael Failla
Ocean Integrated and Breakthough Wellness Centers of New Jersey

Dr. Kaplan nails it in his new book *Awaken the Wellness Within*! In our sick and diseased society, too many people fall for over-hyped drugs, without taking steps to fix their unhealthy behaviors. Dr. Kaplan digs through the popular myths and empowers you to upgrade your own health with Knowledge and Motivation. Read this book, and get yourself and your loved ones on the path to true health!

—Dr. Mark Mandell
Executive Director, Parker Professional Division of Parker University
Chairman of 1994 World Cup Opening Ceremonies Medical Staff

In simplicity there is elegance and in *Awaken the Wellness Within*, Dr. Kaplan takes a revolutionary and powerful new path toward dispelling old myths and actually enabling the reader to know how the body heals itself! Brilliant!

—**Dr. Larry Markson**
Author of *Talking to Yourself is Not Crazy*
Facilitator of The Cabin Experience

Dr. Kaplan's book empowers you to become the CEO of your health!

—**Dr. Luke Henry**
Chiropractic Physician

If I could have only one book on sickness, disease, and longevity, I'd choose *Awaken the Wellness Within*. Dr. Kaplan allows the ready to take control of their health and teaches the patient how to understand the power of the cell. This is one great book.

—**Dr. Thomas Ferrigno, DC**
Bay Area Disc Centers
www.BayAreaBackPain.com

Dr. Kaplan's advice on life, business, and health is priceless. I wish you great success on your new book *Awaken the Wellness Within*. You have been a great coach and mentor in my life. I look forward to teaching this formula and paradigm to all my patients and friends. A great read!

—**Dr. Timothy Peck, DC**

Innovators are often ridiculed for looking at the world in a different way. I don't believe Dr. Kaplan will be ridiculed for this newest work, but he will influence millions of people to start taking control of their own health in a better way with his unique insight and perspective on cellular vitalism.

—**Dr. Jeffrey L Dickhut**

Awaken the Wellness Within will set a new paradigm for health care in our country. His model provides a preventative and empowering model to the patients. Dr. Kaplan's One disease, One Cure philosophy is unique as well as simple. This book is a game changer to the health world. Thank you, Dr. Kaplan.

—Dr. Ralph D. Roles, D.A.C.A.N
Chiropractic Neurologist

Powerful, practical, and solid advice on health and longevity. Apply the knowledge and formulas set forward in this book and you'll fell better, healthier, and younger.

—Dr. Christophe Oliveira DC, DAAMLP
New Jersey Disc Center
DOT Certified Medical Examiner

Dr. Kaplan is always up on the new and relevant research. This is cutting edge stuff. His best book yet. This book is a must-read.

—Dr. Jonathan Donate, DC, MS
Author of *The Neck and Back Pain Solution*

The doctor who revolutionized my practice and improved the level of care I can provide my patients does it again! Dr. Kaplan's books are required reading for every doctor committed to unlocking their full potential and giving their patients the best care!! A must read.

—Dr. Edward Buonadonna BS, DC, F.I.A.M.A.

Awaken the Wellness Within is a revolutionary book that will change the way we view healthcare forever. Thank you, Dr. Kaplan.

—Dr. Eric Nepute
CEO Nepute Wellness Centers

As a health care leader in Jacksonville Florida, daily we are looking for a map to health for our patients. Dr. Kaplan's new book, new paradigm, will help patients get well, stay well and control their health destiny. I will give this book to all my patients. Bravo, Dr. Kaplan.

—**Dr. Royce McGowan**
McGowan Spinal Rehabilitation Center, Jacksonville Florida

Having met and worked with Dr. Kaplan only enhances my feeling towards his new book *Awaken the Wellness Within*. His book awakens the challenge in each of us to be healthy in a world dominated by chemicals. As a practicing doctor with my husband, Dr. Kaplan's lesson of life, love, and health will help change the world, one patient at a time.

—**Dr. Shelita McGowan**
McGowan Spinal Rehabilitation Center, Jacksonville Florida

Dr. Kaplan's new book is a guaranteed best seller. His book makes the diagnosis and treatment of disease easy and understandable. *AWAKEN THE WELLNESS WITHIN* will Awaken your inner healer. This book is a must-read.

—**Dr. Roger Huong**

I've followed Dr. Kaplan and have been a fan for over 30 years. His thoughts, ideas, and paradigms shape our industry. In a world where patients are overmedicated and not fully health educated, this book should be in everyone's health library. This is bound to be another #1 best seller. Great job, Dr. Kaplan. This book is a must-read.

—**Dr. Richard Harvey**

Dr. Kaplan's message will create a new health paradigm.

—**Dr. Reza Nikpour**
Optimum Chiropractic & Health Center, LLC

Awaken the Wellness Within will change the way the world thinks about healthcare. Thank you, Dr. Kaplan.

—**Dr. Russell Nersesov**
www.spinecareclub.com

Awaken the Wellness Within is a timely message for a nation ready to embrace a powerful healthcare revolution.

—**Arnold Kenyon, DC**

As a physician assistant, I am on the forefront of the battlefields of health care. Today's patient must assist the doctors in their quest for health and take a proactive approach. Dr. Kaplan, in his new book *Awaken the Wellness Within*, helps the patient achieve their health goals. A formula so simple, it is great to see a doctor think outside the box. This book is destined to be a best seller while impacting health care professionals and patients throughout the world.

—**Marvin West, PA**

For decades we've searched for a "magic bullet." Dr. Kaplan succinctly explains that the "magic" is within us all.

—**Dr. Jason Helton**

Dr. Kaplan's book *Awaken the Wellness Within* will awaken our innate spirit as well as open the eyes of our nation's healthcare community. This book will change the lives of my patients one cell at a time. Thank you, Dr. Kaplan.

—**Dr. Rich Lohr**

Awaken the Wellness Within is a great read. It is a must-read for health conscious people of all ages. It will change the way you look at your own health and wellness and offer real concrete examples which you can use everyday. Congratulations for Dr. Kaplan! He has done it again!

—**Michael Taylor, DC**

It's rare to find such honest advice in such an accessible format. This book will surely be a classic."

—**Dr. Charles A. Simpson**
Stuart, FL

This is a book that I would suggest to everyone interested in their health and their bodies. The new health paradigm he describes is right on target. Dr. Kaplan explains how we can heal our bodies from the ravages of cancer and more. We all take our bodies for granted until something happens. His explanation of how our bodies are built one cell at a time is amazing. I never quite looked at the human body in the way he describes. He reveals to the reader the key to living a longer, healthier, and better life. He tells, also, how long you live and the quality of your life is in your own hands. Ageless aging is about living without premature aging. I think this book is exactly what we need at this time of binge eating, junk food eating, and neglecting our bodies. A great read.

—**Kathy Zengolewicz**
Intuitive Healer, Author of the #1 bestseller *My Dragonfly Walt*

Dr. Kaplan has zeroed in on the core of good health seemingly long forgotten by Western Medicine—the fact that our bodies were designed to heal themselves. With the knowledge that our bodies can be compromised with toxins, stress, and poor food choices, Kaplan lays out the case for self-care to assure ourselves of increased health and longevity.

—**Maxine Taylor**
Author of three #1 best-selling books including
Move into the Magic and *Earthbound*

This book is *simply beautiful,* as most find living a healthy lifestyle intimidating; making them unable to start a daily practice. You will find your heart touched, your souls rejuvenated, and your feet grounded to making the right decisions for yourself in a world so grossly inundated with poor and overwhelming choices. Dr. Kaplan outdoes himself once again.

—**Dr. Alessandra Colón**
1 Advanced Rehab and Wellness
Woman of the Year Leukemia & Lymphoma Society

I believe things show up when least expected but most needed. That's exactly how I felt when reading Dr. Eric Kaplan's most recent book, *Awaken the Wellness Within*. He brilliantly shares the importance that cellular function has towards one's health. Not only a great read, but Dr. Kaplan explains in simple terms how to reclaim our dis-eased lives in order to heal ourselves one cell at a time. *Awaken the Wellness Within* is filled with up-to-date insight for people like myself who want to end their struggles with chronic conditions. A must-read!

—**Tracey Berkowitz**
Author of #1 Bestseller *Not My Buddy*

Dr. Kaplan's book, *Awaken the Wellness Within*, provides the foundation needed to understand the inner workings of our body. You will finish this book with a greater appreciation for the human body and all its capabilities plus a stronger will to lead a healthier, more authentic life. Dr. Kaplan weaves in his own expertise and experiences to help us find new ways to heal ourselves and slow the aging process. This book is a must-read for anyone who wants to look beyond traditional medicine for the answers to long-term sustainable health.

—**Erin Spitzberg, M.S., R.D.N., C.D.E.**
Registered Dietitian-Nutritionist, Certified Diabetes Educator
Author of #1 Bestseller *Eat Like a Normal Person*

This book encourages patients and doctors to use prevention as a source of wellness. Dr. Kaplan challenges the reader to gain and retain good health by choosing a healthy lifestyle. Rather than rely on modern Western medical approach with chemicals and surgery, he suggests educating ourselves about the body from the cells up to achieve health and longevity. His premise is that our bodies are meant to heal themselves. Ringing true, with a little help, we can heal with ease.

—**Dr. William R. Morris, PhD, DAOM, LAc**

AWAKEN THE WELLNESS WITHIN

A JOURNEY TO HEALTH & WELLNESS

DR. ERIC KAPLAN

Dedicated To & In Memory

This book is dedicated to Steven Kaplan, my older brother who was taken from his family and all who loved him prematurely from lung cancer. Steve would love to save others from the fate he received, and hopefully this book will "Awaken" others to the prevention formula to health care. Steve was a loving brother, father, husband, and grandfather. I will miss him.

My brother's wife, Gloria Kaplan. I am blessed to have her in my life; she is our sister for life.

Contents

Acknowledgements xxiii

Foreword xxv

Introduction: The Health Revolution xxix

Chapter 1: The New Health Paradigm 1

Chapter 2: Body, Heal Thyself 9

Chapter 3: The Body Perfect 21

Chapter 4: There Really Is Only One Disease 29

Chapter 5: Celling Health 47

Chapter 6: The Healer Within 63

Chapter 7: Celling Your Cells, Controlling Your Health 79

Chapter 8: Learning To Live Healthy 91

Chapter 9: Defeating Disease 99

Chapter 10: Cellular Healing Begins Today 113

Chapter 11: Cell City 125

Chapter 12: To Cell With You 139

Chapter 13: Stress Ages Our Cells 153

Chapter 14: Toxins And Disease 175

Chapter 15: Toxic Food Facts 191

Chapter 16: Deficiency And Disease 221

Chapter 17: Your Cells Need Antioxidants 249

Chapter 18: Awakening Our Wellness 263

Chapter 19: The Disease Known As Aging 283

Chapter 20: Cellular Cleansing 299

Chapter 21: Healing And Helping Our Cells................ 309

Chapter 22: Let's Begin To Heal......................... 319

Chapter 23: Chiropractic And The Fountain Of Youth 341

Chapter 24: A Natural Approach To Healthcare 361

Epilogue: Life Exist—LifeXist = The Future 375

References.. 389

Acknowledgements

———◦◉◦———

I want to acknowledge my wife, my muse of 35 years—Bonnie Kaplan—whose patience and understanding has been a blessing.

My two sons, Michael Kaplan and Dr. Jason Kaplan, my future healers. I am hoping the stories in this book will be passed from generation to generation. You both motivate me and inspire me to be my best. I love you both.

Jason's fiancée Dr. Stephanie Lyons—Welcome to the family.

I am also grateful to so many family members I've lost that have inspired me throughout my life, including my parents, Elsie & Mike Kaplan, for always pushing me and making my life and success possible.

To all my grandparents, for their love, belief, and support.

To my aunts and uncles no longer with us—Diane Adler, Herbert "Buddy" Adler, Herbert Punyon, Vivian Daniels, and cousins Doris & Milton Garfunkel, Norman Roth, Lou, Al, Marty and Dick Brenner, Jerome Shapiro, Ruth and Phil Zuck, and Milton "Mickey" Siegal.

Dr. Donald Gutstein was my professor, my mentor, and my friend. He turned boys into men, girls into women, and men and women into doctors. I am grateful for all that I am, realizing this man helped make me the man that I am

To my entire family—aunts, uncles, cousins—for their love and support.

To all my friends, for being my friends.

With special thanks to The Adlers, Alfonsos, Garfunkels, Axelrods, Bards, Beers, Brocks, Bernsteins, Chapnicks, Doughertys, Egittos, Friedels', Goldbergers, Harts, Harveys, Jillsons, Kaplans, Kaufmans, Lawleys, Littenbergs, Mattias, Meyers, Palladinos, Pattersons, Prestons Punyons, Rosens', Rubins, Rubachs, Siegelmans, Siegals, Zweckers, and Zucks.

I especially want to acknowledge the elders of my family, my Aunt Gloria Punyon, she has been there for me my entire life; she is my second mother and always inspired me and believed in everything I ever did.

To my nieces, Beth and Tracy, and my nephews, Richard and Josh, for their love.

To all my aunts, uncles, and cousins, especially the Adlers, Bernsteins, Brenners, Daniels, Garfunkels, Punyons, Siegals, Roths, and Zucks, for their belief in me as a child and their support of me as a doctor.

To all my friends, for being my friend.

To my partner Perry Bard, who pushed me to make this book happen.

To all my teachers, professors, coaches, and mentors too numerous to name, for guiding, tolerating and unselfishly teaching me

To my last remaining uncle, Milton Daniels, and cousins who I love like uncles and aunts—Jack Segall, Linda Siegel, Jerome and Barbara Levine, and Maxine Shapiro.

Foreword

Dr. Eric Kaplan, in his new book, *Awaken the Wellness Within*, implores us to learn more about how our body works and about how healthy lifestyles (including nutrients and exercise) help us to remain healthy. **This message cannot be overstated.** We can choose to do what is right for our body, and thus increase the chance for health and long life, or we can choose alternate paths and pay the consequences. We all have this choice to make, and our fates may depend upon the path we choose. Think wisely about it and make the right decision for health and wellness.

As an academic cardiologist (with decades of clinical practice, clinical research, teaching at a major university, and consultation to/for the agencies and industries that move medicine forward) I may not agree with each and every statement that Dr. Kaplan makes in his book. However, I do strongly endorse his overall aim, and focus, and message.

Having spent time with Dr. Kaplan, we both agree that prevention is the key to health and wellness. Too many people today rely too much and too soon on prescription medications in many circumstances (as even moreso on under-regulated over-the-counter agents and supplements). Activity, diet, and other good-health lifestyles may delay or prevent the diseases that can require drugs or medical procedures. Also, both patients and physicians know less about drugs and their potential interactions than they should, so avoiding or limiting them when possible can be beneficial. However, nutrition and healthy lifestyles alone will not guarantee a disease-free world or disease-free patients throughout their lives, and prescriptions and procedures can be essential, life-saving, and life-preserving. This book is not meant to keep patients away from proper and necessary medical care, but to prevent the need for such, where possible, through good health habits and fuller understanding of the basis for them. Nonetheless, before engaging in any lifestyle change, discuss with your family physician.

The essence of this book is that it challenges both the patient and the doctor to look towards prevention as a source of wellness. This book is about choices. Dr. Kaplan asks the reader to choose a natural healthy lifestyle. He asks the reader to work with his or her doctor or doctors. We live in the greatest country with the best health care potential in the world. But, Dr. Kaplan's book puts the onus of health as much on the patient as it does his or her healthcare provider(s). This is a good thing if he/she follows its path.

Dr. Kaplan is without doubt correct in the overall message he is trying to convey. If we understand how our bodies work – what keeps our cells and organs healthy and functioning properly and what can help them heal from within when something goes wrong – we will almost certainly lead healthier and happier lives and will need to rely on medications and procedures, on physicians and hospitals, less often than our current society does. Accordingly, I endorse Dr. Kaplan's effort in this book to move us towards making better decisions about our lifestyles and to understand why and how this can benefit us all, both individually and societally.

—James A. Reiffel, M.D.
Professor Emeritus of Medicine,
Columbia University, College of Physicians and Surgeons

Recently, I have had the opportunity to work with Dr. Eric Kaplan and his partner, one of my oldest and dearest friends, Dr. Perry Bard. We came together working on two new formulas to aid the body with stress. They are called StressAM and StressPM. One of the principle ingredients of these products is a natural compound found in our bodies called Phosphatidylserine or PS. PS has been extensively studied for its protective effects against stress on our bodies.

As a Neurologist, it is working with the body that so amazes me, inspires me, and enlightens me. I am always looking for a simpler way to help my patients. My life has been dedicated to healing and helping the body reach its potential. For our body to be well, we must handle stress.

Janice Kiecolt-Glaser, professor of psychology and psychiatry at Ohio State, in a recent study focused on 119 men and women taking care of spouses with dementia. The health of the caregivers was compared with that of 106 people of similar ages not living under the stress of constant caregiving.

Blood tests showed that a chemical called Interleukin-6 sharply increased in the blood of the stressed caregivers compared with blood of the others in the test. Previous studies have associated IL-6 with several diseases, including heart disease, arthritis, osteoporosis, type-2 diabetes, and certain cancers. Even more compellingly, both IL-6 and CRP are strongly associated with major depression.

The body consists of a trillion cells that reproduce themselves on a continuous basis. The laws of nature are universal and constant, 24 hours a day, 7 days a week, 365 days a year. We live in a busy world governed by laws, natural and unnatural, and as the population of our world continues to grow, the production and demand for technology will continue to grow. It is because of this increase in demands, that both our bodies and brains must navigate to not only survive but to thrive.

Dr. Eric Kaplan and his new book *Awaken the Wellness Within* works with the laws of nature breaking health down to its simplest level: The human cell. The reader will be taken on a journey of wellness, to "Awaken" the bodies innate healing powers and allow the reader to take charge of their health and their health's destiny.

—Dr. Jay Lombard

Dr. Jay Lombard, Co-founder and Chief Scientific Officer and Medical Director at Genomind, served as the chief of Neurology at Bronx Lebanon Hospital where he led the Stroke Unit. He is also a former clinical assistant professor of neurology at New York Presbyterian Hospital, clinical instructor of Neurology and Medicine at Albert Einstein College of Medicine, and chief of Neurology at Westchester Square Medical Center and the Brain Behavior Center.

He has had numerous television and radio appearances including appearances on Larry King, Dr. Oz, CBS News, Fox News, The Early Morning Show, and others. He was also invited to present at TEDMED 2012.

He is a best-selling author whose books include:

Balance Your Brain, Balance Your Life: 28 Days to Feeling Better Than You Ever Have Freedom from Disease

The Brain Wellness Plan: Breakthrough Medical, Nutritional and Immune-Boosting Therapies to Prevent

Introduction

THE HEALTH REVOLUTION

"The Road to Health is **Always Under Construction**." We are all born healthy and perfect, and then as we age something goes wrong. No longer abundant with health, no longer at our ideal weight, no longer happy, we look within. What went wrong? Well maybe you were duped. We live in a chemical world. Our lives, our bodies, are bombarded with chemicals. With so many toxins thrown at us daily, it's amazing we are healthy at all. Or are we?

A life out of balance will catch up with you eventually—and everyone is out of balance. We generate illness (and wellness) in our lives in various ways. This is one of the tenets of medicine: that health and illness are not only things that happen to us, but also things that we do, a kind of behavior.

This book is about awakening your inner healer, finding the wellness within. This book will focus on cellular health and offer a new paradigm of health and disease. The interaction of all human cellular and physiological systems connects the body and mind in definite but extremely complex ways that innately work in harmony. In essence, there is only one disease: cytopathology.

This is a new type of thinking, a new type of knowledge. It's hard to overstate how far that "obvious" idea has come.

Only a few years ago, medical scientists actually believed that the nervous system and the immune system had nothing to do with each other—how interesting! This seems absurdly short-sighted to the same scientific community today. Of course, it was not the nervous and immune systems that weren't communicating, but neurologists and immunologists! When they finally did start talking to each other, they discovered that their systems of study were totally interconnected—physically, neurologically, chemically, and electrically. The body works as a whole, yet when in comes to disease, usually only one area initially becomes weakened. If someone had heart disease, liver disease, kidney disease, etc., it would be the cells specific to that organ that began to malfunction. When one area or organ weakens, the other areas step up to help the body heal itself. Your body literally goes to war to ward off invaders and bring the body back to health.

Since then, mind-body science has expanded to the point where distinguishing it from physiology is unnecessary and there is now a lot of hard evidence showing the many ways that our physical and mental experiences are intertwined. To *Awaken the Wellness Within*, you have to think healthy thoughts, set healthy goals, be proactive in regard to your health.

We all know that eating right can help you maintain a healthy weight and avoid certain health problems, but your diet can also have a profound effect on your mood and sense of well-being. Studies have linked eating a typical Western diet—filled with dairy, caffeine, red and processed meats, packaged meals, takeout food, and sugary snacks—with higher rates of depression, stress, bipolar disorder, and anxiety. Eating an unhealthy diet may even play a role in the development of physical and mental health disorders such as

ADHD, Alzheimer's disease, and schizophrenia, or in the increased risk of suicide in young people. What we are saying is yes, you are what you eat, where you live.

When it comes to advice about how to live a long and healthy life, there's a lot of confusing, conflicting noise out there. One minute we're told something is good for us—the magic cure to end our fatigue, weight gain, or illness. And the next minute we're told it's entirely ineffective or worse—something harmful that we should avoid. Not to mention, the rapidly increasing rates of obesity, autoimmune disorders, diabetes, and heart disease in our western world suggest that something about the advice we follow and our conventional thinking is simply wrong.

If you've tried diets, exercise programs, and health regimes, but have experienced only short-lived or limited success and you're confused and frustrated about why it's been so hard to achieve lasting results, you're in exactly the right place. To *Awaken the Wellness Within*, it starts with understanding both health and disease and learning it all begins with one single cell.

Jerry Seinfeld, in his best-selling book *SeinLanguage*, says, "Everyone wants to be healthy, but no one knows where to begin." We begin here—now—today. Although he is a comedian, this is a very true statement. Modern medicine has made health and health care so complex. Today in our country, there are so many diseases and so few cures. My goal is to let you know that everything you will need to get well and stay well you already have, that *"the power that created the body heals the body."*

My original working title for this book was *Body by God*, however I didn't want the public to think this was a religious book; it is a book that will help anyone with any disease, or anyone who simply wants to be healthier. Although I do not consider myself a religious man, I do believe in the power of the universe. Regardless of your religion, our maker could not make such a great machine as the human body and have it be flawed. As winter turns to spring,

spring to summer, and summer to fall, nature always prevails. Babies are still born in nine months, regardless of how far modern medicine has come. Two lovers get together and leave in the hands of nature a baby, no studying practicing changes the timeline. No religion or color alters this timeline. Nature has laws and it knows what it is doing. Yet when we get ill, we forget this perfect machine knows what it is doing.

So why is it that we get sick? Maybe we have altered the state of our bodies through additives, preservatives, chemical concoctions that we would not feed to animals, yet we consume daily. No wonder we are a world in chaos, disease like cancer is on the rise, cures are on the decline.

Now imagine if there was really only one disease and one cure. Sounds simple. Well guess what? It is. *Awaken the Wellness Within* follows this new paradigm that there is **only One disease and only One cure**.

ONE DISEASE—TWO CAUSES—ONE CURE

This is a health paradigm made simple. You will learn throughout this book that there is only one disease, two causes of disease, and ONE CURE. This concept will change the way doctors and patients will look at health. Imagine if there was a machine that could cure everything and anything? It now exists. This machine is called the human body; a body made of a trillion cells and that, when working in harmony, has the ability to cure and heal anything.

My wife, the love of my life and muse, said write a book that explains health in easy-to-understand language. This concept of health and disease is scientifically grounded in cutting-edge cellular biochemistry and basic physiology. My life has been a journey; working with my sons on this book has been my dream. Hopefully you will find that this book provides you a simple and natural approach to healing. A concept and paradigm to prevent and/or reverse almost any disease—the ultimate triumph over disease.

My Partner, Dr. Perry Bard, was instrumental in me finishing this book. He stated, "A book like this is needed now more than ever." With ObamaCare on the brink and healthcare costs rising annually, it is a travesty that American people's health continues to decline.

The average person is lost in a glut of complex and confusing health information. When we do get sick, though, not understanding why we are sick or how to become well, we feel like powerless victims, subject to seemingly random infections and genetic predispositions.

As a chiropractor and acupuncturist, my life has always sought natural solutions to health. Why is it today that most Americans feel helpless? Simply because many of our concepts of germs and disease are outdated.

The average American remains stuck in the archaic germ theory. Yet I was not brought up with a fear of germs. Now wherever you go people are scared to even shake hands. Most of the people in the world today worry daily about their bodies being invaded by germs and microorganisms. Yes, disease is all around us, but we beat disease by maintaining healthy bodies, healthy cells. Sounds simple—healthy people don't get sick. We need to focus on building and maintaining the overall health and function of our cells. Disease is not a random event; it is an accumulation of bad habits. The good news is we can choose to prevent it, provided that we know how. Health is determined by what we, as individuals, are willing to do for ourselves; it is our responsibility.

Health is not a game of chance; health is a choice. Whether we realize it or not, the daily choices we make have a direct impact on the health of our cells. When we make the wrong choices our health takes a turn for the worse. The problem is compounded when we blame our genetics, our age, our environment, rather than accepting responsibility for the way we eat, exercise, and live our lives. In truth, the only way to heal any disease is to improve and optimize our cells' function by correcting cellular malfunction, the common denominator of all disease.

Modern medicine has a poor understanding of disease and relies on treating, thus suppressing, the symptoms of disease rather than addressing its true cause. It is scary to believe that most of us die from chronic and degenerative diseases—such as cancer and heart disease—that are "treated" but seldom healed.

I was inspired to write this book after my brother died at the young age of 66 years old. Steve developed lung cancer, but not a common lung cancer. By the time he was diagnosed the jury was already in. Approximately eight months later, after grueling chemotherapy, Steve joined my parents with God. It is very difficult for any doctor to have an ailing family member. I wanted so much to help my brother, cure my brother, but his cancer was so far progressed. Steve was a special person, my big brother; he had the good genes. He was rarely sick and I think had only one cavity his whole life. Yes, he smoked when younger, but quit over 30 years ago. Plus, his cancer was unique, it mimicked mesothelioma. That was actually the original diagnosis. Now, what you must consider is that the right lobe was covered in cancerous tumors, but none on the left. Well how could that be? How could one area be affected and not the other? The more I questioned Steve's dilemma, the more my One Disease theory of cellular malfunction made sense.

As I stated in Steve's eulogy, a person dies twice in a lifetime. Once, when they stop breathing, the other, when we forget their name. My goal is for this book to give Steve a life beyond his years and to extend the lives of my readers.

So I began to ask why some people get cancer and others don't. Why the lung and not liver, spleen, or gallbladder? Why are some parts of the body affected and not all at the same time? How does the body differentiate? Why do some people get better from cancer or any disease and others don't? You will learn that cells in certain areas of the body malfunction, this is called cytopathology. "Cyto" means cell and "pathology" means disease, so cytopathology refers to diseased cells. The medical world may put names on every symptom, but wouldn't it be simpler if they acknowledged that there is only one disease, two causes, and one cure?

The definition for cytopathology may be not fancy or eloquent, and it may even seem too simple to some doctors and scientists; however, in my opinion and the opinion of many of my peers, it is the most profound, precise, and irrefutable definition of disease. The fact is this definition is so simple that no one—scientist, physician or layperson—can deny it. This definition provides the unifying theory of health and disease that the modern medical establishment lacks, which is the reason that modern medicine is unable to address the current epidemic of chronic disease that is now running rampant in our country.

Once cellular malfunction begins, our bodies go to war in a fight for survival; the good cells begin to fight the bad cells. One such example is in chemotherapy; chemotherapy kills all the cells and hopes only the good cells will grow back. The doctors, oncologists, try to attack and kill the specific cancer cells. So as you can see, all disease begins at the cellular level, and this book is about cellular health and healing.

Let's face the facts; concern for our health is something we all have in common. We would all like to live a high-quality, disease-free life no matter how long that life may be. But most of us have no idea that a disease-free life is possible, so our priorities become out of whack, and we form habits that jeopardize our health. Then we ignore the early signs of ill health and, without knowing it, we lay the groundwork for disaster.

My goal is for this book to be an alternative paradigm for health professionals and laymen alike. My goal is for you to think of this book as a guide to health in one easy lesson. Everyone, especially our children, should learn about this cutting-edge approach to health and disease. In the past, health and disease have seemed like mysteries over which we have little control, but no longer. Now we do have control. Knowing of just one disease, two causes of that disease, and the cure lying inside each and every one of us gives us the power to get well and stay well. Take back your life and take control of your destiny!

ONE DISEASE

Cytopathology

TWO CAUSES

Deficiency   Toxicity

ONE CURE

"It is health that is real wealth and not pieces of gold and silver."

—Mahatma Gandhi

Chapter 1

THE NEW HEALTH PARADIGM

There is a new way of health care today in our world, a new change of paradigm. There is only one disease (cytopathology), two causes of disease (deficiency and toxicity), and one cure (treat the cause by healing the weakened cells). Protect the cell, offset disease, and start to "*Awaken the Wellness Within.*"

Now, the "One Disease, Two Causes, One Cure" theory of health and disease may shock the world of medicine. Or do they already know this? I began to think of this concept when watching one of my son's medical school lectures. The teacher was trying to teach these young interns the true cause of disease—its symptoms, its pathways, its causes. Every disease related back to the cell— it sounded so simple. I watched as my son listened to every word, his medical training now starting to make sense. Why have doctors made health so complex?

What if I told you that today modern science has a way to heal cancer, cure most all diseases, and even turn back the clock naturally. There's a lot we can do for ourselves to be happier and healthier—far more than just taking pills. We can observe our lifestyle habits and boost those that need improving.

Exercise, like diet, takes time and discipline—gimmicks won't hasten or change the process. You are building a new and better life, so don't skimp on the materials. Now let's discuss the specifics of your foundation for good health.

1

A study from Harvard Medical School indicated that almost 1/3 of the 9 million Americans over 65 are taking drugs that should never be taken by the elderly.

The Citizen Health Research Group, which is a public-based company in Washington, D.C., found that people over the age of 60 take 40% of all prescription drugs. The average number of prescriptions given to people over 60 is 15 per year; 37% of these people are taking 5 or more drugs a day. How do we educate our children about the difference between good and bad drugs?

The solution to this problem is that the FDA should follow the precedent set by the Commission E, which allows the public to have confidence in homeopathic remedies for sale. Germans can readily buy these over-the-counter remedies in retail stores. In Germany, all physicians have a level of training of these botanical remedies in medical school. In fact, according to a new survey, 80% of German physicians prescribe phytonutrients or plant medicines, which account for 27% of all over-the-counter medicines sold in Germany.

In Germany, Commission E does double-blind human studies on herbal botanical remedies, whereas the FDA in this country only utilizes these standards for pharmaceutical drugs. I find it ironic that last year over one-billion dollars was spent on vitamins in this country, and these vitamins are often being "prescribed" by a salesperson at a health food store who lacks formal, or even limited, training in health care, nutrition, or homeopathy. I am amazed at the number of people who walk in and ask the salesperson what they recommend for ailments such as headaches and arthritis. It is time our country "stepped up" and "looked up" to Germany's model and invest in creating an alternative protocol.

A recent report on 20/20 showed that in Germany, the herb St. John's Wort was recommended for depression 20:1 over Prozac. Yet in this country, Prozac is the number one prescribed medication for depression, at a cost of approximately $1.7 billion a year, in spite of

Prozac's great disfavor by many physicians and consumers because of its sometimes fatal side effects. According to Commission E, there are no known formidable side effects of St. John's Wort in the treatment of depression. Shouldn't we choose the remedy with the least side effects first?

Dr. David Eisenberg's report in the *New England Journal of Medicine* showed that in 1990, Americans made 425 million visits to alternative care providers, which is more than the visits to all conventional care practitioners. It was this wake-up call that finally moved this country away from ignorance about this issue.

We cannot rest on our laurels that we won WWII—over 70 years ago. Instead, we must look at what the Germans and Japanese have accomplished over the past 70 years. They have exceeded us economically and have developed a health delivery system that many professionals believe is superior to ours.

The Industrial Revolution brought us many conveniences. Thanks to washing machines, we don't have to go down to the creek to launder our clothing. We can jump on a power mower to keep our lawns trim. We don't walk or ride our bicycles because now we have cars. We don't climb stairs if an elevator is available. Modern amenities can be wonderful, but they can also deprive us of the vitally needed exercise that was all in a day's work for our forbearers. Without daily exercise, we store our unreleased energy as fat. We lose touch with our physical well-being. We lose touch with the life energy that surges within us.

Only sick people become sick. Once you start to compromise your cells' health, a cascade of events is subject to follow. Once a critical number of cells begin to malfunction, their internal communications and self-regulation systems become debilitated, destabilized, and in some cases disabled. Once the numbers of compromised cells or malfunctioning cells increases, the effects are compounded and disease will occur.

Before anyone can exhibit noticeable signs of any disease, normal cell function has to be compromised significantly throughout the body. Vulnerability to infections, for example, is created by widespread cellular malfunction. An infection indicates that cellular malfunction already has weakened the immune system. Having a cold or the flu is an alarm screaming at you that your body and cells are not well—healthy people resist infections in the first place. Few of us pay attention to these alarms. We think that having a cold or the flu is normal, and that once the symptoms are gone we are well again. How did we get well? Our good cells overcame the bad cells, thus our body healed itself.

We are of the generation that most people expect that their bodies generally take care of themselves, provided they don't smoke, drink to excess, or fall prey to some unstoppable virus or some predetermined genetic disease. Most people believe that as long as they avoid "fattening" foods, they are eating a healthful diet. On all counts, these people are unfortunately wrong.

One of the most important things you need to fight disease and to encourage your health is the knowledge of what caused your disease in the first place and how to heal yourself. This book will hopefully teach you how to prepare and what to pack for a healthy journey through the rest of your life. The small amount of time you will spend reading this chapter and every future chapter will be an investment worth making: It just may save your life. Knowledge is power, and you are about to plug into a tremendous energy source.

A cabinet stocked with medicines, a list of doctors to call, and a head filled with commercial endorsements, medical studies, and drug warning labels do nothing to give you what you need: a true understanding of what makes you sick or how to get well. Without that understanding, you can be caught up in a whirlwind of medical procedures and pharmaceuticals that suppress your cells and treat your symptoms, but, unfortunately, will not treat the cause of your symptoms or disease.

There are no shortcuts to good health, and if we do not accept this truism, we will find ourselves in the position of the young contractor in a story told by Tremendous Jones.

It seems this young contractor was married to a contractor's daughter. The father-in-law wanted to give the young man a boost in his career.

"Son," he said, "I don't want you to start at the bottom where I did. So I want you to go out and build the most tremendous house this town has ever seen, put the best of everything in it, make it a palace, and turn it over to me."

Well, this was an opportunity to make a killing. He hurried out to slap together a building that would survive two fairly stiff gales.

In short order, he was back to dear old dad. "Well, Dad, it's finished."

"Is this the palace like I asked?"

"Yes-siree, Dad."

"Is it really the finest house ever built, Son?"

"Yes-siree, Dad."

"All right, where is the bill? Is there a good profit in it for you?"

"Yes-siree, Dad."

"Very good. Here is your check, and where is the deed?"

As he looked at the deed, the father said, "I didn't tell you why I wanted that house to be the best house ever built. I wanted to do something special for you and my daughter to show you how much I love you. Here, take the deed, go live in the house you built for yourself."

The young gold-bricker crept out a shattered, frustrated man. He thought he was making a fortune at his father-in-law's expense by saving money on inferior materials and short-cuts; he cheated only himself.

The purpose of this book is to empower, inspire, and enable people to take a more natural approach to their health and happiness. We can each enhance our health, happiness, and well-being one cell at a time.

> *"The past is history, the future is a mystery,*
> *but this moment of life is a gift, and that is why we call it*
> *'The Present'."*

I dedicate every moment of my gift, of My Present, to coordinate conventional and alternative medicine into our system so that a sickness-based model will be part of the future. The emergence of alternative medicine is the beginning of a revolution—a health revolution demanded by a public that is "sick and tired" of being sick and tired. We cannot rest on our laurels of being a super-nation if we are not leaders physically, mentally, emotionally, and morally.

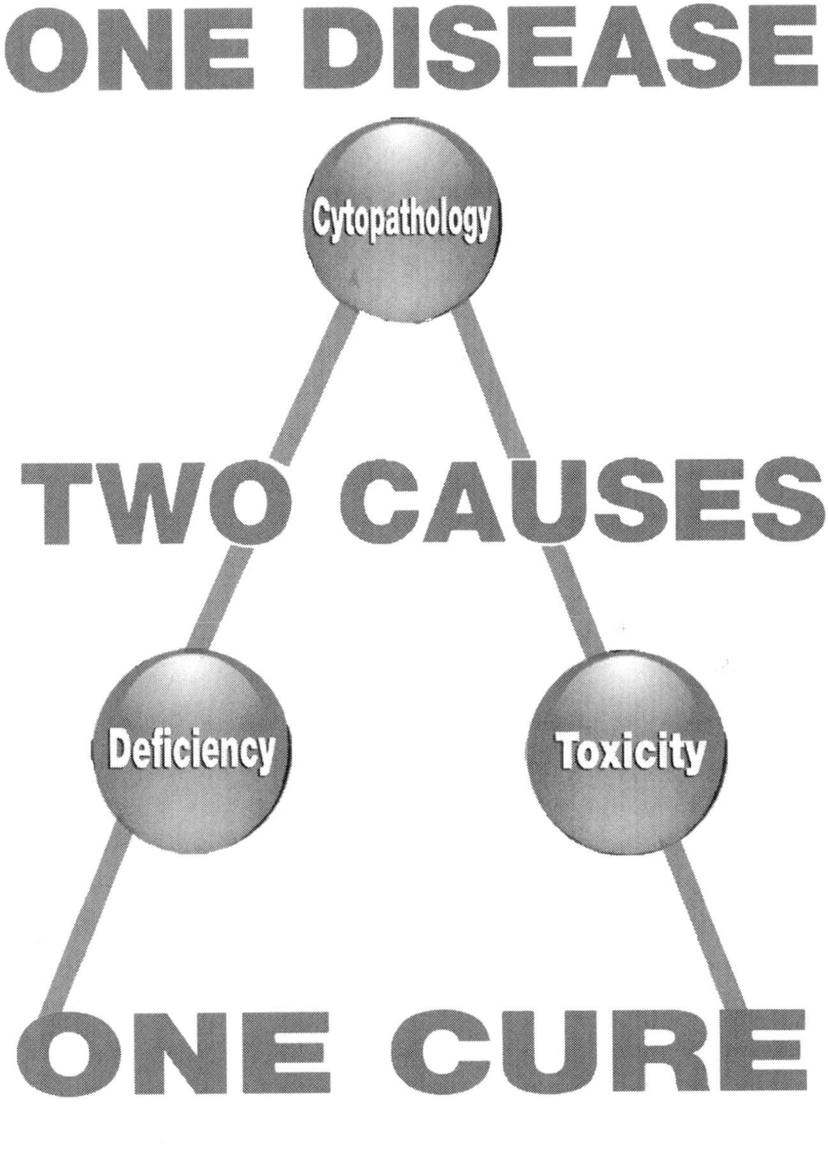
ONE DISEASE
Cytopathology
TWO CAUSES
Deficiency
Toxicity
ONE CURE

"To keep the body in good health is a duty . . . otherwise we shall not be able to keep our mind strong and clear."

—BUDDHA

Chapter 2

BODY, HEAL THYSELF

The beauty of the body, and every cell, is that they both have the power to heal themselves. *The power that created the body has the power to heal the body.* No doctor, no drug, no supplement, no object has ever truly healed anyone on its own. They can only assist the body and only then if they act in harmony with the laws of nature.

In Florida, many of us travel throughout the summer. We begin to plan our summers around Christmas. Before going on our trip, we study maps, we check hotels and airfares, we read brochures, get the proper currency, and research local customs—there is so much preparation. We want the best trip, the best vacation. We want nothing to go wrong. The sad news is we rarely give this much time and attention to our bodies and our health. So my friends, the question I ask you is, "What could be more important than your health?"

Most people take their bodies for granted until something goes wrong. We expect our body to take care of itself, regardless of what we put into it. One of the most important things you need to live a longer healthier life is to have knowledge of your body. You need to understand sickness and how to work toward health. This chapter teaches you to prepare yourself for a healthy journey; a healthy life can make every day feel like a great vacation. Let's prepare ourselves for a good journey and good life as we travel inside the body and learn the future of health care.

The human body has the ability to repair any damage that is not extensively injured beyond restoration. It all begins with the cell—cell health and cell rejuvenation. Heal the cell and you heal yourself. Preserve the cell and you preserve yourself. To be healthy each day, old cells must be replaced with new ones, and each must continue to perform all of its specified functions.

This sounds simple, and it is. The cell is the key to health and longevity. So what have we learned about cell replication, rejuvenating, and healing? When there is damage to your body's cells, the healthy cells from other areas will rush to the affected part, remove the dead cells, replace them with healthy cells, and restore the part like new. As long as the antigen or foreign body causing the damage is removed, the obstacles to healing will be removed.

Do you know what raw materials you need daily to build healthy cells? Do you believe it is possible to build healthy cells with junk food? Foods loaded with chemicals and preservatives like candy, cakes, white bread, salt, sugar, coffee, donuts, pizza, potato chips, French fries, ice cream, and soda. These foods represent a great portion of the American diet, which is why we are considered an overweight nation.

How many of the raw materials that your cells need to be healthy do any of those foods contain? The answer is not many, which is why chronic disease is so prevalent in our country and obesity is on the rise.

The cell is the key to health and longevity. A chronic shortage of vitamins, minerals, water, oxygen, and other nutrients may cause your cells to malfunction. Malfunctioning cells are weakened cells that will give way to shorter telomeres. Throughout this book, you'll learn how it's imperative to maintain and even grow the length of your telomeres to stay young and healthy.

Every day you make health choices when you order fast food, when you smoke, don't exercise, or drink too much. You also make health choices when you get proper rest, exercise, take supplements, read positive material, and serve others. Life and health are about the right choices. When we make the right choices, our cells stay strong and our telomeres remain long.

Cells are created and maintained by extremely complex actions and interactions, but nature, in its infinite wisdom, knows how to take care of that complexity. We call this innate intelligence.

Your job from this chapter forward is simple: Make certain your cells get what they need and do not expose them to what could harm them.

This book will teach you how to nourish your cells and maintain a happy life. Your body, your castle, will always work to protect your cells. Cellular health is the key to total health. A healthy body has healthy cells. Sick or malfunctioning cells will lower our immunity and make us vulnerable to sickness and disease. When you protect your castle with strong cells through a strong cellular membrane, it can ward off antigens. Antigens are also known as foreign invaders. They are not welcome in your kingdom. As long as the antigen causing the damage is removed, the obstacles to healing will be removed. Now that you sit on the throne of your kingdom and know you are in charge, protect your castle, your kingdom, for your cells are your servants. They serve you daily and ask only to be treated fairly with respect. What kind of king or queen are you?

Each cell has an outer cell wall—the membrane—whose purpose is to keep out toxins, bacteria, viruses, and other harmful substances while still allowing nutrients to reach inside where they are needed. The membrane also prevents healthy and necessary substances from leaking out of the cell, while still allowing waste products to be excreted. These membranes are made of fats. You will learn throughout the book that there are good and bad fats. Bad fats slow the body down, make the cells vulnerable, and weaken our bodies. One of the key parts of cells are the powerhouses called mitochondria. They create energy and assist the cells in producing all the body needs, such as neurotransmitters, hormones, and antibodies. Your cells also have electrical and communication systems that help to keep everything working in balance. Cells have many important jobs to perform during every second of every day; anything that interferes with these tasks is a threat to our cells and eventually our total health.

The fact is that any toxin or any nutrient deficiency will affect the body's cells. Simply, a chronic shortage of vitamins, minerals, water, oxygen, or other nutrients may cause your cells to malfunction. You may be unaware that this malfunction is happening, particularly at the early stages, but a chronic shortage of even one nutrient eventually makes you sick. So what are you beginning to learn? You are learning the cell is the key to our health, and the cell must be void of toxins. You've also learned that cells require certain foods and vitamins or they become deficient. When shortages are chronic, the body stops repairing and self-regulating; cells then deteriorate into a diseased state. The earlier detected, the easier corrected.

Health, when understood, can be simple. It's a tragedy that modern medicine has chosen to insulate itself into every aspect of life, medicalizing everything it can find and often forgets to understand the cause of disease. Disease is simply caused by the malfunctioning of cells.

It is unfortunate that today we live in a chemical world. A world filled with chemical toxins in our food, cleaning products, even our water. Yet, we look to treat our bodies with many of these same chemicals. Every drug known to man and woman has side effects. Yet, natural phases of life, like menopause, have become diseases to be treated with chemicals. Temper tantrums in children are being redefined as mental disorders to be treated with chemicals. Childbirth has been distorted so that in America nearly a third of all deliveries are done by caesarean with all the attendant risks of major surgery and the drugs that go along with it.

Wholesale use of vaccines, rather than allowing the body to go through a natural process to fight disease, has resulted in immense harm, including the suggestion that 1 in 88 children develop autism.

The Center for Disease Control and Prevention's latest autism report shows rates of the disorder are on the rise, up 23% from the previous estimate. The news has sparked experts to advise parents they should learn the signs that may signal a problem with their child's development because the earlier the intervention, the better.

According to Dr. Paula Ballie-Hamilton, who wrote the book *Toxic Overload*, a U.S. study found that children who received vaccines containing a preservative called thimerosal, which is almost 50% mercury, were more than twice as likely to develop autism than children who did not. Although mercury has been removed from regular childhood vaccines due to growing safety worries, it is still present in other vaccines children might get.

Compound this by the fact that learning disabilities affect as many as 15% of otherwise able schoolchildren. Almost 1 in 5 children today is on some form of medication; we need to reduce their sugar and caffeine, provide them with more exercise, and help them develop healthier cells.

It's even sadder that the most important medical truth of all is being ignored. The body is an incredible self-healing and repairing device. More often than not, if left alone, healing takes place. The body is a marvelous self-healing mechanism. It contains the knowledge of how to function properly and bring itself back into balance. Our job is to learn to align ourselves with the natural healing processes of nature. A healer may help to bring us into alignment, but it is ultimately up to us to integrate and sustain the results of the healing. Being able to reach out and receive help is crucial to healing, but equally important is the ability to follow through with good self-care. In the long run, developing and exercising our ability to self-heal will bring the most lasting and significant change.

As stated above, no doctor and no drug have ever truly healed anyone. They can only assist if they act in harmony with the Laws of Nature.

Our innate system is designed to heal itself. All we need to do is to remove toxins, replace deficiencies from the body, and allow the miracle of life to take place; this can be accomplished with or without the help of others.

Let's look at some examples:

If you happened to cut any part of your skin with a razor while shaving, the body knows exactly where that cut is, and if the damage is not serious, your body will close back the wound by using specialized cells to stop and repair the skin so well that you will not be able to tell the difference and will probably shave the same area the next day. This miracle of healing takes place without any outside assistance.

If you cut your finger with a sharp object, the wound heals itself, and if the damage is not extensive, the repair job is so perfect that after a few weeks you can't even remember which finger was hurt. Even the fingerprints are reconstructed.

If you break a bone, the doctor may set and cast the bone, but it's your body that identifies exactly where that break is and heals the bone in four to six weeks.

If you bruised your knee or your foot by excessive impact on abrasive surfaces, your body will remove the old skin, and over time it will develop new skin to replace the old cells.

Even if you walked barefoot for a while, you may not have noticed it, but the cells in your soles are constantly removed due to friction, and healthy cells keep on growing over the area.

This is the power of the self-healing body. It has the power to maintain natural health and natural healing. Even if we abuse our body, it tries to heal itself unless the damage is extensive and we continue making mistakes for years. Severe illnesses are largely a result of our complete ignorance on both the physical level (diet, poisoning by toxins, lifestyle) as well as on the mental level (bad mental hygiene and discipline). Pain and suffering are just signals to our conscious mind that we have to change our ways. When we do make changes, in the right direction, we recover. When we follow the flock and resist nature, we suffer. This is the law of nature. The self-healing process goes on all the time, and in every part of your body.

The biggest mistake you can make is to accept someone's advice that your condition is incurable. If you accept such advice, your fear effectively sabotages the self-healing process, which is under complete control of your consciousness on all levels, including the subconscious functioning of your body and mind. Fear blocks any logic, dramatically reducing your self-healing ability.

After being poisoned and paralyzed with cosmetic injections, containing botulinum toxin, my wife and I were told we would probably live the rest of our lives in wheelchairs and on ventilators. We were told we would never live as we once lived and that our lives would be compromised. There is no cure for botulism, and my wife and I received enough botulinum toxin type A to kill 2,800 people each, according to the CDC. A toxin so strong there is no known cure.

Well, I shot an 84 yesterday on a tough golf course, and my wife planted flowers at our house in Georgia. Yes, we have beaten the odds, and, yes, we did not listen to the doctors who said we would never get well. We believed in the power of our bodies to heal. We have learned, firsthand, that there is nothing in the universe to be afraid of except our ignorance and its consequences. Unfortunately, most people doubt everyone and everything except their ignorance of their bodies.

The idea of having an incurable or chronic condition comes from our limited understanding of the healing and aging processes and from the arrogant attitude of people who claim to be health authorities but have never seen a true recovery or cellular transformation.

The bottom line is this: Your body will heal itself. It is our basic nature. The body is inherently healthy and self-healing and always strives to maintain or reestablish optimal healthy conditions.

Certain naturals laws have to be followed and applied to achieve and maintain optimal well-being, vibrant energy, and freedom from illness. These laws include meeting the body's inherent, natural needs while respecting its boundaries by avoiding all toxic influences that will cause our cells to malfunction, a precursor to any disease.

The concern for our health and cellular well-being is something we all must share in common. We all would like to live a high-quality, disease-free, long, and happy life. Genes tell our bodies how to develop from one single cell into an entire human being. Genes are the blueprints for this structure and function of every cell in our bodies. Although we inherit genes from our parents, how we maintain and care for our genes determines how well our cells will work.

Over our lifetimes, our cells may deteriorate and mutate naturally, by awakening our inner wellness we can preserve these cells and increase our life expectancy; however, we must focus on eliminating man-made free radicals that accelerate or distort this natural process. A lifestyle that minimizes the damage to our cells is crucial. Important steps are to avoid toxins and restore any deficiencies our body may have. Many people assume that their family history of disease or "family genes," predispose them to a life of sickness and disease. They figure why not drink and smoke because they're going to die early anyway. The great Mickey Mantle felt that way. He felt he was predisposed to die young, so he lived his life with ruthless abandon. It was only later in his life that he wished he had taken better care of his body. He did so much, but could have done so much more.

The truth is while genetic predispositions do put us at risk for disease, what a person chooses to do to protect the health of their cells and genes plays a more important role in whether or not disease developed. Choice, rather than simply genetic inheritance, is the key.

We must focus on how we play the game, not just the cards that we're dealt. In a game of poker, the total number of possible hands is 2,598,960. The great news is you don't have to be dealt the best hand to win. If you play your hand, your body will heal itself. If we get out of our own way and allow it, it heals itself. It's our basic nature. Anybody who tells you anything other than that is trying to sell you something, no matter what you have been told. Don't give up on yourself and don't buy into the lines like "oh well, you've had a good life" or "at your age" or, the worst of all, "there's nothing further I can do, I suggest you finalize your affairs." They actually told my wife and me this. How dare anyone have the audacity to tell you to give up! It's up to you. Do you want to get better? Make things better? It's human nature to make things better, evolve, and grow.

Required for health are pure air, pure water, moderate sunshine, regular exercise, good spinal health, adequate rest and sleep, juicing. Things like detoxing or fasting when ill, a diet of whole, organically grown foods, eating foods in proper combinations and amounts for optimal digestion, emotional poise, spinal adjustments, and nurturing relationships will allow our bodies to heal. The same laws of nature need to be followed to reestablish health and ageless aging.

We are what we eat and drink, what we feel, and what we think. When we feel perfectly healthy, all physical, mental, spiritual, and emotional aspects of our life are working in total harmony and balance. To eliminate poor health, we should commit ourselves to take full responsibility for our bodies and look to adapt our lifestyles, our inner thoughts and emotions, our environment, and our diets accordingly, so that our body's cells, and consequently our general vitality levels and functionality, can be restored. If we make these changes one cell at a time, we turn on our natural ability to fight off infection and disease. Thus, our cells will regain proper control, which will allow them to self-heal. The human body is such an amazingly capable living being if given the right external and internal conditions in which to flourish. Our job is to give the body what it needs when it needs it.

The big secret of health and longevity is the body's ability to connect to the powers of nature that reside in each and every one of us. We just need to tune ourselves into them and let them manifest throughout every cell in our body. This is how the body self-cleans, self-cures, and self-maintains us and keeps us in the best possible shape.

The body is truly a perfect machine that works every day, regardless of how you treat it or what you put into it. Imagine treating it well and giving it the nourishment it wants and needs. Let's pack our bags and continue our journey to a new land where health is abundant and healing takes place every second of every minute of every hour of every day for the rest of our life; this is the gift of life, the gift of a self-healing body.

Dr. Kaplan's Ten Essentials of Self-Healing

1. **Proper diet**—Fuel the cells.
2. **Exercise**—Energize the cells.
3. **Self-awareness**—Awareness of your body, emotions, and thoughts.
4. **Knowledge**—Knowledge of your body, the role that your cells and beliefs play in the functioning of your body, and ways to bring greater health to all levels of your being.
5. **Motivation**—A strong enough desire to have greater health, happiness, and well-being to motivate you to take action.
6. **Self-love**—The ability to love and appreciate yourself.
7. **Courage**—The courage to move out of your comfort zone and make the changes in your life that are necessary.
8. **Taking responsibility**—Taking responsibility for your life and your health and being responsible for your decisions regarding your diet and health care as opposed to relying solely on the opinion of authorities.
9. **PMA (Positive Mental Attitude)**—You must be positive regardless of the negativity around you. Stress shortens your telomeres and weakens your cells.
10. **Self-care**—Taking practical steps to heal your cells is essential, but without the first nine essentials, you won't be consistently effective.

"*If we are creating ourselves all the time, then it is never too late to begin creating the bodies we want instead of the ones we mistakenly assume we are stuck with.*"

—DEEPAK CHOPRA

Chapter 3

———◦◦◦◦———

THE BODY PERFECT

We learned in the last chapter that the body is an incredibly sophisticated creation; just look at some of its amazing abilities. We have a heart that beats on the average of 72 beats per minute—100,000 times a day and over 30 million times per year—and it never takes a day, hour, or even a minute off.

We have a body so perfect that it can repair itself continually at the rate of 2 billion cells per day. If you cut yourself, the body knows exactly where the cut is and how to form a clot to stop the bleeding. The body also knows how to send more cells to heal the skin.

The continuous renewal of the body is not limited to just the tissues of our skin. Over 98% of our body is replaced in less than one year. More specifically, we change

- Our skin about every 20 days
- Our stomach about once a month
- Our liver about every 6 weeks
- Our skeleton about every 3 months

This means that if you did not like yourself yesterday, don't worry because today is a new day and you are a new you. Every year, we recreate ourselves. We are changing all the time; you just need to decide to change for the good.

The cells in our body contain telomeres that become shorter every time our cells divide. Eventually, the telomeres become too short, and we die. But what if that didn't have to be true? What if we could not only keep our telomeres from becoming shorter, but we could actually help them become longer? This process is possible, and I call it ageless aging.

We must also learn to have respect for our body, a body that performs miracles every day. The body is perfect when at ease. When the body is not at ease, it is at dis-ease, which leads to disease. The key is to keep the body and all of its parts working in harmony. Just look at the perfection of the body:

- Our brain has about 8 billion cells and virtually limitless capacity to store and process information.
- Our brain contains 100 billion neurons, with each neuron capable of transmitting an impulse of 80 times per second.
- Our circulatory system consists of 60,000 miles of blood vessels.
- Our heart not only beats 100,000 times per day but pumps at least 46 million gallons of blood by the time we are 70 years old.
- Our nervous system consists of about 7 miles of nerve fibers with the capability to send messages at a rate of 100 yards per second.
- Our kidneys contain about 1 million filters (nephrons) that will have removed 1 million gallons of waste products from your blood by the time you are 70 years old.
- Our body consists of about 600 muscles, 200 bones, and 20 square feet of skin
- Our eyes contain about 100 million receptors
- Our ears contain 26,000 fibers

Let's say you're cutting up celery for a salad when the knife slips and you cut your finger. Do you immediately think you're going to bleed to death? Or perhaps you come down with a cold. Do you think that it will never go away—that this cold is going to kill you? No, of course not. We all innately know that little things like a cut, a scrape, a bruise, or a cold will eventually heal themselves. Why is it that sometimes we trust our bodies, and at other times we lose faith? This book is about the power of the human body, a machine so magnificent that everything needed to carry on life resides within it. The body is a self-healing organism. Now imagine you wanted to build a new body, where would you begin, how would you put this magnificent, self-healing machine together? The answer is simple, one cell at a time. To live a longer and healthier life, you must start with the cells of the body. Our bodies consist of trillions of cells, some better and healthier than others. Not all cells are the same. Every cell has its function or role to play, but they all work together to form and support the whole body. If one cell is unhealthy, it can affect all of the rest of the cells. To *Awaken the Wellness Within* we must clean house of all our bad cells and only produce clean, happy, healthy cells.

To turn back the clock, we must only produce clean, happy, healthy cells. If we replace our bad cells with healthy cells, our body gets stronger. When we are sick, we rest so our cells can heal and rebuild better, stronger, and healthier cells. Cells are the key to health and ageless aging. If you help your body build healthier cells, you can turn back the clock and experience ageless aging.

Awakening the Wellness Within begins with cell health. We must protect and preserve each and every cell in our body. If a cell is not working at full capacity, it will put our body in a weakened state. If we want to live longer and healthier, we must heal our bodies; and all healing begins with our cells.

Cellular healing will make remarkable things happen to the body, along with the mind, when we give our bodies healthy food, proper exercise, and avoid toxins. The body's amazing innate intelligence and wisdom, present in every cell, begins to manifest health immediately. When the quality of the food entering the body is higher than that of the tissues, the body begins to discard the lower grade materials to make room for the superior materials, which it uses to make new and healthier cells and tissue.

Your body will use whatever materials you give it, but if you want the best, give your body the best. When we are deficient in any vitamin, mineral, or any necessary material, our bodies make changes to overcome the deficiency. The body is very selective and always aims for improvement—thus better health.

How long you live, and the quality of your life, rests largely in your hands. "Ageless Aging" is about how we can live without aging prematurely. Looking good and aging well are not accidents of fate. Instead, they mostly depend on two things: your lifestyle and how much you make use of some of the recently discovered tools for protecting your body against degeneration.

The essence of ageless aging is to remove the factors that cause cells to malfunction and premature aging. We do this by protecting and preserving each and every cell in our body. A scientific approach focuses on treating cells and maintaining their health, aiming at longevity by attempting to extend their maximum lifespan. This is why telomeres will be mentioned in detail throughout this book. They are the key to the aging process. Scientists have deeply explored the processes of aging and degeneration in very specific terms—from the wrinkling of skin to the disruption of a cell's genetic material, which is implicated both in aging and in the development of cancer. Science is discovering specific and effective remedies for counteracting these processes of aging and degeneration.

The key to living better, longer, healthier—to *Awakening the Wellness Within*—depends on your intelligent and effective use of the ground-breaking research that is now available to all of us. In this book, you'll learn about much of this research and the new ways to heal ourselves and slow the aging process that have recently come to light. You will learn the importance of the cells and their telomeres thanks to the scientific research. These scientists, formulators, doctors, and educators are leaders in cellular health and ageless aging, exploring all levels of modern aging technology and scientific disciplines. We no longer have to only imagine the ability to cure disease and age with health, grace, and dignity—we can take action.

This book is about "**Awakening the Healer Within**", which starts with cellular health. This book is about taking charge of yourself and healing yourself naturally. Throughout this book, we will continually learn to how to protect our cells and how to preserve our telomeres. As you learn more about cellular health and the cell's end plates (telomeres), you will see how we begin to unlock the secrets of health and aging. This natural approach is dependent on the numerous scientific discoveries that have taken place, mostly within the last 50 years. These discoveries include a growing understanding of the role that the cells and their telomeres play in regard to our immune system, as well as the rate at which we age. You will learn how antioxidants can be used to prevent age-related damage on a cellular level, which will strengthen our cells and improve our immune functions. This, coupled with specific nutrients such as antioxidants and the free-form amino acids, can be used to alter the chemistry of our cells. We need to think young as well as feel young. Through cellular health and longer telomeres, we move into a paradigm of ageless aging that studies show can assist the body's ability to remove wrinkles, firm up sagging muscles, improve one's energy—and, of course, live a longer, healthier life.

Healing takes time. Consider the Chinese Bamboo Tree. The Chinese Bamboo Tree is a remarkable tree. The Chinese plant the seed for the tree, water it, fertilize it, but the first year nothing happens. The second year they continue watering and fertilizing it, but still nothing. The third year nothing. The fourth year they continue to water and fertilize it, with no evident results. Then during the fifth year, in six weeks the Chinese Bamboo Tree grows 90 feet in just those six weeks. If during any of those six years they hadn't watered or fertilized the seed daily, there would have been no Chinese Bamboo Tree.

So be patient; we will change our bodies one cell, one day at a time. Every day, researchers are becoming more aware of how specific pathways between the mind and body enable your feelings, attitudes, and expectations to play a major role in determining the rate at which you age or don't age. To get the best results possible and get maximum benefits from what is currently known about aging and cellular health, we need to integrate natural law and modern science into a single power for ageless aging. When used together, you will not only look and feel better, you will also go a long way toward preventing degenerative cellular diseases like cancer, heart disease, and stroke. These diseases, the top three causes of death in our country, are wreaking havoc on our health, well-being, and medical system. Once we change the paradigm and begin treating the cause of disease, we will have moved much closer to healing all disease. So you can sit back and be a victim of the health system or be proactive and take your health back in your own hands. To *Awaken the Wellness Within*, you must understand that health is an inside job.

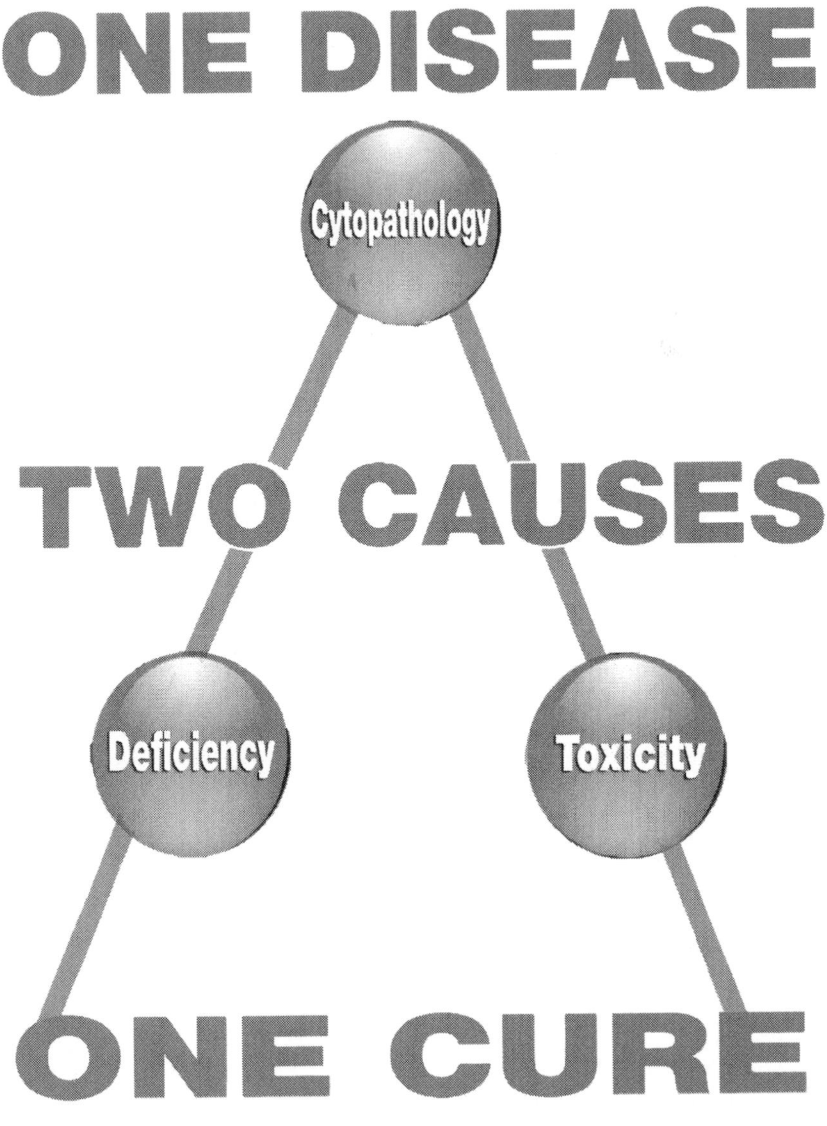
ONE DISEASE
Cytopathology
TWO CAUSES
Deficiency
Toxicity
ONE CURE

"A healthy outside starts from the inside."

—ROBERT URICH

Chapter 4

THERE REALLY IS ONLY ONE DISEASE

At this stage in the book, we have learned the importance of our cells and that to ***Awaken the Wellness Within***, we must awaken our cells' potential. Since I became a doctor, I have asked myself the same five questions every day:

- *What is health?*
- *What is disease?*
- *Why do people get sick?*
- *How can disease be prevented or reversed?*
- *How can aging be prevented or reversed?*

As I continued to study the cell, these answers started to fall into place. Throughout this book, we will study the power and importance of the cell and how to harness this power. To answer all of the above questions, we must continually go back to the basics.

The concept of only one disease will simplify health care, simplify disease, simplify health, and make clear the path to ageless aging.

The secret to health is now exposed. Give your cells what they need and protect them from what they don't need and you'll be healthy. Cells malfunction only if they suffer from a lack of nutrients (deficiency) or toxic damage (toxicity). By making the choice to prevent disease, by avoiding the two causes of disease, you improve your potential to live agelessly. Health depends on the choices we make. Taking care of your cells is the smart choice.

We have been conditioned our entire lives to think of many different diseases with many different names, rather than recognizing what is common to all disease—cellular malfunction, which leads to diseased cells—cytopathology. If you have cytopathology, your telomeres will shorten, and you will age.

This theory requires you to look at health, disease, and ageless aging in a completely different way. Using the concept of one disease dramatically simplifies how we perceive disease in general; however, by following this new paradigm, it will make us focus on the cause of all disease and not just treat its subsequent symptoms.

If we understand the root cause of disease and aging, then we can cure disease and slow down aging. Once you grasp the concept of one disease, you will then acknowledge that disease and aging are the results of a large number of malfunctioning cells—widespread cytopathology. It all begins with one cell. I find this theory so simple that it would be difficult for any scientist, physician, or layperson to deny it. This theory provides a simple unbiased explanation that health, disease, and aging can be reversed by understanding and treating the cause, by treating and focusing on the cell.

The assault on our health care system has begun. Over the next few years, insurance companies, pharmaceutical companies, HMOs, and other healthcare profiteers will spend billions in advertising and billions in lobbying to convince us that we have the best healthcare system in the world. Nothing could be further from the truth. We have claimed a reputation for quality health care by deceit. We are not the best in the world; we are 37th on the list. How is it possible that we pay more money than any other country in the world, have the best doctors, the best hospitals and surgeons in the world, and we don't even rank in the top 20 of all the industrialized nations in the world?

If it's broke, it's time to fix it

The problem is not the healthcare delivery system—we are a world filled with great doctors and great technology—the problem is that we have a sickness-based model, not a health model. If you keep people healthy, you cut healthcare costs. We should focus on wellness care, not symptom care. Correct the cause and you cure the disease.

We must start healing ourselves

If there is only on disease (cytopathology) and two causes (deficiency and toxicity), what is the cure? *The power that created the body heals the body.* Sounds simple, but it is a fact of nature. As a doctor, I learned that many are trained to believe that they know your body better than you do. If you get sick, you should hand yourself over to the medical world so a drug can heal you. This is the same type of way you might bring your broken-down car to a mechanic. With little or no input from you, if the exchange goes well, voila! You're all fixed up and ready to roll.

Your body is a self-healing organism. By bypassing its natural self-repair process and handing all your power over to a medicine alone, you might be ignoring the very thing you need to heal. This is not a revolutionary idea. As doctors, we learn that the body can heal itself. Our physiology texts teach us that it is brilliantly equipped with natural self-repair mechanisms that kill the cancer cells we produce every day, fight infectious agents, repair broken proteins, keep our coronary arteries open, and naturally fight the aging process. This is why some patients do get well. The drugs did not heal them; they allowed the body to conquer the enemy, by allowing the body to repair the malfunctioning cells.

The greatest power in the universe is your life force! The energy that keeps you alive also powers every bit of your healing! Will you use it to your full advantage or ignore and squander it, erroneously assuming your healing power is to be found elsewhere?

Your body is constantly working as best it can to preserve and improve its vital domain: repairing its parts when needed, regenerating, rebalancing, and optimizing all of its functions. This healing force is vigorous and thorough—under favorable conditions.

Our bodies consist of 50 to 100 trillion cells. Of which 4 to 5 trillion cells die each day, and they are regularly replaced, so our goal is to replace bad cells with good ones. Your body is capable of repairing itself with amazing capacity. It is not the doctor who is healing you. It is the human body systems that are capable of healing you. The creator designed you for living well.

The heart is a pumping motor. It pumps the blood all over the body through a network of pipes. Blood carries food and oxygen to the heart and other parts of the body. These pipes are capable of carrying 4–5 liters of blood. The blood travels along 100,000 kilometers of blood pipes, which is equal to about 2.5 times around the equator. The blood contains 25–30 billion red cells, and 2 million red cells are made every second. You have a total of 1 trillion white cells for fighting germs and infections. You make 10 billion new white blood cells each day. Your heart pumps 13,640 liters of blood and, your heart beats 100,000 times each day.

Your brain is a super computer and can process up to 30 billion bits of information per second. The brain is equivalent to 9,656 km of wiring and cabling. Your internet of nerves contains about 28 billion neurons. A neuron is a tiny computer that interprets information received through your five sense organs. Each neuron is a tiny self-contained computer, capable of processing one billion bits of information. Neurons also communicate with other nerves through a network of 160,935 km of nerve fibers. The brain and network of nerves are one of the fascinating human body systems.

You're a food-processing chemical factory

The food we eat must be broken down into smaller molecules before our body cells use it. Our digestive system is a chemical processing unit that breaks down the food and also excretes the waste. It is a piping structure consisting of stomach and intestine. The stomach produces up to two liters of hydrochloric acid. There are 500,000 cells in your stomach lining that are replaced every minute.

Your untiring breathing machine

You inhale 6 liters of air per minute or 8,640 liters a day through the lungs. You breathe 28,800 times a day. Breathing is a vital process by which you take oxygen into the blood. After being on a ventilator, I know firsthand how important the lungs are. Like the rest of your body, they continually work, even while you sleep. The more you think about your body, the more you must realize how perfect it is.

You are a marvelous creation by the creator. All the discoveries made by the man are created as a thought in our brain. Our thoughts transform into reality. Your brain is more than a super computer. You have an amazing capacity to fight the disease and rejuvenate the body. Whatever you are searching for elsewhere is within you. By looking elsewhere for health, you have distanced yourself from the body's own healing power. You cannot be ignorant of the power within you. Science has proved that it is not genes or DNA but your beliefs that are responsible for your behavior and destiny. As we continue to read on, we will discover this innate capacity, explore and experience it.

With rare exceptions, your cells contain the perfect instructions for all manner of self-healing; it happens automatically. All that is needed is that we intelligently cooperate when our body calls for rest, meditation, or healthy foods so that it can accomplish its tasks without interference. This means stepping out of the way and conserving energy so that our fullest energy potential is available for the healing work.

Our innate body intelligence knows best—it trumps our own meddling mind and our futile tinkerings every time! To be healthy you must trust your body's wisdom—let it do its work and your "healing miracle" will take place in its own time. Healing can be fast or slow depending on you and your lifestyle; however, we must be patient to accept that the body is always doing its best and knows what it is doing.

When we are sick or injured, the body's actions are 100% focused as it goes about its business of restoring health. Occasionally, we may need some form of emergency care to facilitate the natural healing of the entire organism; this should be done without interfering with the body's self-correcting actions. If we cooperate with the body, providing the optimum conditions for health, the healing job will be accomplished in minimal time.

Squandering our self-healing power is a tragic mistake made too often by too many. We only delay healing and prolong suffering when we attempt to "fix" or "treat" the body with too many drugs or modalities. The body heals not *because of* but *in spite of* such interventions! Allowing our innate power to do its work, while we patiently ride out the health restoration process, is a beautiful experience; it is always the most prudent approach. Best of all, it's free!

Healing is as easy as lying down, closing your eyes, and letting the God within take over. Sleep is the most powerful healing remedy! The body is a self-healing marvel!

Every day we nearly run out of nerve energy and, as is nature's way, we fall asleep. This nerve energy is our vitality—it is our most precious commodity, bar none! Nerve energy powers our nervous system, our organs, and the self-healing processes and it comes from rest and 100% nerve supply. A pure functioning nervous system is the source of our vitality!

Proper nerve supply is your fountain of self-healing energy; you must make sure you get what your body needs. This is what makes chiropractic care so crucial to any healing regime. We need to try a natural approach to health before we bombard our system with medicine and other toxins.

Researchers have shown that most healing takes place when we sleep. The more you get proper sleep, coupled with proper nerve supply, the more your vital energy will build up for all of your mind-body functions. Rest, meditation, and sleep charge your nerve cell "batteries" and fill up your nerve energy "storage tank." It's like putting "money in the bank." When your nerve energy "bank account" is full, you will feel like a million bucks and be enabled to heal as quickly as possible! Keep your nerve energy strong via sleep and rest, a simple nutrient-rich raw food diet, and a restful healing program and your body will heal with great vigor!

Sleep and chiropractic care are the two key components of nerve energy. Healing does not come from drugs, stimulants such as nutraceuticals and superfoods, "energy drinks" with caffeine, "energy work" therapies, or activities of any kind. Often, they deplete our precious nerve energy through stimulation. Never squander your nerve energy, especially when you are in need of healing, which is all about building up and conserving nerve energy so that the body can use it for the most important tasks at hand. The ultimate healing approach is to take water, fast, and bed rest.

Do you feel tired, irritable, cranky, upset, or depressed? Is your mind unclear and your ability to reason muddy? Are you healing too slowly or getting nowhere with your health quest? We cannot do anything well when we are short on sleep. Sleep and sleep some more until your energy is restored and you feel renewed—then you will be on your way to vibrant health!

You can get something from nothing! Do nothing, intelligently: go to sleep when your body is tired or ailing. When it needs to accomplish extraordinary work, it demands more sleep. The "do nothing" cure is the smartest thing you can do when you need healing. Make it your first resort, not your last! After all, it is free! All else is usually a waste of time, energy, and money!

You can spend a fortune going to all the best doctors in the world. I have been there. Our bodies and our bodies alone healed us from botulism of which there is no known cure.

Take this million-dollar advice: eat right, exercise, drink plenty of water, maintain a good attitude, and at the end of the day go to sleep and allow your body to charge up with healing energy and heal. Nothing else but your own body can heal you! That's 90% of everything you need to know about healing right there. Now combine a good night's sleep with some morning exercise and your telomeres will say thank you.

Remember, you have the self-healing power! Sleep, proper diet, and exercise are key elements. I call them the "magic elixir of life," "the rejuvenator," "the invigorator," or the "healer within." Your body's cellular system is your personal power plant, your healing sanctuary, the ace up your sleeve, and nature's great gift!

When your body is in need of healing, it will communicate to you with many signs that are generally in the form of pain and suffering. These are signals to you that you have to change your ways, change your lifestyle, and remove the source of the sickness that is causing the pain and suffering.

Some doctors do not treat the source, but rather deal with you symptomatically. They may prescribe painkillers to hide or remove the symptoms (pain and suffering). You might think you are healed, but you are not. Often these substances are toxic in themselves and create other serious problems.

The right step to take is to change your life—take control of your lifestyle, and remove any causes of the disease. Nature will go to work in your self-healing body and will bring about a miraculous recovery. Your body has an innate desire to self-heal because it wants to be in good health and remain healthy. Self-healing takes time. Your body is improving itself moment by moment and day by day. Be patient, committed, and diligent. When you change your lifestyle to include healthy habits, you'll attain health. There are no shortcuts to health.

If there is **one disease, two causes, and one cure**, let's begin to focus on the cure: healing our cells by removing either the toxin or deficiency. With this paradigm it's easier for you to begin to heal yourself by healing your cells, giving you longer telomeres and a longer life. It's important to remember that if our cells are deficient of a food source or a vitamin, then we need to add that supplement to our diet, not to heal the cell, but to give the cell what it needs to heal. Supplements don't heal; the body heals itself.

We are a society that is quick to take drugs but slow to get involved with vitamins and supplements. We do not have a health-care delivery system in this country; we have a sickness response system. We treat disease but fail to provide an avenue or philosophy of wellness or health. We must change the model to a health-based model. This can be done by educating the public to the avenues of health and implementing and utilizing a natural approach.

Treatment through phytonutrients or herbs is not new. Digitalis is provided by the foxglove plant and is the basis of one of the most prevalent heart medications utilized during the past century.

Penicillin, our most powerful antibiotic, was developed from moldy bread and only truly introduced in our country in the 1940s. We survived millions of years without antibiotics. The science of antibiotics is relatively new, and we doctors are learning more about antibiotics every day. Let me share with you the timeline behind antibiotics.

Antibiotic Timeline

1929 Alexander Fleming discovers penicillin in laboratory experiments

1933 First clinical success with an antibiotic (sulfanilamide)

1938 First clinical success with penicillin

1942 Alexander Fleming warns about the emergence of antibiotic-resistant staphylococci

1950s Rise of penicillin-resistant staphylococci

1950s Japanese researchers find new resistance factors in dysentery-causing bacteria

1952 A Japanese researcher isolates the first organism resistant to several different antibiotics

1955 Almost 12% of 474 milk samples from around the United States contain traces of penicillin

1969 Epidemic of antibiotic-resistant dysentery (Shigella) in Guatemala infects 112,000; 12,500 die

1970s Outbreak of antibiotic-resistant staphylococci sweeps through Europe, Unites States, Australia and Greece

1976 Penicillin's-resistant gonorrhea spreads to east and west coasts, responsible for one-third of the cases of sexually transmitted diseases in Los Angeles

1977–1979 310 cases of new antibiotic-resistant salmonellosis in Great Britain; 2 die

1988 The streptococcus resistance for rheumatic heart disease causes an epidemic of the disease in Salt Lake City

1990 Penicillin-resistant gonorrhea rises by 60%

1990s Penicillin can control only 10% of staphylococci it used to kill

Ayurvedic medicine, Chinese medicine, mind and body medicine, chiropractic medicine, naturopathy, homeopathy, and aromatherapy are just some of the alternative therapies utilized and recognized throughout the world.

Homeopathic remedies are generally dilutions of natural substances from plants, minerals, and animals. This is based on the principle of like cures. Homeopathy was founded in the late 18th century by German physician, Samuel Hahnemann. Dr. Hahnemann came to a breakthrough during an experiment in which two times a day he ingested cinchona, a Peruvian bark well known as a cure for malaria. Soon after Dr. Hahnemann began his experiment, he developed fevers common to malaria. As soon as he stopped taking the cinchona, his symptoms disappeared.

He theorized that taking large doses of cinchona created symptoms of malaria in a healthy person, but the same substance taken in a smaller dose by a person suffering from malaria might stimulate the body to fight the disease. His theory was born out of years of experiments with hundreds of substances that produced similar results. Based on this work, Dr. Hahnemann formulated the principles of homeopathy:

1) *Like cures like (law of similar).*
2) *The more the remedy is diluted, the greater its potency (law of infinitesimal dose).*
3) *An illness is specific to the individual (holistic model).*

Dr. Hahnemann believed that each case of disease is radically and rapidly annihilated and removed only by a medicine capable of producing within the human body the most similar and complete manner of the totality of the symptoms.

One of the most powerful forms of alternative care is the use of antioxidants. Antioxidants have been recognized as great disease deterrents and health enhancers. We can live without food for days or weeks, but the primary substance of life is oxygen. In each of our bodies, we have stable and unstable oxygen molecules.

In 1954, Denham Harmon, MD, PhD, of the University of Nebraska College of Medicine, founded the free radical theory and its effect on the aging process. There is a common denominator that causes aging and all of the conditions that occur as we grow older. It has been estimated that approximately 10,000 times per day every cell in our body is exposed to free radicals that are destructive to our cells. If our telomeres are in jeopardy, our cells are in jeopardy.

Throughout this book, I will show you ways that we will battle aging and disease—caused by free radicals such as cancer, heart disease, and atherosclerosis—through a proper lifestyle that combines exercise and a diet filled with antioxidants. Antioxidants are germane to cellular health and longevity. There are both stable and unstable oxygen molecules in your body; both have a purpose and are essential to life. Specialized unstable oxygen molecules (free radicals) are essential in that they enable our bodies to fight inflammation, kill bacteria, and control the tone of smooth muscles. These oxygen molecules regulate the working of internal organs and blood vessels.

One key to healthy, longer telomeres is the ability to maintain control of free radical balance. If the production of free radicals is exacerbated by exogenous (outside) sources such as stress, poor diet, smoking, drinking additives, and preservatives, then the body needs free radical scavengers known as "endogenous antioxidants" that gobble up the free radicals, preventing them from damaging the body. If the body becomes overwhelmed by free radicals, this shift in balance causes the unstable oxygen molecules to shift from the body's allies into molecular predators. These predators then begin to wreak havoc by attacking both healthy and unhealthy parts of the body. Heart disease, various cancers, cataracts, and many other diseases are the result.

The ability to divide forever and never age describes our ancestral germ line, but it also describes a much less pleasant type of cell line—cancer.

In today's world, we are all aware of cancer. Cancer begins when something goes wrong in a cell, causing it to lose control over its growth. It begins to divide repeatedly, ignoring chemical signals that tell it to stop; however, the telomeres continue to shorten in these cells, and eventually the cells reach a stage where they can no longer divide, at which point they enter a crisis mode.

In the vast majority of cases, when this crisis is reached, the cells will enter senescence and stop dividing; however, very occasionally, they will find ways to re-lengthen their telomeres. When this happens, a cancer cell begins to divide not only uncontrollably but indefinitely, and this is when cancer becomes truly dangerous.

In most cases (85-95%), cancers accomplish this indefinite cell division by turning on telomerase. For this reason, forcing telomerase to turn off throughout the body has been suggested as a cure for cancer, and there are several telomerase inhibitor drugs presently being tested in clinical trials.

So, anti-aging scientists must be out of their minds to want to turn the telomerase gene on, right?

No! Although telomerase is necessary for cancers to extend their lifespan, telomerase does not cause cancer; this has been repeatedly demonstrated. At least seven assays for cancer have been performed on telomerase-positive human cells: the soft agar assay, the contact inhibition assay, the mouse xenograft assay, the karyotype assay, the serum inhibition assay, the gene expression assay, and the checkpoint analysis assay. All reported negative results.

Famed telomere researcher Dr. Bill Andrews states, "As a general rule, bad things happen when telomeres get short. As cells approach senescence, the short telomeres may stimulate chromosome instability. This chromosome instability can cause the mutations normally associated with cancer: tumor suppressor genes can be shut off and cancer-causing genes can be turned on. If a mutation that causes telomerase to be turned on also occurs, the result is a very dangerous cancer.

Paradoxically, even though cells require telomerase to become dangerous cancers, turning on telomerase may actually prevent cancer. This

41

is not just because the risk of chromosome rearrangements is reduced, but also because telomerase can extend the lifespan of our immune cells, improving their ability to seek out and destroy cancer cells.

It's fairly obvious that long telomeres in human beings are not correlated with cancer. If that were true, young people would get cancer more often than the elderly. Instead, we usually see cancers occurring in people at the same time they begin to show signs of cellular senescence—that is, at the same time their immune system begins to age and lose its ability to respond to threats. Extending the lifespan of our immune cells could help our bodies fight cancer for much longer than they presently can."

It is essential to maintain a balance between stable and unstable oxygen molecules. Research now clearly indicates that antioxidants can offset many diseases derived from diet, lifestyle, environment, and activity patterns. This breakthrough enhances our ability to control not only the quantity but the quality of our lives. James Fries, MD, a professor of preventative medicine at Stanford University School of Medicine points out that there is a significant difference between chronological age and biological age. An individual may be chronologically 60 years old, but biologically have the health of a 45-year-old, and vice versa. Imagine having the ability to turn the clock back or even slow down the clock. The public is moving toward antioxidant therapy and away from antibiotic therapy. Is this a radical approach? I don't think so.

Today, treatment of chronic disease accounts for approximately 85% of the national healthcare bill. We wait for illness to develop and then spend huge sums of money trying to treat the symptoms, rather than recognizing the cause. It is no different than driving down the highway and having the oil light go on. It would be simple to mask the warning sign by removing the bulb because the car will continue to function properly for a while. But by not treating the cause and simply removing the symptom, a true correction will never occur.

In 1988, Surgeon General of the United States, C. Everett Koop, MD, released a report on nutrition and health that pointed out that dietary imbalances are the leading preventative contributors to premature death in the United States. He recommended the expansion of nutrition and lifestyle modification education to all healthcare professionals. When he and I first met, he was concerned with how many former employees of the FDA now work for drug companies. Drugs in our country are big business, probably our leading export. Most drug companies are public companies, which means that their stock only goes up if they sell more drugs. Drugs can treat sickness, but only the body has the ability to heal. The sickness model our country is utilizing is not working, and we need to change the paradigm.

Dr. Lowell Levin, a professor at Yale University, said, "It sounds like a joke. But the hospital is no place for a sick person to be. The increased use of potent antibiotics is one of the reasons for the ever-present life-threatening hospital infection. As more and more potent antibiotics are developed, increasingly resistant strains of microbes evolve."

According to the *Archives of Internal Medicine*, published in October 1995, preventable prescription, drug-related diseases, and death costs us a whopping $77 billion a year.

If a cell is deficient, it becomes weakened. The key is to heal the cell, and we do that by providing the cell with the food it needs. We must not try to trick the cells with drugs but heal them by treating their deficiencies. My paradigm is to treat the cause of sickness and aging, and we do that by treating the cell, attacking and removing the cause and not just masking the symptoms.

In Germany, phytonutrients, or botanical medicines, are approved as over-the-counter drugs by a government body known as Commission E, which is comparable to our Food and Drug Administration. Commission E provides physicians with strict guidelines on natural remedies, such as when to prescribe these remedies, for which conditions, the expected effectiveness, and safety precautions. These natural substances are manufactured to pharmaceutical standards, are government regulated, and are clearly labeled as to approved dosage, possible side effects, contraindications, and toxicity. It examines all of the modern scientific evidence available on botanical remedies and has issued over 300 monographs on herbal medicines, 200 of which have been approved as safe and effective.

Yes, genes and germs trigger cellular malfunction and disease. But this happens only after the body is subjected to deficiencies or toxicities, which are always the common denominators of any and all disease. Eliminate these factors and you eliminate disease.

When we have a chronic deficiency of essential nutrients, this leads to cellular malfunctions. When the cells are compromised, a decline in overall health occurs. Replenishing these cells with the essential nutrients supports bioenergy production and leads to optimal cell health.

Proper supplementation may begin with FDA guidelines, but that is not where it ends. Your optimum dosage is determined not only by how vitamins and minerals interact with your body but by how they interact with each other. I recommend that you do some experimentation under your physician's guidance until you arrive at a formula that is right for you. As we learned from the bamboo tree, healing takes time. So no matter what your state of health is in, don't be discouraged.

One of the common denominators in people with bad health habits—whether it is smoking, drinking, the lack of exercise, or overeating—is that they are looking for a detour or escape route from a new, healthy lifestyle. They hunt for reasons to return to their old ways, and in some cases manage to find them. Discouragement is a major pitfall in any health regime, but remember your body is working hard to help you heal. Faith means having faith in not only God but the body that God created.

Let me tell you a story about discouragement.

It seems that one day the devil was going out of business, and he decided to sell all his tools to whomever would pay the price. On the night of the sale, they were all attractively displayed. Malice, Hate, Envy, Jealousy, Greed, Sensuality, and Deceit were among them. To the side, though, lay a harmless wedge-shaped tool that had been used more than the rest.

Someone asked the devil, "What's that? It's priced so high."

The devil answered, "That's Discouragement."

"But why is it prices so much higher than the rest?" the onlooker persisted.

"Because," replied the devil, "with that tool I can pry open and get inside a person's consciousness when I couldn't get near it with any of the others. Once discouragement gets inside, I can let all the other tools do their work."

We probably confront some form of discouragement every day. How we handle this emotion determines whether we succeed or fail in reaching our goals. Discouragement is only a pit stop—it's not the pits unless you allow it to be.

We now know there is only one disease and disease is a result of deficiency or toxicity. Remove the cause and you can heal the cell. Discouraged? I have never been more optimistic.

"You're in pretty good shape for the shape you are in."

—DR. SEUSS

Chapter 5

CELLING HEALTH

We now know the body is a self-healing organism, and we have learned many ways to keep our bodies healthy. Unfortunately, most people do not know their bodies are weak, that their cells are malfunctioning, until it's too late. By the time my brother was diagnosed with lung cancer, the cancer had spread throughout his entire lung, and during this process he was not aware of this. We must know the shape we are in; it begins with a basic blood test, having our weight and blood pressure checked. If you are overweight your cells are stressed. Cellular health starts with you.

What is your concept of health? Not being sick? How about being symptom free? Generally, people will equate the absence of pain with the presence of health. You must look at this closely and challenge this paradigm first. People who have heart attacks, cancer, or strokes were evidently developing serious problems long before the body told them so, before their body broke down. WHO, the World Health Organization, defines health as, "a state of complete physical, mental, and social well-being and not merely the absence of disease or infirmity."

The state of health or disease in your body is the expression of success or failure experienced by the body in its efforts to adapt to environmental challenges. Health is metabolic efficiency. Sickness is metabolic inefficiency. Nobody is totally healthy or totally sick. Each of us is a unique combination of health and sickness, as our body continually fights off viruses and toxins. Each of us has a unique combination of abilities and disabilities, both emotional and physical, and the ability to overcome anything put in our path.

Talk to Americans about health and the topic generally switches—immediately—to health care, ObamaCare. It makes sense. Health care, ObamaCare, is our *Titanic*.

In what other country do you spend 20% or more of your total economy on a dysfunctional system that ranks you 50th in the world for lifespan (according to the CIA). In the U.S. we have a "system" where appendectomies in the same market can cost $1,500 or $100,000, and debt collectors sit interviewing patients in ERs. With health care simultaneously critical to individual survival and bafflingly bizarre, no wonder people first want to talk about health care.

Health is a much bigger issue than health care. Health is a social, political, and economic issue that speaks to national survival. A healthy economy requires a healthy population. A healthy population is also a resilient population that can grow an economy and help create the kind of society people yearn for.

The huge increase in lifespans in the world through the last century occurred primarily because of improved public health—better sanitation, nutrition, education, and vaccination.

The WHO definition of health matters for many other reasons. Physical and mental health is greatly affected by how people eat, move, rest, and socialize. Social well-being and social support keep people living longer.

Maintaining an optimal level of health wellness is absolutely crucial to live a higher quality life. Cellular health matters. Health matters because everything we do and every emotion we feel relates to our well-being. In turn, our well-being directly affects our actions and emotions. It's an ongoing circle. Therefore, it is important for everyone to achieve optimal cellular health in order to subdue stress, reduce the risk of illness and ensure positive interactions.

The Centers for Disease Control and Prevention (CDC) estimate that up to 90% of all illness and disease is due to stress. Stress can kill the good bacteria and yeast that live in your intestines and keep your immunity and digestive health strong.

As the good bacteria and yeast die off, the bad bacteria and yeast are able to take over. Body Ecology teaches that this creates an imbalanced inner ecosystem, which can set the stage for illness and disease. Each day, we are surrounded by poisonous substances that affect our cells and bodies.

Life and conception

To truly understand health, we need to go to the beginning. The life of a baby begins long before he or she is born. A new individual human being begins at fertilization when the sperm and ovum meet to form a single cell. We have the joining of the male sperm and the female ovum. The zygote is the result of the biochemical embrace of 46 chromosomes, 23 from each parent. As the sperm fertilizes the ovum, the zygote starts to develop after implantation in the uterine wall. This is what is called a blastocyst and where stem cells can be extracted. An amazing hormonal dance starts. By five weeks there is a neural tube and the beginnings of the heart and other organs. This is the launching of the embryonic period. The embryo is no bigger than the tip of a pen.

By six weeks, things are happening fast: there is an eye spot, the beginning of a distinction between upper and lower jaw, and even an arm bud. The embryo can move its back and neck. Usually, a heartbeat can be detected by vaginal ultrasound at around 7 weeks. The heartbeat may have started around six weeks, although some sources place it even earlier at around 3 to 4 weeks after conception.

To me, life itself and the process is a miracle. We begin with one cell and soon we have this tiny mass of cells wherein a primitive nervous system is already connected to a primitive heart so as to tell it to start doing its job. How exactly does this happen? The first heartbeat is, in a sense, the transition between something with dividing cells and something that has a systemic integration—organs communicating with other organs.

Life begins with one cell. This book will help you realize, recognize, and actually accept that all sickness comes from one cell, and ageless aging is accomplished by preserving the integrity of the cell. The essence of this book's message is healing and preserving the cell.

Our health begins when our life begins, and our life begins at conception. Life as we know it is a miracle. Something so simple, and yet so amazingly complex. Imagine we start when an egg and a sperm come together, then a new life, a new energy form, is created. Simple cell division takes place for a short period of time, but soon the first very special system in our body develops. It's called the neural-streak because it will become the brain and the spinal cord. The first system to form is the brain and the spinal cord because from that system all the other systems will develop. All development is controlled by the nervous system. That's why it's the first system. The nervous system communicates with all parts of the body.

The brain may simply be the bossiest part of the body: It tells virtually every other part of your body what to do and how to do it. Whether you're aware of it or not, awake or asleep, your brain is at work. It works 24 hours per day, 7 days per week, never taking any time off. The brain not only controls what you think and feel but also how you learn and remember. It also controls every function in your body, even the way you move your body. The brain works through your conscious and subconscious minds. Consciously, the brain reacts to your request but also to things you might be less aware of, such as the beating of your heart and whether you feel sleepy or awake are controlled by your brain.

Think of the brain as a central computer that controls all the functions of your body, and the nervous system is like a network that relays messages back and forth from it to different parts of the body. It does this via the spinal cord, which runs from the brain down through the back and contains threadlike nerves that branch out to every organ and body part. The brain is germane to cell health and reproduction. The brain carries the energy of life throughout the body.

When a message comes into the brain from anywhere in the body, the brain tells the body how to react. For example, if you accidentally touch a hot stove, the nerves in your skin shoot a message of pain to your brain. The brain then sends a message back telling the muscles in your hand to pull away. Luckily, this neurological relay race takes a lot less time than it just took to read about it. The brain works with amazing speed. We must keep these pathways free and clear, any obstructions in our spine will cause a deficiency and allow the cells to malfunction. We must keep the pathways of our brain and spinal cord free to maintain optimum health.

In essence, this book will focus on these two areas repeatedly:

- Healing the cell
- Preserving the cell

It is important to understand that an infection is an expression of symptoms and symptoms are our bodies' way of telling us our cells are being attacked, literally at war. Healthy cells can fight off disease. Unhealthy cells succumb to disease. An infection in our bodies indicates that cellular malfunction has already weakened our immune system. Having a cold or the flu is an alarm; it is our cells, our immune system, screaming for help. They scream in the form of symptoms. Symptoms that were caused over time through toxicity to the cell, deficiency, or both.

Remember, if your cells are healthy, you will be able to resist infections in the first place. We so often are busy living our hectic lives that we fail to pay attention to these alarms, these symptoms, these warning signs. We think that having a cold or the flu is normal, and that once the symptoms are gone we are well again. Not necessarily so.

The level of your health and immunity determines whether or not the presence of a cellular malfunction is present. If your body is attacked by any toxin or microorganism, this may result in an infection. You were beginning to be sick before you came down with the infection. A healthy doctor can see patients in the hospital and not get sick. Otherwise everybody, every visitor, every doctor who is exposed to any given "bug" would become sick, which is simply not the case. Strong cells lead to a strong immune system and this book is about protecting your cells and having them become healthier and stronger. The stronger the cells, the stronger and longer the telomeres of the cell are, the better we age.

The common theory is that we "catch" diseases, that people become sick only after their body is already compromised. Disease, which we now know as cellular malfunction, comes first; active infections and chronic problems follow. Otherwise, when one child in the classroom gets sick, why doesn't every student get sick as well? The healthy ones stay healthy; the weakened ones get sick.

How often have we heard, "But he/she was born with asthma and suffered from it as an infant." "She/he was in the best of health, took great care of himself/herself, and then suddenly got breast/prostate cancer?" Although we hear these kinds of statements frequently, the theory is flawed. The paradigm that a person is a powerless victim of disease to me is just not acceptable and modern science proves this. Sometimes these children were born with the pathways to their organs blocked, through spinal subluxation. Chiropractic care, when administered to children at a young age, can offset many of these ailments by allowing the body to heal itself by restoring the deficiency. An increase in chronic childhood disease is part of the reason parents today seek alternative health care for kids.

Healthy people simply do not get sick. Healthy people have healthy cells. Make certain your cells obtain what they need to flourish, and they will stay healthy. Choosing health means learning how to supply your cells with what they need while keeping them free from what they don't need. Cells have great powers to take care of themselves, to reproduce themselves, to repair themselves, to stay healthy unless they are overwhelmed by toxins, poor diets, unhealthy habits, or environmental hazards. Your daily choices determine whether your cells stay healthy or get sick. Your daily choices will affect your telomeres, whether they grow or shrink or whether they are short or long. This book is about choices, your choices to live a longer healthier life. It begins here and now; it begins with the cell.

Most of us were not raised to think this way. We grew up in a society where it was not abnormal for someone close to us to have a chronic disease. We have been taught by society and television that that disease is a normal part of the aging process. That taking drugs is normal. This is not true. Throughout time, the two causes were there all along, gradually wearing down cellular competence and creating an opportunity for disease to wear down the body's cells, thus lowering our immunity system. The more toxins in our environment, the more we must protect our cells.

We learned that as a part of the body's normal maintenance and repair process, old cells are constantly being replaced with new ones. This is why as we progress through this book we will learn the importance of protecting our telomeres. Simply stated, if the new cells are not built with the proper raw materials they need, they will be deficient and eventually become unhealthy and weak. If the cells become weakened with age, this is a result of the telomeres becoming shorter. If the cells telomeres get shorter, our cells become weaker and we become weaker.

Cells that are not able to perform their normal tasks, including routine cellular repairs, will be vulnerable to sickness and disease. Once this happens, the body will be vulnerable to a breakdown in the body's self-regulation systems. We are all prone to weakened cells because of the diets we eat, the water we drink, and the toxins we come in daily contact with. Cells are rarely deficient and toxic when first created, unless the mother was in a toxic or weakened state. If not tended to, then we will most likely continue to be sick and toxic unless we remove the cause. When we have a large number of cells either not functioning at 100% or malfunctioning, we will be in a weakened state. Weakness is a sign of weak cells with shortened telomeres.

How do we know when a child is sick? When they curl up and have no energy. When they don't want to go out and play. Hopefully, we are now aware that any number of things can affect a person's health adversely. A cell that is already deficient, one bombarded with toxins, will be prone to any pathogenic organism. How often do we feel weakened after a long trip or a long plane ride? Were we sick when we got on the plane? Or if we got sick, did everyone on the plane get sick? Perhaps we entered the plane with weak cells, which were then bombarded by germs and other micro-organisms? Almost any attack to a compromised immune system can be the straw that breaks the camel's back.

What is disease?

We've talked about health, now let's talk about disease. **There are only two causes of disease, either cellular toxicity or cellular deficiency.** In dealing with toxins, how strong an invader is in our body and if the cell is healthy enough to remove it. If deficient an invader can be traumatic to your cells.

Toxins come in many different disguises. They can be in common food or household chemicals. They can enter the body in the form of bacteria or virus, which can be infectious. The most important factor in disease is the resistance of your body to disease. Your immunity system will determine how strong your body is to fight off the invader from within and that varies from person to person. The stronger your cells, the stronger your immune system.

Cellular health, or strength as we discussed, can come from any type of toxin or nutritional deficiency. Any cell can be altered if the cell has too much or too little of any of nutrient. For example, too much sugar is bad for the cell. Too little omega-3 will cause a cell deficiency, which will affect the cell's outer wall.

The key to cellular health is balance. Imagine how simple it is:

One disease: *Cytopathology*
Two causes:
    1. *Toxins to the cells, creating malfunction.*
    2. *Deficiency of the cells, causing weakening and malfunction.*

Cells can also be damaged by poor nutrition, thus creating a deficiency or nutritional imbalance. For example, too much sugar harms your cells. Too few omega-3s harms your cell's outer wall. The key to cellular health is balance.

Understanding health is very simple—one disease, two causes. The disease is cytopathology and the causes are toxins and cell deficiency, most often caused by nutritional imbalance.

Once cellular health and integrity is affected, our immunity weakens, and the weakness of one cell will continue to spread. When this becomes rampant, disease sets in.

Germs and disease

When we eat sugar and nutrient-deficient diets, expose ourselves to toxins, lose sleep, fail to exercise, and fail to adapt to stress, our immunity becomes depressed and we open the door to infection. Then we blame the germ, when really we are the one to blame. Rather than being obsessed with germs and rushing for flu shots and antibacterial soaps, optimizing cellular health and improving our immunity would be a far better approach. The perspective that germs cause disease is so ingrained in us that many have difficulty making the shift to the new way of thinking, but to avoid infection, we must do exactly that. In truth, only sick people get sick. The problem is we spend decades making ourselves sick, all the while thinking we are healthy.

The popular misconception is that microorganisms (germs) cause infections. Yet, why is that the same doctors that visit patients in hospitals don't get sick?

If germs alone were the true cause, the microorganisms would have to produce the same effect all the time, which is not the case. Not everyone who is exposed to a particular organism gets sick, and not everyone who gets sick does so to the same degree. In truth, whether or not someone develops an infection depends on the balance between several factors, namely the virulence of the organisms, the number of organisms and, most importantly, their state of immunity. We live in a sea of microorganisms, but they do not make us sick until we alter the natural balance between them and us. Our normal coexistence with germs rather than a germ-free environment ensures our health.

This book is for those that want to be healthy and age gracefully.

Are you tired of your doctor prescribing you a pill for every illness? Are you sick of the side effects from your pills and potions? A revolution is happening in health care that will reduce prescriptions and the side effects we suffer. I believe that a holistic approach is essential for being happy and healthy—having good sleeping, eating, thinking, and exercise habits. Sadly, many people only take a natural approach to their gardens and pets, but not for their own health and happiness.

There is only one disease: *Cytopathology*

When cells malfunction, the body is no longer able to maintain homeostasis (balance) by regulating and repairing itself. This is the essence of disease—no matter what you call it or how it happens.

Because only one disease exists, all we need to do is prevent the causes of that one disease.

There are only two causes of disease:
1. *Deficiency*
2. *Toxicity*

A person cannot be sick unless a large number of cells are malfunctioning. The first steps on the path to disease are taken when, for whatever reason, a single cell begins to malfunction, and then another cell and another. When the number grows large enough, we may begin to feel symptoms, perhaps experiencing a pain here, a discomfort there, or a lack of energy. By the time your cells and health have deteriorated into a diagnosable chronic disease, no cell may be left in your body that is still functioning optimally. A simpler and more effective solution is to focus on the process—the one disease—and to ask what causes it. When you understand disease as a process, rather than a "thing" to be cut out or suppressed, then you see why surgery and drugs, virtually the only tools of the physician, are limited in what they can do.

Deficiency and toxicity, regardless of their cause, increasingly compromise the functioning of cells, making a person steadily more vulnerable to developing a diagnosable disease. By the time you contract a diagnosable disease (whether we're talking about the common cold, allergies, cancer, or heart disease), you have probably been "sick" for a long time. You have suffered enough cellular damage from deficiency and toxicity that cells throughout your body are malfunctioning. You are sick long before you get sick. By the time symptoms are produced, cellular malfunction has become widespread, cell-to-cell communications have been disrupted, and the systemic manifestations are the symptoms. Remember that disease does not just randomly happen; it is a process of accumulation of toxicity or deficiency. Health, not disease, is the natural state of human existence, but forgetting this point is easy when we see all the disease around us. In today's world, we live of fear of germs and disease, yet diseases like cancer are on the rise. There was a time in my life when it was a rare exception to hear of someone having cancer. Now cancer seems common in most conversations and almost everyone knows someone who has had or has cancer. We are not curing disease; we are now living in fear of germs and think germs alone are the cause. We must remember that our parents and generations before them have made it here without so much fear.

Jay Leno stated it best when talking about our obsession with germs and the fears parents today deal with in regard to our children's health and safety. I was born in 1952; it is amazing I am alive and healthy.

TO ALL THE KIDS WHO SURVIVED THE 1930s, '40s, '50s, '60s and '70s!

First, we survived being born to mothers who may have smoked and/or drank while they were pregnant.

They took aspirin, ate blue cheese dressing, tuna from a can, and didn't get tested for diabetes. Then, after that trauma, we were put to sleep on our tummies, in baby cribs covered with brightly colored lead-based paints.

We had no childproof lids on medicine bottles, locks on doors or cabinets.

And we rode our bikes with baseball caps, not helmets, on our heads.

As infants and children, we would ride in cars with no car seats, no booster seats, no seat belts, no air bags, bald tires, and sometimes no brakes. Riding in the back of a pick- up truck on a warm day was always a special treat.

We drank water from the garden hose and not from a bottle.

We shared one soft drink with four friends, from one bottle, and no one actually died from this.

We ate cupcakes, white bread, real butter, and bacon. We drank Kool-Aid made with real white sugar. And we weren't overweight.

WHY?

Because we were always outside playing . . . that's why! We would leave home in the morning and play all day, as long as we were back when the streetlights came on.

No one was able to reach us all day. And, we were OKAY.

We would spend hours building our go-carts out of scraps and then ride them down the hill, only to find out we forgot the brakes. After running into the bushes a few times, we learned to solve the problem.

We did not

- Have Play Stations, Nintendos or X-boxes

There were

- No video games
- No 150 channels on cable
- No video movies or DVDs
- No surround-sound or CDs
- No cell phones
- No personal computers
- No Internet
- No chat rooms

WE HAD FRIENDS and we went outside and found them! We fell out of trees, got cut, broke bones and teeth, and there were no lawsuits from those accidents.

We would get spankings with wooden spoons, switches, Ping-Pong paddles, or just a bare hand, and no one would call child services to report abuse.

We ate worms, and mud pies made from dirt, and the worms did not live in us forever.

We were given BB guns for our 10th birthdays, .22 rifles for our 12th, rode horses, made up games with sticks and tennis balls, and although we were told it would happen, we did not poke our eyes out.

- We rode bikes or walked to a friend's house and knocked on the door or rang the bell, or just walked in and talked to them.
- Little League had tryouts and not everyone made the team. Those who didn't had to learn to deal with disappointment. Imagine that!!

These generations have produced some of the best risk-takers, problem solvers, and inventors ever.

The past 50 to 85 years have seen an explosion of innovation and new ideas.

We had freedom, failure, success, and responsibility, and we learned how to deal with it all. So what happened? Now we live in fear of germs of disease and yet have made no changes in our approach toward health. This book is about changing your approach to health and disease. There is only one disease—cytopathology. There are two causes of disease—toxins to the cells or deficiency of the cells. And there is only one cure—*the power that created the body heals the body.*

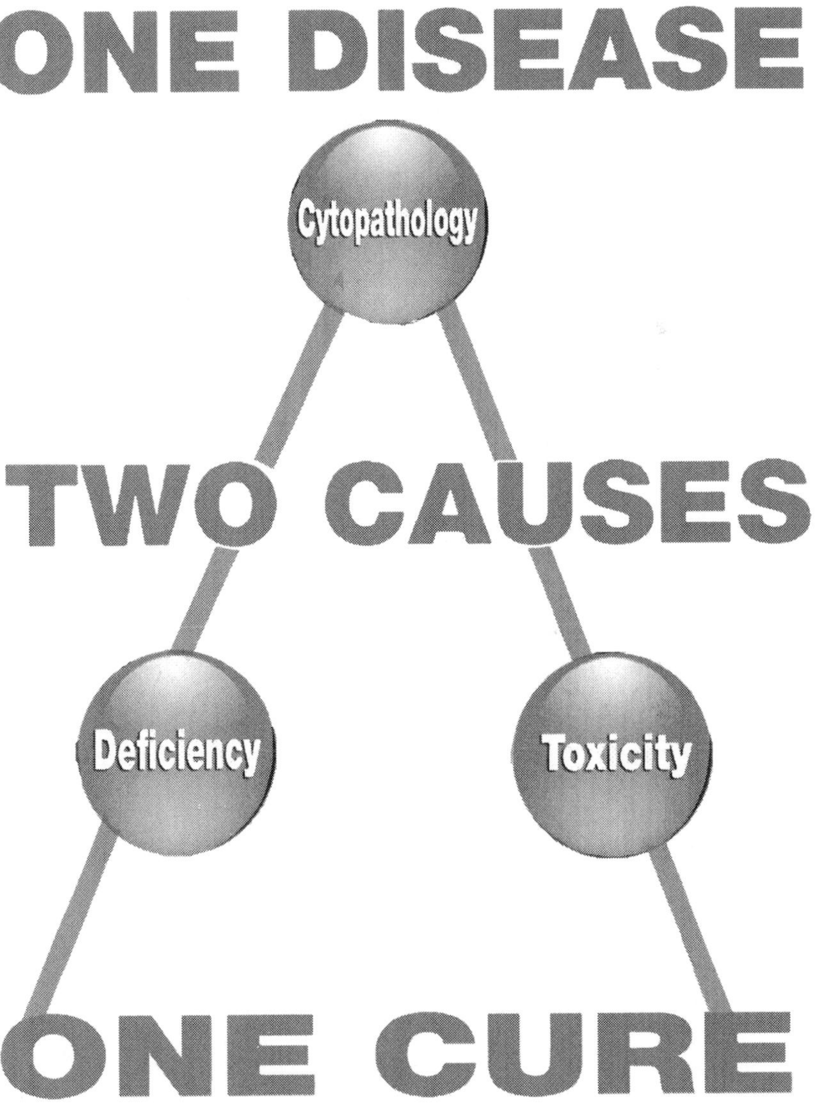
ONE DISEASE
Cytopathology
TWO CAUSES
Deficiency
Toxicity
ONE CURE

"*Good health is not something we can buy. However, it can be an extremely valuable savings account.*"

—ANNE WILSON SCHAEF

Chapter 6

THE HEALER WITHIN

As I look back at my life, it is hard to imagine that I have been a doctor for 38 years. This was not always a blessed journey. My wife had colon cancer and was given 6 months to live, yet she survived and shares with me my spirit for health. We both overcame botulism and it was feared we would live our lives in a wheelchair, on ventilators, if we lived at all. Not once but twice in our lives we were given a terminal sentence, we were told there was no cure. Yet, I sit here today and write this book more impressed with the power of the human body and the human spirit than ever before. Our bodies were built for survival; *the power that created our bodies has the power to heal our bodies.*

Life is for living, laughing, loving, and learning, not just whining, worrying and working. The one thing I promise you about life is you will not get out of it alive. Friends, life is for the living and we have lived, grown and survived. Now 63, I jog, golf, take walks with my wife, and consider myself in the best shape in years. I have been a doctor for 38 years, but a student of health my entire life.

It was early in my training as a chiropractor and an acupuncturist, that I began focusing on alternative health care. My goal was to build the bridge between Eastern and Western medicine. Owning five clinics in Palm Beach County Florida, working with families like the Trumps, gave me the vehicle. I began to add medical doctors to my staff in 1987; my offices employed an orthopedist, neurologist, psychiatrist, physiatrist and an osteopath. My sons were raised on the paradigm of combining Eastern and Western medicine. Is it by accident today that I have one son interning in medical school and the other a practicing chiropractor? I don't think so. Being brought up on the best of Eastern and Western medicine, they simply both made their own choices. My goal is for a convergence of both Eastern and Western medicine to provide the best care in the most natural format, to prevent disease, and treat the cause of the disease (not just the symptoms) by understanding there is only one disease, we focus less on the disease and more on the cause.

Eastern medicine has been around for centuries; the Chinese have been doing self-healing techniques utilizing natural remedies for thousands of years. Antibiotics for that matter did not become available in our country until 1945, yet why is eastern medicine called alternative? As I mentioned, I believe the treatment with the highest risk should be the alternative.

I discussed earlier how my sons motivated me to write this book. Being around a house of doctors is no easy task. We continually challenge each other and often we each learn something new. As stated prior, my beliefs of the one disease theory were augmented by one of my son Michael's lectures. While listening to his professor, preparing these future medical doctors for their licensing exam, I was pleased to hear how he educated his students by simplifying disease and death. He stated most causes of death are actually caused by the brain, the heart, and the kidneys. When one of those organs begins to fail, or stops working, that is when death most likely occurs. Example: Does someone die from cancer? No. Cancer may destroy their organs, their bodies, but they will survive until the kidneys fail, the brain stops working, or the heart stops beating.

When understanding this theory, you must ask yourself what causes the organs to fail? But if we dig deeper—what are the organs made of? The answer—cells. So in essence, chronic diseases like heart disease and cancer are a cellular disease. All disease, all organs, all tissues begin the same; they all begin with one cell. Then doesn't it make sense for all disease to start the same way as life?

My talks with my partner, Dr. Perry Bard, a leader in the chiropractic field, one of the brightest men I have ever worked with in chiropractic, pushed me to keep digesting more and more material on cellular health anti-aging and telomeres. I shared with him my theory that is both simple and direct, that there is only one disease, two causes and one cure. His first reaction was "brilliant." He stated, "This theory just simplifies medicine and health as we know it."

If we change the paradigm of health care, better understand disease and aging, recognize cellular health and importance, we can *Awaken the Wellness Within*.

Simply stated then, when cells malfunction, the body is no longer able to maintain homeostasis (balance) by regulating and repairing itself. Thus the body is no longer at ease, and dis-ease is now present. This is the essence of disease, no matter what you call it or how it happens. Because only one disease exists, all we need to do is prevent the causes of that one disease. How do we do that? We protect the cells.

Healthy people do not get sick; only sick people become sick. Once you start to compromise health, a series of health events start to follow. It begins with one cell. Once a critical number of cells begin to malfunction, internal communications and self-regulation of the body's organs and systems become debilitated and destabilized. This malfunction started with just one cell. Thus, if only one cell is sick and other cells become weakened, our internal communication system, our innate intelligence, sends our symptoms. The greater number of cells that are compromised, the more the effects of the cells malfunction becomes compounded. Before anyone can exhibit noticeable signs of disease, normal cell function has to be compromised significantly throughout the body. Vulnerability to infections, for example, is created by widespread cellular malfunction. An infection indicates that cellular malfunction has already weakened the immune system. One weakened cell—malfunctioning, affecting and weakening other cells—is the cause of any and every disease. **Thus, one disease—cytopathology (sickness).**

What is the cold or the flu? It is the body weakened by symptoms. Through symptoms, the body sends out an alarm screaming at you that you are not well. It literally tells you your cells are tired, deficient. It forces you to bed, to rest, to build newer healthy cells. Healthy people resist infections in the first place, otherwise how could the husband be ill and the wife and children healthy, or vice versa. How could doctors and nurses walk around hospitals and not catch every contagious illness?

Symptoms are alarms, and most of us pay little attention to these alarms. We think that having a cold or the flu is normal and that once the symptoms are gone we are well again. That is not necessarily the case.

The level of your health and immunity determines whether or not the presence of a microorganism results in an infection in your body or if your cells are healthy enough, strong enough, to combat the antigen (anything foreign to the cell is an antigen). You are already sick, your cells have already become weakened and compromised prior to you coming come down with an infection. Disease (cellular malfunction) comes first; active infections and chronic problems follow.

To state that a person, any person, is a powerless victim to ill health or disease, is a flawed theory. This way of looking at disease comes from living in a society that does not have an accurate understanding of disease or of what is required to create and maintain health.

This book is about *Awakening the Wellness Within* to turn back the clock of time to when life was easy, when life was fun. What made it easy and fun you might ask? The answer is healthy cells. As the cells weaken, the bodies weaken. The essence of this book is that disease and aging begin with the cell. I have spent my life studying health, and all roads led to the cell. Now we know how to make cells healthier, happier, and younger again.

Symptoms mean sick cells

To embrace my One Disease theory, you must constantly understand dis-ease, its cause, and its origin. Once we begin to feel symptoms, regardless of the outcome of any test, we are most likely already sick. Does this make sense to you? If the test is normal but the symptoms are still present, does this mean you are well?—or a hypochondriac? No, it simply means there is time; your cells are fighting, and the bad or sick cells are not in control yet. You must accept the warning of symptoms, and prepare for the storm ahead.

Symptoms tell us that the cells are in distress and that our our body needs help. Now why just mask these symptoms? If we mask the symptoms, your brain and body may be fooled, but only temporarily. Even if you mask your pain with a pain killer, the cause of the pain is still prevalent. Drugs may reduce your symptoms, but your cells will continue to malfunction and eventually die. The goal is for your new cells to be better and stronger. We all need to listen to the body's warning signals so that we can evaluate our own health—and conversely the decline of our health.

The problem with most Americans is we simply do NOT listen to our bodies. We ignore the early symptoms, the mild symptoms, until the problem becomes so serious it demands attention. A cut that is not treated will possibly become infected. If you ignore your open wound, your infection will progress until the infection travels. We are quick to treat open wounds because we can see them, but we ignore the internal wounds—like acid reflux, a mild cough, shortness of breath, or tooth pain—until the problem becomes so severe we seek medical attention.

Let's review: Symptoms are caused by cellular malfunction, thus the one disease theory. It is time modern medicine accepts this theory that there is only disease and the fact that there are two causes of disease:

1. Toxicity
2. Deficiency

So the key to health is finding out whether our cells are toxic or deficient.

How healthy are you? How strong, how healthy, do you feel? How is your energy level? As you are reading this, are you suffering from any symptoms? Symptoms are the body's way of getting your attention. They are warning signs and are evident in your day to day life. Simply put, if you are tired, lack energy, feel terrible and just don't look good, your body is fighting disease. Symptoms tell you when your body is absorbing too many toxins for the cell to handle or is so deficient the cells cannot reproduce healthily.

Below are some of the most common symptoms/warning signs. If you are experiencing any of the below, it means your cells may be toxic or deficient. Treat the cause, you cure the disease.

When we have malfunctioning cells, we have cytopathology and symptoms; both go hand in hand. One of the key symptoms and the cause for most doctor visits is decreased energy.

Sick people have low energy levels

How do we recognize when our child ill? They just lie around, watch TV, and simply lay there. So a good mom goes over and feels their head to see if it is warm. If they are warm or hot, they have a fever. Now if it is a virus, do you give the child antibiotics? No, because modern medicine accepts the fact that antibiotics don't heal viruses. So how do we get better? Simple; the body again heals itself by removing toxins—through eating well, and with supplements.

Within your cells and muscles are mitochondria, which are to muscle cells and other cells what the piston and cylinders are to the gasoline engine. It is in the mitochondria that energy is extracted, just as the energy of gasoline is extracted in the piston and cylinders. This bodily process is almost heatless, but it produces free radicals of oxygen—a primary cause of aging. It is the concentration of free radicals in the mitochondria that contributes to a significant loss of endurance and strength in aged muscle; this in effect will shorten our telomeres. So you can see if our energy is low, our cells may be abundant with free radicals.

Free radicals can be helped with antioxidants and we will go into more detail throughout book on how to heal our cells. But consumption of foods and vitamins alone is not the key to good health. Your cells, your mitochondria, your telomeres love exercise. So if you want to *Awaken the Wellness Within*, you must exercise.

Exercise and your cells

Exercise helps decrease your chances of developing heart disease and keeps your bones healthy and strong.

We know that exercise increases your immunity to illnesses, exercise helps the cells eliminate waste and remove toxins.

- Physical activity may help flush bacteria out of the lungs and airways. This may reduce your chance of getting a cold, flu, or other airborne illness.
- Exercise causes changes in antibodies and white blood cells (the body's immune system cells that fight disease). These antibodies and white blood cells circulate more rapidly, so they could detect illnesses earlier than they might have before; however, no one knows whether these changes help prevent infections.
- The brief rise in body temperature during and right after exercise may prevent bacteria from growing. This

temperature rise may help the body fight infection more effectively. (This is similar to what happens when you have a fever.)

- Exercise slows down the release of stress-related hormones. Some stress increases the chance of illness. Lower stress hormones may protect against illness.

Although exercise is good for you, be careful not to overdo it. People who already exercise regularly should not exercise more intensely just to increase their immunity. Heavy, long-term exercise (such as marathon running and intense gym training) could actually decrease the amount of white blood cells circulating through the body and increase stress-related hormones.

Studies have shown that people who go from a sedentary ("couch potato") lifestyle to a moderately energetic lifestyle benefit most from starting (and sticking to) an exercise program. A moderate program can consist of:

- Bicycling with your children a few times a week
- Taking daily 20–30 minute walks
- Going to the gym every other day
- Playing golf regularly (my favorite)

Exercise can help you feel better about yourself, just by making you feel healthier and more energetic. So go ahead, take that aerobics class or go for that walk. You'll feel better and healthier for it.

There is strong evidence to prove that taking immune health supplements, along with exercising, lowers the chance of illness or infections.

Time to get moving

In general, it's fair to say that research has shown that regular, moderate physical activity can be beneficial to your immune system.

If you are just beginning to exercise more often, here are some tips:

- Take your time. Your immune system and the rest of your body will need time to adapt to regular exercise.
- Start at a duration and intensity level you can easily manage. For some that may be 30 minutes, and for others it may be 10 minutes.
- Keep in mind that positive changes in your immune system are just one small additional benefit you will get from regular exercise. There are many other health benefits as well, such as improved cardiovascular fitness and endurance, and improved flexibility, muscle strength, and balance.

For people who exercise regularly, here are a few pointers:

- Light and moderate exercise won't be harmful, and in some cases may make you feel better when you are feeling a little under the weather.
- It's okay to have a heavy workout, but it's not necessary to do a heavy workout every day. Your body and immune system need a chance to rest and return to a normal state.

For athletes and those who train hard

As a doctor, I have worked with many pro athletes and organizations like the Miami Heat and Montreal Expos. Athletes are true competitors, true warriors. Athletes must learn to listen to their bodies. Today's pro athletes are better at this, as they know the repercussions of career-threatening injuries.

- When you are following a heavy training regime, keep an eye on your health (e.g., watch for signs of feeling worn out or cold/flu symptoms) and try to minimize other risk factors for colds and viruses.

- Research has shown that consuming carbohydrates before a heavy training session may help to ward off drastic immune changes, making you less susceptible to colds.
- Other research has shown that vitamin C may also help to ward off drastic immune changes.

If you are feeling unwell, it may be best to delay your heavy training session until you are feeling better. Lauren Cox, ABC News, reported, "People who run every day do it to keep their hearts strong, spirits up, and waistlines trim, but how many could guess that sweating it out on the treadmill may actually fight aging?

"A new study in the journal Circulation shows that vigorous exercise may be inducing a natural anti-aging effect that goes right down to our DNA.

"People who exercise have better health and live longer; however, the mechanisms are not completely understood," said Dr. Ulrich Laufs, lead author of the new study and researcher at the University of Saarlandes in Saarbrücken, Germany "You'd be amazed at how little we know about the mechanism of exercise on the cellular level.

"In his small study of 104 people, Laufs and colleagues found that 50-year-old adults who had exercised vigorously over a lifetime—such as marathon runners or endurance athletes—appeared biologically younger, sometimes decades younger, than healthy people the same age who were not active.

"The American College of Sports Medicine and other medical institutions agree that exercising can prolong life by protecting against diseases.

"But research has not been able to point to an actual anti-aging effect in exercise, or detail exactly how exercise protects against some diseases even among people who are otherwise thin and healthy."

Exercise aids in lengthening telomeres

Research has shown us that cells love exercise, and exercise aids the cells. To *Awaken the Wellness Within*, we must awaken our cells. Our cells and their end plates (telomeres) can also determine our current state of health. This simple fact was proven by studies that showed how exercise has a direct effect on our telomeres. To awaken our inner healer, we must awaken our telomeres and preserve them. One of the great discoveries in cellular health is with telomeres. Telomeres are key genetic material that act as a biologic fuse or time clock telling us how much life is left in our cells. The older we get, the shorter our telomeres get and the older and sicker our cells behave. The older and sicker our cells behave, the older and sicker we become!

Oxidative stress, metabolically generating free radicals, is now a broadly accepted theory of how we age and develop disease. Oxidative stress results in DNA damage, and inhibits DNA repair. DNA repair is the mechanism that fixes the damage caused by environmental impact.

As stated, one of the most common complaints made to doctors in our society is a lack of energy—fatigue. Low energy levels go directly to the cell's ability to heal, restore, and reproduce. Low cellular production is one of the first things affected as our cells malfunction and become diseased. If you do not have the energy you used to have, aging is not the problem; You are getting sicker, and you have cells under duress. Symptoms like forgetfulness, loss of energy, loss of sex drive, loss of muscle mass, and gain of fat are all symptoms of the disease we call aging. And at the center of all this is the telomere and its length.

Exercise is a fountain of youth—a fountain of health

I remember meeting the great Jack LaLanne when I was lecturing in Ohio at the Arnold Schwarzenegger Classic. I sat with my good friend Dr. Gerald Mattia, one of the leading sports chiropractors in the world. We were at the same table with Hall of Fame Baseball player and friend Barry Larkin and the great Jack LaLanne. LaLanne also gained recognition for his success as a bodybuilder, as well as for his prodigious feats of strength. Arnold Schwarzenegger once exclaimed, "That Jack LaLanne's an animal!" after a 54-year-old LaLanne beat then 21-year-old Schwarzenegger badly in an informal contest. On the occasion of LaLanne's death, Schwarzenegger credited LaLanne for being "an apostle for fitness" by inspiring "billions all over the world to live healthier lives," and, as governor of California, had earlier placed him on his Governor's Council on Physical Fitness. Steve Reeves credited LaLanne as his inspiration to build his muscular physique while keeping a slim waist. LaLanne was inducted to the California Hall of Fame and has a star on the Hollywood Walk of Fame. (Wikipedia)

So here I was sitting next to Jack, and we spoke of health and healthy cells. He told me he exercises over 4 hours each day, and then he added, "I hate it, but I'm Jack LaLanne, and I feel great every time I'm done."

Writer Hal Reynolds, who interviewed LaLanne in 2008, notes that he became an avid swimmer and trained with weights, and describes his introduction to weight lifting:

He found two men working out in a back room who kept weights in a locked box. When he asked them if he could use their weights, they laughed at him and said, "Kid, you can't even lift those weights." So he challenged them both to a wrestling match with the bet that if he could beat them, they would give him a key to the box. After he beat them both, they gave him a key and he used their weights until he was able to buy his own.

He went back to school, where he made the high school football team and later went on to college in San Francisco where he earned a Doctor of Chiropractic degree. He studied Henry Gray's Anatomy of the Human Body and concentrated on bodybuilding and weight-lifting. (Wikipedia)

LaLanne blamed overly processed foods for many health problems. For most of his life, he advocated primarily a meat and vegetable diet, eating meat three times per day with eggs and fruit in the morning and many servings of vegetables in the afternoon and evening. For six years he was a vegetarian. In his later years, he appeared to advocate a mostly meatless diet but which included fish and took vitamin supplements.

He also added, "I know so many people in their 80s who have Alzheimer's or are in a wheelchair or whatever. And I say to myself 'I don't want to live like that. I don't want to be a burden on my family. I need to live life. And I'd hate dying; it would ruin my image.'"

LaLanne summed up his philosophy about good nutrition and exercise: "Dying is easy. Living is a pain in the butt. It's like an athletic event. You've got to train for it. You've got to eat right. You've got to exercise. Your health account, your bank account, they're the same thing. The more you put in, the more you can take out. Exercise is king and nutrition is queen: together, you have a kingdom."

I loved his philosophy and looking at this man in his late 80s you knew he was on to something.

I have found during my 38 years as a doctor that most energetic athletic people simply age better.

"As most people grow older, they develop an increased likelihood of developing chronic diseases such as heart disease and diabetes. People who exercise regularly have been shown to have a lower rate of developing those chronic diseases," explained Wojtek J. Chodzko-Zajko, a member of the American College of Sports Medicine and head of Kinesiology and Community Health at the University of Illinois at Urbana-Champaign. "But individuals differ widely in how they age. I think we're a long way from understanding all of it," he said.

Laufs and his colleagues decided to tackle the problem by studying exercise's chemical influence on telomeres—caps, that act as a sort of buffer at the end of chromosomes that protect DNA from damage. A young cell typically has long telomeres, but telomeres begin to degrade and fray as the cell ages. Older people typically have shorter telomeres in their cells. If telomeres in a cell are too short, the cell dies.

Detecting how exercise affects your DNA

Laufs first did a series of experiments with mice and showed the more that the mice exercised, the more their bodies' biochemistry protected their telomeres from deterioration. The mice also helped researchers pinpoint exactly how exercise rejuvenates cells in the cardiovascular system.

The researchers then analyzed the blood chemistry of endurances athletes and non-active, but otherwise healthy people who were either in their 20s or 50s.

Human and mice endurance athletes of any age showed the same chemical signs that exercise was protecting their telomeres. But 50-year-old athletes had significantly longer telomeres than relatively healthy people their same age.

Ageless aging is about healthy cellular reproduction. To reproduce new healthy cells, the cells must be healthy and strong.

Remember the boundless energy that we had as children? We could run and play all day, never feeling tired or depressed. Contrast this to the anxiety, depression, low energy, and fatigue so many of us feel during the day. So what do we do? We head to Starbucks for a quick pick me up. Needing several cups of coffee just to keep going is not the answer.

In China, the most successful doctors are those who treat the fewest patients. They "treat" people with natural, noninvasive techniques before illness develops.

My goal for you in this book is that you will learn that we still have not reached the limit of human longevity and that an average healthy lifespan may soon be 100 to 120 years for many people. Just as our ancestors could not even imagine the many discoveries of modern science, from traveling to the moon to the development of antibiotics, we too cannot imagine all the new discoveries that will impact the human condition to allow us to live longer and healthier lives than any of us thought possible.

"*Health is the greatest of all possessions;*
a pale cobbler is better than a sick king."

—Isaac Bickerstaff

Chapter 7

CELLING YOUR CELLS, CONTROLLING YOUR HEALTH

Recently, I had the pleasure of appearing on the Dr. Oz Show. What a delightful man; what a unique experience. Prior to the taping, we sat and talked about the changing landscape of health care in our world today. Dr. Oz, a Harvard-trained surgeon, believes in prevention. He believes in alternative health care. We agreed that the best way to treat disease and to reduce healthcare costs was to change the paradigm of treatment. We must stop just treating symptoms and start attacking the cause. Often the cause is our environment, the foods we eat. We live in a toxic world. The first key is to rid your body of these toxins. Dr. Oz believes an educated patient is the key to our success in this country.

Cellular health and anti-aging starts with attitude and nutrition, not with drugs or potions. Great nutrition is essential to aging gracefully. To age well you need to eat well. Eating the right kind of food will have an immediate impact on the way you look—and on the way you feel.

Energy, vitality, and zest for life come from within—from a body and brain supplied with the essential nutrients needed for optimum performance.

Good nutrition is also vital for skin tone and muscle tone—every cell in your body needs essential nutrients to regenerate and repair. Eating the right things has a huge impact on the way your skin looks and how well it copes with the passing of time. Enjoying what you eat is such an important part of eating healthily. Here, you won't find recommendations that you eat something just because it's the latest anti-aging wonder food.

Now imagine being paralyzed, being told you may never walk or breathe on your own again. I have the strength and the stamina to run, hike, play golf, and take leisurely strolls with my wife of 35 years. Each and every day, my wife and I only look to attract what is good, what is natural in the universe. I began my quest with my first book, *Lifestyle of the Fit & Famous*. Hopefully our next president, Donald Trump, who sits on the cover of my book and calls it "**The Taj Mahal of health books**" will repeal ObamaCare and offer a system for Americans that works. Regardless of your political conviction, all Americans should be entitled to good health care. My book delivered a strong message on health and wellness that is still recognized as a leading resource of information on alternative health care and natural, healthy living. My entire life has been spent trying to find a simpler and easier way to achieve health and wellness and to educate the public. With this book I believe I've found the solution to better health.

I have come to learn that there are no mistakes in life—only lessons. The key to being a good educator, a good communicator, is to find common ground with the student. Now if you've read this far, I have your attention. If you've read this far, you want more out of life. Like you, I share in this mission.

This is now my fifth mainstream book. I have written 20 manuals for doctors, so in essence, this is my 25th publication and my most important book. The health model of our country is in question; it is time for a better, safer model.

One of the most profound conclusions I have reached is that health is a choice; virtually no one ever has to be sick. The potential for human health and longevity is far greater than we are now achieving. Scientific studies describe populations who lived longer and healthier lives than we do, simply because their societies made dietary and lifestyle choices that supported human health. With just a little knowledge and effort, we can do the same. We can choose health, but first we must educate ourselves.

Seventy-five percent of the aging process is determined by things under your personal control, and diet is a big one.

Seven Primary Strategies to Slow the Aging Process

1. Boosting blood flow (maintaining healthy arteries)
2. Reducing inflammation
3. Reducing oxidation
4. Boosting insulin sensitivity
5. Healing and strengthening our cells
6. Protecting our Telomeres
7. Improving our nerve flow and removing any nerve interference

There is only one disease

The most difficult aspect of this revolutionary theory is that this book requires you to look at health and disease in a completely different way. Using the concept of One Disease dramatically simplifies how we perceive disease in general.

To simplify disease, we must first have an understanding of what disease is. In order to do that, we need a basic understanding of cells. Every plant and animal on earth is made of cells—the smallest unit of life. Fossil records show that the earliest forms of life were single-celled organisms.

Likewise, we learned earlier that each human being started as one cell—a single cell encoded with all of the information needed to develop into the vastly complex, multi-trillion-celled organisms that we are today.

The facts remain that each of us is made of trillions of cells. Not all of these cells are the same. Humans have over 200 different types

of cells (nerve cells, blood cells, muscle cells, bone cells, etc.), forming many different types of tissues that enable us to eat, breathe,
feel, move, think, and reproduce. Together, cells combine to form
the building blocks of biological structure and function. All of these
cells communicate with each other 24/7, and we rely on these cells
working together in harmony in order to keep us alive and well.
Healthy cells make healthy tissues, which are highly resistant to disease and physical injury. Unhealthy cells create unhealthy tissues,
which are quite susceptible to both disease and injury.

Sickness and disease are specific to the cells in question. If you
have a lung disorder, it is the lung cells that have weakened and are
under attack. It will need the liver cells and heart cells to come to its
rescue. If someone has heart disease, they have sick heart cells. Yet, if
someone had a heart attack, they could get well and their cells could
heal. Medications give the body the time to build the strength to aid
the weakened cells.

There is only one disease: *Cytopathology*

When cells malfunction, the body is no longer able to maintain homeostasis (balance) by regulating and repairing itself. This is
the essence of disease, no matter what you call it or how it happens.
Because only one disease exists, all we need to do is prevent the causes
of that one disease. So if there is only one disease, what is the cause?

There are only two causes of disease:
   1. *Deficiency*
   2. *Toxicity*

Cellular malfunction, we have learned, is the essence of disease.
But why does it happen? We get sick when cells become compromised and begin to malfunction. This can happen in many different ways, and the biochemistry of these cellular malfunctions can be
exceedingly complex.

Cancer is simply a malfunction of cells, where the bad cells overcome the good cells. Jennifer Loros, PhD, a professor of biochemistry and genetics at Dartmouth medical school says, "A cell's natural cycle has checkpoints when it determines whether it's in a healthy state and should divide or is damaged and should repair or kill itself. Cancer can occur when the normal checkpoints in the cell cycle are misregulated somehow and the [unhealthy] cell starts dividing. Usually, a powerful protein called P-53 will trigger tumor suppression if damage is detected at the checkpoint, causing a potential cancer to stop dead in its tracks."

Recently, Loros's research team found that cell damage can trigger the body's biological clock to reset itself. She suspects that protective proteins might fool these cells into thinking they're at the time in their cycle when cell division doesn't occur, thus averting cancer in the making.

Dr. Oz recently aired a show in which he revealed the facts about some cancer mis-information that is commonly accepted, when in fact knowing the truth may save our lives. How many of us think cancer is *not* contagious? Well, it seems some cancers can be contagious! Cancer genes can be passed to you not only from your mother's side of the family but from your father's also! How can knowing the truth save our lives?

As Dr. Oz explained that when you know the truth and you know your risks, you can take advantage of the kinds of foods and activities that are known to be essential to prevent cancer from developing or to catch it early for cure. His three guest medical experts explain these facts:

We don't get cancer. We provoke cancer. Dr. William Li, MD, Cancer Researcher, President and Medical Director of the Angiogenesis Foundation says that every single person absolutely has microscopic cancers growing inside them. He explains that the human body is made up of more than 50 trillion cells that are continuously dividing to keep us healthy. But if just one of those cells makes a mistake or "mutates"—then presto!—we have formed a potentially microscopic cancer. The good news is that most of these abnormal cells will never become dangerous because our bodies have excellent defenses against cancer. Our immune system is one defense and another defense is our body's ability to resist blood vessels from growing into and feeding cancers.

So, what causes these harmless microscopic cancers to develop into full blown cancer? Dr. Li says doing things that provoke the development of cancer! Like getting too much sun and exposure to cigarette smoke, first or secondhand. Excessive alcohol and too much processed meats can have an adverse effect on the cells. The body has a hard time digesting the preservatives and nitrates in processed foods and they actually accumulate in our bodies, becoming carcinogen. Anything that dwells in the body that can provoke cancer cells is bad for you.

But on the other hand, as Dr. Li explains, we can actually add things to our life that can boost our body's cancer defense systems. Like exercise and getting enough restorative sleep. And eating foods that contain anti-angiogenic properties (starving cancer cells) like fruits and vegetables with high nutrient and antioxidant compounds. Dr. Li even explained that Gouda and some other types of hard cheeses like Edam, Jarisberg and Emmentaler contain vitamin K2, a special type of vitamin k which is a byproduct of the bacteria of the fermentation process of the cheese. This vitamin K2 inhibits angiogenesis meaning it stops blood vessels growing into and feeding cancer cells, literally starving them.

It is all about the cells, in fighting not only cancer, but all disease.

So now you know. Thus deficiency and toxins will stimulate the growth of cancer cells.

Cellular malfunctions can be broken down into two basic causes: deficiency and toxicity.

- **Deficiency** means that cells are lacking something that they need in order to function the way they are designed to function.

- **Toxicity** means that cells are poisoned by something that inhibits proper cell function.

Either one of these factors—and usually a combination of both—can and will cause disease.

We discussed how the body continuously loses and replaces cells every day. The body's cells generally die for two reasons: first, because they do not get everything they need; second, they get poisoned by something they decidedly do not need. Humans can live long and healthy lives if we do two things right: provide our cells with all of the nutrients they need and protect our cells from toxins. To the extent that we can accomplish these tasks well, we can significantly extend the length and the quality of our lives. In the real world, these two tasks are never accomplished perfectly. As a result, cells suffer, we age, the quality of life is diminished, and we die. The variable in this sequence is how fast we allow this to happen.

> Gen. 6:3 Then the LORD said, "My Spirit shall not strive with man forever, because he also is flesh; nevertheless his days shall be one hundred and twenty years."

So what happened?

Life expectancy is the average expected lifespan of an individual.

Deep in their heart, everyone wonders how long they will live. This is a question everyone asks at some stage in their life—How long will I live? When will I die? Life expectancy statistics are based on the average number of years of life remaining at a given age.

Today humans have an average life span of 31.99 years in Swaziland and 82 years in Japan. The oldest, confirmed, recorded age for any human ever born is 122 years of age; some people are reported to have lived longer, but there are no records to confirm these claims.

The great variations in life expectancy statistics worldwide are mostly caused by differences in public health, medical care, and diet from country to country. Climate also has an effect on what age you will live to, and the way data is collected can also be an important influence.

There are also variations between different groups within single countries. For instance, significant differences occur in lifespan expectancy between males and females in France and many other developed countries, with women tending to outlive men by five years and over. These gender differences have been steadily decreasing in recent years, with statistics showing male life expectancy improving at a faster rate than that of females.

Yale University takes pride in their cellular research. The Department of Cell Biology at Yale draws on a rich history rooted in the medical school's early forays into the fields of anatomy, microscopy, and histology. Their website tells the story: In 1858, Rudolph Virchow articulated what became the accepted form of the cell theory, Omnis cellula e cellula ("every cell is derived from a [preexisting] cell"). He founded the medical discipline of cellular pathology, which posited that 'disturbances in cells' are the fundamental bases of human disease.

All diseases are disturbances at the cellular level (Rudolph Virchow, 1858) To treat disease; we must understand its cause. To understand the cause of a disease, we must understand the alterations that occur at the level of individual cells.

With the elucidation of the human genome, we have greatly enhanced our potential for pinpointing the molecular aberrations responsible for even genetically complex diseases. However, identifying mutant genes or altered patterns of gene expression by themselves are insufficient to turn this information into understanding or new therapies. The functions and cellular contexts of these gene products must also be understood, assays developed to enable their study, and models put in place to test new therapies. Thus, genomics and informatics will increasingly rely on cell biology and cell biologists.

Further, not all diseases are genetically based (infectious disease, for example) nor do all affect processes that can be easily revealed by gene expression patterns.

As the study of cell biology will become increasingly important to the study of disease, the study of the cellular basis of human disease has already produced some fundamental insights into cell biological principles.

The Yale School of Medicine website lists the following major diseases elucidated, as a result of systematic cell biological analysis:

- Familial hypercholesterolemia (defective cellular uptake of lipoproteins; led to the development of "statins", widely taken to reduce cholesterol levels)
- Cystic fibrosis (chloride transport proteins are misfolded and retained in the endoplasmic reticulum, failing to reach their site of action at the cell surface)
- Lysosomal storage diseases (defective transport of hydrolytic enzymes)
- Alzheimer's disease (defective processing of amyloid plaque precursor protein)
- Hypertension (defective endocytosis of sodium channels)
- Hypertension (defective formation of junctional complexes in kidney epithelial cells)
- Muscular dystrophy (defective plasma membrane-associated cytoskeleton)
- Bullous pemphigoid (failed adherence among skin cells due to cytoskeleton defects)
- Pigmentation defects (defective maturation and transport of melanin granules in melanosomes in the skin)
- Several forms of cancer (defective transport of growth factor receptors, aberrant cell migration, defects in mechanisms of epithelial cell polarity, defects in cell cycle regulation)
- Virus infections (endocytosis, membrane fusion)

- Deafness due to mutations of myosin genes that control mechanotransduction in cells of the inner ear

The Yale School of Medicine can be considered as the birthplace of modern molecular cell biology. To this day, Cell Biology remains one of Yale's great strengths, and Cell Biology at Yale remains one of the top handful of centers anywhere in the world for research in the field.

It's time to build a better you

Now that you have a sense of your state of health and have identified many of the early warning signs of cellular malfunction and disease, we can begin to build the foundation of a new lifestyle:

- Keep a daily diary of your energy levels each morning—tired, good, great.
- Keep a food diary every day for a week, writing down everything you eat and drink. How much of your diet is eaten raw? Do you buy truly fresh, organic vegetables and fruits? Is the meat you eat treated with antibiotics and hormones? Do sugar, white flour, salt, dairy products, and processed oils weigh down your diet? Do you buy genetically modified food and cleaning products?
- Keep track of the amount and kind of exercise, movement, or other physical stimulation (saunas, etc.) you participate in during the week.
- Keep track of how much you sleep each day, per week.
- Daily, consider the products you use on your body: Are the ingredients in your deodorant, toothpaste, shampoo, makeup, and skin cream natural and nontoxic?
- Take a look at the products you use to clean your house. Consider, too, the furnishings, including your rugs. List the

sources of emissions within your house, including your carpets, furnace, hot-water heater, and stove.

- Take stock of the stress in your life.

- Think about the doctors you visit, the treatments or tests that you approve of, the medicines that you take. Are they doing you more harm than good? Are your doctors and your medical treatments addressing all your pathways to health, or is their focus narrow and incomplete?

- When was the last time you saw a chiropractor to check for nerve deficiency?

- Do you take vitamins or other supplements consistently, and are they of high quality? Do they contain cheap, ineffective ingredients such as carbonates and oxides, or toxins such as artificial colors?

Either you are going about the process of getting well and staying well, or you are going about the process of getting sicker. Healthy people do not get sick. Keep trying new things until you discover what works for you.

After you have identified some of the problems in your lifestyle—ways in which your body is becoming deficient or ways in which toxins threaten you—begin today to make changes; begin today to *Awaken the Wellness Within*.

A real understanding of the relationship between health and disease cannot be achieved through knowledge of germs, inherited genes, medicines, or surgery. Keeping up with these subjects is complex and doesn't really help people to take care of themselves. What we need right now are solutions for good health. The time is now to simplify: You must take control of your life, and to do this you must understand what your cells need, how they work, and what causes them to malfunction. Your cells are what provides good health and makes your life possible. Healthy cells equal a healthy life. If we protect and nourish our cells, we will take control of our health and our destiny.

"*He's the best physician that knows
the worthlessness of the most medicines.*"

—BENJAMIN FRANKLIN

Chapter 8

LEARNING TO LIVE HEALTHY

In the United States, we are told we have the most modern and most sophisticated health care in the world. But do we? We pay more money for health care than any country in the world, and yet we are not even in the top ten in health and longevity of all the major industrialized nations. How is it that we have the best doctors and the best hospitals, yet we have a shorter life span, more cancer, more heart disease, more diabetes, more back problems, and more arthritis than most of the so-called less fortunate countries throughout the world? We may have beat the infectious diseases, but the internal diseases—the ones that are not visible, the slowly progressive diseases such as those I have mentioned—are killing and crippling millions each year.

This is because our model on health and disease has never changed. It's been said that doing the same thing, the same way, but expecting a different result is insanity. By accepting there is only One Disease and Two Causes of any disease we can change the model of health in our country.

If we pay the most toward health, we need to be the healthiest. My dad always said there are three ways to lead:

1. One is by example
2. Two is by example
3. Three is by example

We need to lead the world in health by setting the example. To do this we can no longer follow a sickness model—a symptom model. The problem exists because we are led to believe that all of our problems can be fixed with a pill or a potion. So we begin to, what I call, "chase the symptoms." This simply means we take medication and then we wait and wait and wait to see if the problem will go away. Finally, the problem scares us enough or becomes painful enough or interferes with our lives enough that we run to a physician, any physician, and say, "Okay, doctor, I'm ready. Fix me." It doesn't work that way. In fact, the longer you wait to have a problem corrected, the more damage occurs to your cells occur.

It's inexcusable that so wealthy a country should be inhabited by so many people who are poor in health. Inexcusable, but true. Fred L. Allman Jr., MD, points out that, "over one million American workers call in sick on any given day, with the result being more than 330 million workdays lost every year because of health-related causes."

And if you think that you know the number one health hazard facing Americans today, you may be surprised by Dr. Allman's findings.

"Physical deterioration of the body is the worst disease in the United States today. It is so prevalent that if you are 25 years of age or older, then there is a 50% chance you are suffering from some form of disease. Deterioration may occur very slowly—so slowly, in fact, that it may go undetected for many years and not become readily apparent on physical examination by a competent physician."

The saddest part about this state of affairs is that deterioration can be slowed dramatically by a healthy lifestyle. I have often wondered why doctors have traditionally placed so little emphasis on nutritional paths to optimal health.

One thing is certain: You won't find the magic elixir of well-being in a capsule, pill, or injection. Despite the billions of dollars we pay to the drug industry, doctors' offices are crammed, primarily with people looking for more medication. It is crucial for you to understand that drugs are only for the control of symptoms, and that drugs alone cannot cure disease.

My philosophy is based on the belief that the body is a self-healing organism. *The power that created the body can heal the body.* The most that properly prescribed drugs can do is aid the body's defense system against disease.

Understanding the true meaning of wellness

Our life is a journey with many winding roads, enclaves, and detours. It takes far more than dedication and discipline to succeed on this journey than on any other journey we have embarked upon. It is a journey that leads us to make many decisions we must sit and labor over. We must consider ourselves travelers. We must sit and review the maps of life as we proceed to our final destination. We must utilize the proper information and material at our disposal to help us make these decisions.

The curse of our society, and sometimes our being, is that we must seek something we do not have. We seek wealth when we are not wealthy, we seek happiness when we are not happy, we seek health when we are not healthy. We don't live in a society that dictates our diet, mental attitude, thoughts, or goals. We exist in a free society scientifically superior to any other. So why do we continue to fail?

Our libraries are overflowing with books and periodicals on health and well-being. Yet we find ourselves continually on another road, another path, searching again to find the secrets of health. We live on a Ferris wheel going round and round, up and down. In God's infinite wisdom, He created no two human beings the same. I cannot count how many times I'd have a patient come to me who is 75 years old, the picture of good health, only to learn in his history that he is a chronic smoker. Of course, he smoked non-filtered cigarettes for 50 years of his life.

Common sense dictates to us that smoking is not good for our health. Yet here stands a man 75 years old, vibrant, healthy, active, who continues to smoke. I am sure we all know at least one person who can sit down at a table and eat to his heart's content yet never gains a pound. I have found in my journey on the "highway to health" and through my clinical experience as a chiropractic physician that no two people are the same.

In spite of the fact that some people have lives that "look" healthy, burnout is the disease of the '90s. We now have automobiles that map our course, televisions with giant screens, the best stereo equipment, dishwashers, clothes washers, and refrigerators that make ice cubes for us. We have self-cleaning ovens, self-defrosting freezers, and garage doors that open with the touch of a button. Then, after a long, automated day, we are rocked to sleep in a water bed. So why are we so overwhelmed by stress that we have to invent a term like "burnout?" I believe the answer is that while we have plenty of outside help, we have ignored the need for inside help. And this is the gap my book was written to fill.

To *Awaken the Wellness Within*, we must look within. I can't overemphasize the importance of "inner winning." In *Think and Grow Rich*, author Napoleon Hill gives many case histories of successful people. Few of these people were born beautiful, rich, or incredibly talented. The one thing these individuals had in common was a burning desire to succeed. Take the story of Edward C. Barnes, who was determined to become a business associate of the great Thomas Edison. Barnes was not a scientist, nor was he a wealthy man. And there were two obstacles to his goal:

1. He had never met Edison.
2. He lacked the train fare to New Jersey where Edison lived.

Barnes could have given up, in which case you wouldn't be reading about him right now. Instead, he made his way to a startled but impressed Edison who said, "He stood there before me looking like an ordinary tramp, but there was something in the expression of his face which conveyed the impression that he was determined to get what he had come after. I had learned from my years of experiences with men that when a man really desires a thing so deeply, that he is willing to stake his entire future on the single turn of a wheel in order to get it, he is sure to win. I gave him the opportunity he asked for, because I saw he made up his mind to stand by until he succeeded."

Subsequent events proved Edison correct. Edison had perfected a new office device that was to become known as the Edison Dictating Machine. At the time he met Barnes, he was having difficulty getting his people to market the invention. His sales force simply wasn't enthusiastic. Barnes took over the job and sold the machine so successfully that Edison gave him an exclusive contract to sell, market, and distribute the Edison Dictating Machine. The rest is history.

Our body is perfect. God created us with a body far greater than anything else He could ever reward us with. God gave us a body that consists of trillions of cells, and He gave us the ability to duplicate ourselves in the amazing confines of reproduction. I have come to understand the human body as an amazing machine. Each and every one of us possesses this machine. A machine that consists of a heart, lungs, a brain, and millions of pores that are constantly acting as a cooling mechanism. Our digestive system has the ability to turn simple food into healthy new blood and bones. It helps the muscles have strength, and gives the bones stability. How did this body teach the muscles and bones to work together? God has given us, within this magnificent body, a power called Innate Intelligence. This power that creates the body and operates the body has the power to heal the body.

It is known that Babe Ruth, "The Sultan of SWAT," was successful at hitting 714 lifetime runs. A total that many felt would never be equaled; a feat so spectacular that even today, years after his death, he is still a legend to every child or every person who ever enters the game of baseball. But he was also the man who struck out a record of 1,732 times. The point here is that we will be remembered more for our successes than our failures.

Another man who is remembered for his victories rather than his defeats is Abraham Lincoln. I think of Lincoln primarily as the president who brought our country through a bitter civil war; the man who ended slavery. I also knew that he did not begin life with the trappings of success. I was stunned to read the following concerning Lincoln:

1816 Forced from home
1818 His mother died
1831 Failed in business
1832 Defeated for State Legislature
1833 Failed in business again
1834 Elected to State Legislature
1835 His sweetheart died
1836 Suffered a nervous breakdown
1838 Defeated for Speaker of State Legislature
1840 Defeated for Elector
1843 Defeated for Congress
1846 Elected to Congress
1848 Lost reelection
1854 Rejected for job of Land Officer
1855 Defeated for Senate
1856 Defeated for Vice President
1858 Defeated for Senate
1860 Elected President of the United States of America

Here was a person with a dream so strong, no failure could dampen it. We were all taught about his greatness. Now I understand that Lincoln's greatness stemmed from his perseverance. In 28 years of politics, he had four times as many defeats as victories. Most men would have decided that life was unfair and given up. Because Lincoln remained true to his goals, he eventually won the most important race of all. In 1860, not only was he elected as President of the United States, but he went on to become one of the greatest presidents our country has ever known.

These people all shared an incredible perseverance and an inner desire that kept them motivated.?

There are millions of people who believe they are fated to suffer from conditions ranging from obesity to poverty by forces beyond their control. Nothing could be further from the truth. God created men and women in His own image, and that image is not one of failure. God created us to succeed, but it is up to us to follow His plan. "God's gift to man is life, and man's gift to God is what he does with his life."

*"Take care of your body.
It's the only place you have to live."*

—Jim Rohn

Chapter 9

DEFEATING DISEASE

If the power that created the body heals the body, why do we get sick in the first place? I have studied this question my whole life. This is why I am here to educate you on the theory that there is only One Disease. We now know that disease occurs as a result of two causes. In dealing with toxins, you have to look at how strong the invader is in your body and if the cell is healthy enough to remove it. If deficient, an invader can be traumatic to your cells. Toxins come in many different disguises; they can be in commons food or household chemicals. They can enter the body in the form of bacteria or virus, which can be infectious. The most important factor in disease is the resistance of your body to disease. Your immunity system will determine how strong your body is to fight off the invader from within, and that varies from person to person. The stronger your cells, the stronger your immune system will be. Cellular health, as discussed, can come from any type of toxin or nutritional deficiency. Any cell can be altered if the cell has too much or too little of any of nutrient.

Cells can also be damaged by poor nutrition, thus creating a deficiency or nutritional imbalance. For example, too much sugar harms your cells. Too few omega-3s harms your cell's outer wall. The key to cellular health is balance.

Understanding health is very simple—one disease, two causes. The disease is cytopathology, and the causes are toxins and cell deficiency, most often caused by nutritional imbalance.

Once the cellular health is affected, our immunity will weaken and the weakness of one cell will continue to spread. When this becomes rampant, dis-ease sets in, and dis-ease will lead to disease.

Most doctors are only interested in fighting off the germ, virus, or the invader and its effects with the use of drugs or surgery. But this will only treat the symptom. The more alternative or natural physician is interested in making our bodies stronger and healthier to fight the invader off from within, using our body's own normal responses. Now I find it odd that natural medicine—like chiropractic, acupuncture, and nutrition—is considered alternative care. Alternative care should be the care that contains the most risk, the most side effects. Shouldn't drugs and surgery be the alternative care if natural remedies don't work?

Disease is a form of darkness in our lives. What is darkness? Simply the absence of light. In the same sense, what is disease? Simply the absence of health.

Dis-ease

When the body is no longer at ease, it is at dis-ease. To understand this paradigm, One Disease, One Cure, you must first always look to cellular health. Each cell must perform specific tasks daily in order to collaborate effectively with other cells in the body. If all of your cells are healthy, the body functions at optimal levels, thus you will be and feel healthy. The fact is simple: if all of your cells are healthy, you are healthy. If your cells are sick, you are sick. If a cell starts to malfunction, it is less able to perform its assigned tasks, which is where problems can begin. When such malfunction occurs in a large enough number of cells to impair the body's ability to self-repair and self-regulate, disease occurs. Hopefully this book will awaken your cells and teach you how to maintain optimum health.

As perfect as we humans are, the fundamental concept of disease is simple: Disease is the result of a large number of malfunctioning cells throughout any area of the body. Sickness=Malfunctioning cells.

So what causes our cells to malfunction? There are many factors may conspire in contributing to the malfunction of our cells and the many different ways in which they can malfunction. In the end, though, cellular malfunction creates the measurable abnormalities that we call disease. Therefore, no matter which cells malfunction, or why they malfunction, the malfunction of the specific cells to any area of the body is the one disease, cellular malfunction.

If we take care of our cells' health, good health is at our fingertips. A person cannot be sick unless a large number of cells are malfunctioning. The first steps on the path to disease are taken when, for whatever reason, a single cell begins to malfunction, and then another cell and another. When the number grows large enough, we may begin to notice. We begin to experience symptoms. For some, symptoms are far ranging—often experiencing a pain here, a discomfort there, or a lack of energy. By the time your health has deteriorated into a diagnosable disease, your cells are now fighting for their respective lives.

I often find it amusing when someone tells me that outside of their current health problems they are in excellent health! Healthy people are healthy, sick people are sick. If you are diabetic, are you healthy? Disease is a breakdown of cells to the body's weakest link.

Toxic living versus nontoxic living

Imagine if Iran, Cuba, Russia, or China stated that they were planning to poison our food, our homes, our workplaces or, for that matter, the entire planet? We would be outraged. We would be sitting by our televisions, waiting for updates on our lives and planet. Yet this has happened to each and everyone one of us and few of us are outraged. We are constantly told that small amounts of toxins are safe. The fact is— a toxin is a toxin. Chronic disease is rampant because these small amounts of toxins, when added together, are disabling our detoxification systems, exceeding our body's innate capacity to detoxify them, and bioaccumulating in our tissues to disease-causing levels.

Some toxins, such as estrogenic chemicals (from pesticides, plastic bottles and canned foods), tobacco, and medications are not safe even in amounts so small they cannot be measured by the usual techniques. Every day we eat food, breathe air, and use products containing these and other harmful toxins. Some exposure is virtually unavoidable but most exposure is by choice. We have to start making different everyday choices about what we put on and in our bodies and what we expose ourselves to in the workplace. We need to change our perspective that small amounts don't matter. *"It is the little things in life that make the big difference."*

Toxins interfere with normal cell function, thereby causing malfunctions. Most people know that toxins are dangerous. Toxins in our environment can impose an undue external burden on us, while poor digestion, lack of exercise, and negative thoughts and emotions can increase our toxic loads internally.

Our bodies do have the ability to detoxify, but our detoxification mechanisms require essential nutrients to function properly. Inadequate nutrition causes a cellular deficiency that deprives our bodies of the raw materials necessary to detoxify, so toxic levels build and negatively affect cellular health. To "Awaken" our inner healer, we must avoid toxins and remove those that are present in our diet and homes.

I am of the belief that in our society today, toxic overload is abundant and is having a bigger effect than it should because our deficient diets do not supply the nutrients necessary to operate and maintain our detoxification mechanisms. Not only is our toxic overload the highest in our history, but our ability to process and eliminate these toxins is impaired due to the many drugs we take for the symptoms that the toxins have provided.

We know that excessive toxic exposure causes cells to stress, thus they begin to wear down and malfunction. When this happens, disease is simply a matter of time. Whenever dealing with toxins we must know how toxic they are and where we are exposed—where they are, how they get there, and how we can minimize our exposures to them. The toxin pathway into our lives provides insight into the toxic aspects of our daily lives—in our food supply, water supply, homes, and personal products (including many soaps, shampoos, and toothpastes).

Fortunately, the world is changing and natural, healthful alternatives are available. Toxic exposure is an unfortunate fact of life; we must provide our bodies with the nutrients to better equip our bodies to eliminate these toxins.

Toxic overload simply means the toxic input exceeds our ability to process it. Understanding this approach can help us to reduce toxic exposure to manageable levels by teaching us to recognize and avoid toxins in our daily lives.

We are exposed to toxins in various ways: in the air we breathe, the water we drink, the clothes we wear, and the food we eat. In our modern world, we are exposed to these environmental toxins all day, every day.

In our society, toxic overload is having a bigger effect than it should, because our deficient diets do not supply the nutrients necessary to operate and maintain our detoxification mechanisms. Not only is our toxic load the highest in history, but our ability to process and eliminate these toxins is impaired. Unfortunately, toxic exposure is a fact of life, and the body is designed to deal with it to some degree. Our problem is toxic overload, i.e., when the toxic input exceeds our ability to process it, causes major trauma to our cellular ecosystem. Understanding the foods we eat and the environment we live in, as well as the products we use, can help us to reduce toxic exposure to manageable levels in our lives. By teaching you to recognize and avoid toxins in our daily lives we begin to *Awaken the Wellness Within*.

Poisoning our cells

The battle against toxins in our cells and our lives is ongoing. We can begin at the supermarket and how we shop.

Much of the toxic trouble we face begins before the food hits our tables. The Genesis of our food often begins prior to the food leaving commercial farms. Farming practices today are different than years ago when quality was the key. Today it is about quantity. In today's world, many agricultural practices are dependent on chemicals to make for a larger crop, such as chemical fertilizers, insecticides, herbicides, and fungicides. These chemical toxins are utilized to produce larger quantities of food regardless of the fact that these chemicals reduce the nutritional quality of the food and deplete the soil of nutrients needed to produce future quality crops.

Research has shown that chemical fertilizers, which are supposed to put nutrients into the soil, often end up causing nutrients to be removed from the soil. The most common types of chemical fertilizers that support high food production, add three major nutrients to the soil: nitrogen, phosphorous, and potassium. The problem, however, is that these plants require many other nutrients absorbed from the soil, such as zinc, calcium, magnesium, selenium, germanium, chromium, manganese, nickel, and molybdenum. Chemical fertilizers alone do not supply these nutrients. By not replacing these nutrients and by growing more food on the same land year after year after year, critical nutrients are continually lost from the soil, leading to nutrient-deficient soil, nutrient-deficient crops, nutrient-deficient farm animals, and nutrient-deficient human beings. Deficiency of our land equals deficiency in our diet, which causes deficiency to our cells.

In her 1976 book, *The Living Soil*, Lady Eve Balfour describes an 18-year experiment on three farms with similar soil profiles. One of the farms was managed organically, one chemically, and the third was a mixture of the two. During this eighteen-year study, the soil on the organic farm was found to have the highest mineral content. Not coincidentally, the dairy herd on that farm was healthier, produced more milk, and had higher reproductive capacity.

The use of chemical fertilizers triggers a series of problems as plants struggle to cope with deficient soils and toxic attacks. Plants grown in nutrient-deficient soils are less healthy and more vulnerable to insects, molds, fungi, viruses, bacteria, and weeds. The susceptibility leads to the use of other agricultural chemicals, such as pesticides, herbicides, and fungicides to protect sick plants. These toxic chemicals create "dead soils," killing not only the undesirable organisms but also the helpful organisms (earthworms, insects, bacteria, and fungi) that are responsible for taking minerals out of the soil and converting them into forms that plants can use. When these bacteria and fungi are killed, the plants no longer receive adequate nutrition.

Insecticides, fungicides, and herbicides accumulate in the soil to a level where they inhibit plant growth. These poor growing conditions have spurred the development of new kinds of plants, such as hybrid and genetically modified crops.

In creating genetically modified plants, which humankind has never eaten before, we may have (unknowingly) altered the nutritional value of the plants, as well as made them more toxic or allergenic. More and more genetically modified foods are contaminating the food supply with novel and unnatural varieties of organisms.

105

Our bodies are toxic

Man-made toxins are so prevalent today that they are impossible to avoid, regardless of where you live or what you do. Over the last one hundred years, we have introduced tens of thousands of man-made toxins to our environment, thus changing it dramatically. Our bodies are not designed to deal with these levels and types of poisons that are accumulating in our tissues faster than we can rid ourselves of them.

Environmental toxins are not our only problem. We also generate powerful toxins inside our bodies. Unless we can minimize our exposure and maximize our bodies' detoxification systems, we will become sick. An extreme overload of any toxin may even kill us.

Chronic exposure to small amounts of seemingly harmless toxins presents a problem more dangerous than people realize. Even in trace amounts, toxins can build up and overload our cells, causing malfunction. The average American is building up (bioaccumulating) between three and five hundred manmade chemicals, most of which did not exist prior to World War II and have never before been in human tissue. Therefore, the combined toxic effects of these chemicals are impossible to calculate.

Henry Schroeder, MD, a former professor of medicine at Dartmouth Medical School and author of *The Poisons Around Us*, wrote that "five toxic trace metals: antimony, beryllium, cadmium, lead, and mercury are involved in at least half the deaths in the U.S. and much of the disabling disease."

In all, more than one 100,000 chemicals are now in commercial use, at least 25% of which are known to be hazardous; many others have never been tested at all!

In the 19th century, less than 1% of all deaths in the United States were caused by cancer, and even at the turn of the 20th century, only 3% of the population was affected. Today, more than 4 in 10 people will develop cancer in their lifetime, and 1 in 4 will die from cancer.

What are you celling me?

Today and every day moving forward we must watch what we put into our bodies. Often we care more about how we look than how we feel. In my parents' generation, they smoked cigarettes to look cool. Today, cosmetic injections are in—because it's not cool to look old, or is it?

If you're reading this and you are thinking about wrinkle-reducing injections, my recommendation to you is to think **twice**!

Before engaging in any procedure, you must weigh the risk versus the reward. If someone came to you with a syringe filled with anthrax and told you it would make you look younger, would you let them inject you? Of course not. Now suppose someone comes to you with a syringe of botulism toxin and tells you it will make you look younger and remove wrinkles; would you let them inject your face? Last year over seven million Americans said yes.

How have so many people been persuaded to receive injections of this deadly toxin? Because we naively trust pharmaceutical marketing, our government, and the healthcare delivery system to protect us. We don't ask questions about the materials doctors use to make us look younger.

Since the FDA approved it for cosmetic use in 2002, Botox has become a household word and many people have been injected with the drug at the site of a facial line to paralyze the nerve and make the skin appear wrinkle free. This FDA-approved and licensed botulinum toxin type A is derived from the waste of the bacterium Clostridium botulinum, the same toxic byproduct that causes botulism food poisoning. Botulinum toxin is the most poisonous substance known to man. Because of its extreme potency and lethality, the ease of production, transport, and misuse, botulinum toxin is considered a bioweapon. A single gram of crystalline toxin, evenly dispersed as an aerosol and inhaled, would kill more than one million people. The name Botox is cute, but remember it is short for botulism toxin.

Since aerosol dispersement is difficult, terrorists might instead use botulinum toxin to deliberately contaminate food sources. Development and use of botulinum toxin as a biological weapon began during World War II. Terrorists attempted to use botulinum toxin as a bioweapon in Japan in the 1990s but these attacks failed, either due to faulty microbiological technique, deficient aerosol equipment, or internal sabotage. After the Persian Gulf War, Iraq admitted to having produced and loaded into bombs and military weapons enough concentrated botulinum toxin to kill the entire current human population by inhalation. You may not sleep as well tonight after you know that the whereabouts of those toxic weapons is still unknown.

At one time, food poisoning from botulism was considered a dinner table threat in most American households. Since the toxin is rendered inactive when heated at boiling temperature for ten minutes, the only way a human may contract the bacteria through food is when contaminated sources are not properly heated before consumption. This used to be the case with improper home canning processes that were common before so much of our food came packed full of preservatives.

Botulism-causing Clostridium botulinum bacteria and their spores are found in fruits, vegetables, and seafood worldwide. The bacteria and spores themselves are harmless, but as the bacteria grows, it produces a dangerous substance called botulinum toxin that may enter the human body through contaminated food or exposure in an open wound. Once the toxin is in the body, it irreversibly binds to nerve endings where the muscles and the nerves join. The toxin blocks the release of acetylcholine, thereby rendering the nerves unable to send signals to the muscles to contract. Weakness and paralysis starts in the head and moves downward through the body, affecting the person's ability to breathe. About 8% of those who contract botulism will die.

Millions of people have been injected with Botox and most do not realize that the serum is a weaker version of botulism bacteria. Any toxin regularly injected into the body must have side effects; however, to look young we often turn our back on what is good and what is not.

Cosmetic procedures gone wrong is the quiet epidemic sweeping America that no one in the drug industry wants you to know about. Few of us realize we could be risking death when we ask doctors to help us preserve our youth. My wife and I learned from our mistake, and we want to share our insight with you. For those who are thinking of cosmetically altering your appearance, do your research and ask questions about what is going into your body.

Prior to November 23, 2004, no one in the world had ever been poisoned by fake Botox or injections of raw botulinum toxin. The dosage we received should have been fatal. We were both 100% paralyzed, and the prognosis was not good. I am thankful to Dr. Dennis Egitto, his hand-picked team, and the Shepard Center for our miraculous recovery. There is no cure to botulism. We learned first hand that the "power that created the body can heal the body."

Thankfully, in our case the injections were not fatal and good triumphed over a bad situation. I have learned that our mental attitude dominates our physical condition. Yes, brains are superior to brawn! The power of our mind, spirit, and soul is stronger than any muscle in our body; and the stronger our spirit becomes, the more we empower our body to heal.

As a doctor, I thought I knew the risks, but no one ever expects to face the consequences. Any surgical procedure comes with risk. I now tell my patients, "The difference between major and minor surgery, is that minor surgery happens to someone else."

Because of our programming, we have come to believe that there are good drugs and bad drugs. We must realize that drugs are drugs, no matter what the label says. Every drug has side effects. I never thought I was risking my life with drugs. Like every other naive person in the world, I thought if something was approved by the FDA, or a procedure was performed in a doctor's office, or regulated and monitored by the state, it would be okay. Yet, according to a Harvard study, over 100,000 people die annually as a result of their doctor's care. According to the Cyclopedic Medical Dictionary, "Iatrogenesis is any adverse or physical condition induced in a patient through the effects of treatment by a physician or surgeon." Iatrogenesis is now the fourth leading cause of death in our country behind cancer, heart disease, and stroke. Taking a drug is taking a risk. If you remember or learn one thing from this book, remember that **ALL DRUGS ARE DANGEROUS AND THEY ALL HAVE SIDE EFFECTS**.

If you have already been damaged by drugs and medical procedures gone awry, perhaps this book will help you find encouragement in the midst of your suffering and injustice. Friends, you cannot continually inject yourself with any toxin and not expect side effects.

In order to get the best results possible and get maximum benefits from what is currently known about aging and cellular health, we need to integrate natural law and modern science into a single power for ageless aging. When used together, you will not only look and feel better, you will also go a long way toward preventing degenerative cellular diseases like cancer, heart disease, and stroke. These diseases, make up the top three causes of death in our country and are wreaking havoc on our health, well-being, and medical system. Once we change the paradigm and begin treating the cause of disease, we will have moved much closer to healing all disease.

1. **Let go of the past.** Before any of us can create a better future, we must let go of the pains in our past. Failing once does not mean we will fail forever. Even if we fall flat on our face, we are still moving forward. We need to get up and brush ourselves off. Learn from the past, but don't hold on to it or let it stand as

an obstacle between you and your future. I had to let go of my past or I would have remained diseased. I am no longer mad at myself for what happened. I learned from my mistake and have come to cherish my life.

2. **Success stays forever.** Just as important as learning from and overcoming past failure is recalling past success. Hold on to everything good in your life. Memories are magic, memories create miracles. No matter who you are, you have succeeded at something in your past. Don't forget those moments. You have earned those memories. They are your right of passage. Use them. Replay them to remind you that you can achieve your goals.

- No matter what your state of health, you can always get healthier.
- No matter what your state of wealth, you can always get wealthier.
- What you think about can actually come about.
- We live in a world abundant with resources. There is nothing in life that is not possible.
- The sky is not the limit; it is only as far as you can see.
- The universe, like each of our physical and economic potentials, is infinite.
- If you can see the invisible, you can do the impossible.

We will discuss the toxic overload our cells are bombarded with on a daily basis and how to cleanse and protect our cells more in upcoming chapters. To *Awaken the Wellness Within* we must adapt a cellular lifestyle or protecting and preserving our cells.

"The bottom line is, I'm blessed with good health. On top of that, I don't go around thinking, 'Oh, I'm 90, I better do this or I better do that.' I'm just Betty. I'm the same Betty that I've always been. Take it or leave it."

—BETTY WHITE

Chapter 10

---◈◉◉◈---

CELLULAR HEALING
BEGINS TODAY

We learned in the past chapters, that health is more than just the absence of disease. Insurance companies push the doctors to give a name for every illness ache or pain, a diagnosis to each and every ailment. Without a diagnosis, your insurance company will simply not pay your claim.

For example, if you have a headache, the word for the diagnosis is cephalgia. To have one disease is too simple. How could insurance companies ever refuse your claim for a pre-existing condition?

Doctors are trained that to recognize disease it must be diagnosable. What this means is that you're not sick until the day the physician can diagnose something. Once they come up with a diagnosis, your insurance company will pay. No diagnosis, no pay. Are you beginning to see a trend?

The absence of diagnosable disease is not a fair definition of health. Why wait until your cholesterol levels are out of whack before you do something about it? If we are trending high, we must recognize the body's weakness before it becomes a disease. Modern medicine has no way of recognizing or diagnosing disease when your health is in its initial decline. Remember, it only takes one weakened cell.

The cell's first line of defense against disease is the cell membrane, the security wall that surrounds the cell and carries out many important functions. Healthy cell membranes, built from appropriate materials, protect the cells from harmful invaders such as viruses. Malfunctioning membranes allow bacteria, viruses, toxins, and other harmful substances to damage the cells. The key to a healthier, happier cell is a strong membrane.

Our cells come into contact daily with chemicals in our environment. The connection between diet and increased toxicity and health disorders is evident. It's vital to understand how and why it occurs so that we can avoid or reduce it from our diets and our lives.

If we have weak cell membranes, we'll be vulnerable to these outside agents. Toxins find their way into the human body through contact from external sources, including via the respiratory pathway from polluted air, from consumption of contaminated food, or via the skin.

Toxins can also be generated internally in the body. There are a variety of chemicals in drugs, additives, and in processed foods. Chemical allergens are toxic inside the body. Toxicity weakens the cells due to the accumulation of any substance to excessive levels within the human body.

In our journey through this book, we'll learn how to protect your body and protect your cells. As we age, if we allow the cells to weaken, our telomeres become shorter and our cells become weaker. With properly functioning cells, you have strong resilience to various kinds of stress—physical, chemical, biological, and emotional.

The body is a self-healing organism and that gives us the ability to make daily repairs to our cells, the ability to build healthy new ones, and the ability to efficiently remove pathogenic microorganisms and toxins from our body. We then reach homeostasis and become an optimally balanced person with integrated mental and physical equilibrium. Achieving good cellular health gives our society the ability to produce healthy offspring, to live a healthy life. If we protect these cells, we can literally *Awaken the Wellness Within*.

Health is the state wherein all cells are functioning optimally and our body is at balance or homeostasis. Our goal is to keep cellular malfunction to a minimum. Even in healthy people, cells are constantly being damaged, dying, and being replaced at a rate of almost two billion per day. Our bodies produce more than 10 million new cells every second as we constantly rebuild our tissues. How healthy each of these new cells are will be the key to ageless aging. If we replace sick cells with sick cells, we'll never recover. As cells die off, are we replacing them with healthy cells or sick cells?

We must treat disease before it becomes diagnosable. Sickness and disease do not just happen, they accumulate. We must learn that symptoms are warning signs and are the start of disease. In today's current paradigm of health care, doctors are trained that to recognize disease, it must be diagnosable. What this means, by definition, is that you are not sick until the day the physician can diagnose something.

Let me offer you an example. A normal fasting blood glucose target range for an individual without diabetes is 70–100 mg/dL (3.9–5.6 mmol/L). The American Diabetes Association recommends a fasting plasma glucose level of 70–130 mg/dL. Personally, I think 130 is high. We need to watch our numbers before a disease like diabetes is diagnosed.

Now let's discuss cholesterol. Mayo Clinic considers below 200 mg/dL to be desirable, and above 240 mg/dL is considered high. What if your cholesterol is 199? Is it time to watch what you eat, exercise, and change your lifestyle? The answers are yes, yes, and yes.

My first book, *Lifestyle of the Fit & Famous*, talks about the impact sugar and carbohydrates have on our bodies. If you are overweight, you may be sugar and carbohydrate intolerant. This intolerance will cause your cells to malfunction and may first appear as low blood sugar. Yes, we get low blood sugar sometime before high blood sugar, hypoglycemia, which is a precursor to diabetes.

In our journey through this book, you will learn how to protect your body and how you must protect your cells. If we allow our cells to weaken as we age, our telomeres are prone to become shorter, thus our new and existing cells become weaker. With properly functioning cells, you have strong resilience to various kinds of stress—physical, chemical, biological, and emotional. The body is a self-healing organism that gives us the ability to make daily repairs to our cells, the ability to build healthy new ones, and the ability to efficiently remove pathogenic microorganisms and toxins from our body. When this occurs we are able to reach homeostasis and become an optimally balanced person with integrated mental and physical equilibrium.

Achieving good cellular health gives our society the ability to produce healthy offspring and to live a healthy life. If we protect these cells, we can turn back the clock on aging.

Health is the state wherein all cells are functioning optimally when our body is at balance or homeostasis. Our goal is to keep cellular malfunction to a minimum. Even in healthy people, cells are constantly being damaged, dying, and being replaced at a rate of almost two billion per day. Our bodies produce more than 10 million new cells every second, as we constantly rebuild our tissues. The health of these new cells will be the key to ageless aging. If we replace sick cells with sick cells, we will never recover. As our cells die off, are we replacing them with healthy cells or sick cells?

Who succumbs to disease?

Our fast-paced, time-poor lifestyles push the idea that faster is better. Our work habits, phones, Internet, cars, and computers get faster and faster. A faster-working pill is presumed to be a better-working pill. Unfortunately, there is no such thing.

A life out of balance will catch up with you eventually, and everyone in today's world is prone to be out of balance. We do generate illness (and wellness) in our lives. This is one of the tenets of medicine—that health and illness are not only things that happen to us, but also things that we do, a kind of behavior. The interaction of all human physiological systems connects the mind to the body in definite but extremely complex ways.

To heal our bodies, to create homeostasis, and to protect our telomeres we must take care of our cells. The world needs to know that when it comes to health, faster doesn't necessarily mean better.

Not only does modern science now understand the simplicity of disease and its causes, it also understands how to use that knowledge to turn back the clock naturally. There's a lot we can do for ourselves to be happier, healthier, and live younger—far more than just taking pills. We can observe our lifestyle habits and boost those that need improving.

Defend your castle

Your body is your castle; your cells reside in your kingdom. It's your job as king or queen to protect your castle and your responsibility to take care of its residents—your cells. No matter how clean our environment may be, we share our living space with many microorganisms. If you could examine with a microscope the room you're now sitting in, you would clearly see the millions of creatures you are living with.

So, in this sense, a human being is a besieged castle. It goes without saying that to protect this castle under assault, a failsafe plan is necessary. Human beings were created with the perfect protection that they need; they are not defenseless against these enemies. We were created with innate micro-defense systems in the human body, protecting it from all sorts of dangerous organisms and fighting to defend it on multiple fronts.

We can compare the human body to a fortress under attack. Just as the defense of a fortress besieged by enemies is very well planned, so the human body has a perfect defense system if we keep our cells healthy and our body in balance.

We protect our castle with a strong line of defense, maybe we build a moat and maybe we put our archers on the walls. The cell, when not distracted by toxins or weakened from lack of nourishment, knows how to defend your castle. As stated, the cell's first line of defense is a healthy cell membrane. The cell membrane controls everything that goes in and out of the cell. Making certain only the right things go in and out of the cells is critical. Think of it like a drawbridge. If you protect your cell, you protect your castle.

You must feed the members of your castle with the foods to give them strength from outside invaders. Real foods support the health and function of your cells whereas processed foods do not.

Here's one example: Whole grains (such as wheat, oats, millet, and quinoa) are seeds that contain all the ingredients necessary to create a new plant—to create a new life. Anything that can create life, can sustain life. These nutrients that are necessary to create life are also necessary to sustain the cells of your castle.

Foods that are nutritious but nontoxic come from the following categories:

- Organic foods produced naturally without any man-made chemicals, such as pesticides, herbicides, fertilizers, preservatives, antibiotics, hormones, processed animal feed, etc. These foods are generally higher in nutrients and lower in toxins than non-organic (commercially produced) foods of the same type.
- Fresh foods harvested at their peak of nutrition (ripeness) and consumed shortly thereafter. Food that is harvested too early does not gain any more nutrition (even though it may

continue to ripen); in fact, nutrition begins to decline. Some foods deteriorate more quickly than others, but the point is that you want to eat your food as soon after harvesting as possible. The more the food sits around (during harvesting, storage, transportation, and distribution) the more nutrition it will lose.

- Unprocessed foods minimally altered from the way that nature provides. Avoid foods that are overcooked, peeled, cut, ground, dehydrated, frozen, canned, etc. Unprocessed foods are whole, complete foods, rather than just part of a food—whole grains instead of flour made from grains, for example, or potatoes with the peel still on.

Life would be simpler, healthier, if we could all revert to hunting, gathering, growing our own food, and eating it fresh and raw; however, that is not being realistic. So we must learn to evaluate the foods that are available to us and make choices that are both healthy and realistic.

Even foods that are truly fresh and ripe can nevertheless be nutritionally destroyed if you prepare them improperly. Our biological ancestors usually did not cook or process their foods. Foods were eaten fresh and raw. The healthy Hunzas ate 80% of their diet raw. Their foods not only had more nutrition to begin with (because of traditional farming techniques and rich soils), they also did not typically diminish that nutrition by cooking. Nobel laureate Linus Pauling believed that the mostly raw, mostly vegetarian, unprocessed diet of our biological ancestors provided a level of nutritional quality far superior to the food supply available today.

The bulk of the modern American diet comes from processed foods that have been deliberately altered from the way nature provided. This altering includes trimming, peeling, chopping, blending, mashing, commercial refining and cooking. While some degree of processing may be necessary, there are many degrees of processing—from the simple slicing of a carrot for your salad all the way to the grinding and bleaching of wheat in order to make white flour. The most significant causes of malnutrition, other than commercial farming and distribution techniques, are cooking and processing.

Although the health benefits of raw foods need emphasis, a few words of caution are important about raw animal products (such as eggs, meat, fish, and poultry). Even though nature intended us to eat raw foods—animal products included— today's hazards of bacterial, viral, and parasitic infections make raw animal foods dangerous. Also, raw animal foods must not touch other foods intended to be eaten raw.

Even just a few generations ago, people typically ate more raw food than they do now, and the trend toward cooked and processed foods appears to be worsening. According to U.S. Department of Agriculture statistics, over the last century average consumption of fresh apples declined by more than three-fourths, fresh cabbage by more than two-thirds, and fresh fruit by more than one-third. During that same period, consumption of processed vegetables went up hundreds of percent and consumption of processed fruits went up by about 1,000%.

You monitor the health of your castle, your kingdom, by the health and happiness of your cells. If your soldiers, your cells, are experiencing any of the symptoms below, they are in a weakened state and thus your castle is vulnerable.

- Fatigue
- Aches and pains
- Skin problems
- Allergies
- Digestion troubles
- Sleep difficulties
- Susceptibility to infections

- Weight issues
- Mood, thought, or behavior problems

We protect our cells by protecting their outer membrane, or their armor. Despite our society's obsession with and fears about fats and oils, these nutrients are an incredibly important part of a healthy diet.

Each of the trillions of cells (your army) in your body is surrounded by a permeable cell membrane. Fats and oils are the primary building materials used to create those cell membranes. The cell membrane is critically important because all the nutrients your cells need and all the toxic waste products they must eliminate need to pass through it. If you eat the right kinds of fats and oils, your cell membranes properly regulate the passage of materials; eating the wrong kinds causes your cell membranes to work against you. When your cell membranes are not working correctly, your cells will malfunction, which can manifest into just about any disease you can imagine.

Essential fatty acids are the term used to describe the "right kind" of fats and oils. They are essential because the body needs them but cannot make them, so we must obtain them from food. These essential fatty acid molecules have a specific shape that is critical to the way they work in forming cell membranes—like bricks that fit perfectly together to build cell walls.

To put healthful oils in your diet, eat plenty of omega-3 foods and use high-quality olive oil and flaxseed oil. Also, beneficial fatty acids can be found in organic, fresh, unprocessed food in its natural state, such as raw seeds, raw nuts, and avocados. High-quality eggs, meat, and fish are also good sources of fatty acids. Keep in mind, though, that essential fatty acids are readily damaged by heat. Use the minimum heat necessary to cook these foods. Supplement your diet with a high-quality essential fatty acid supplement.

A life out of balance will catch up with you eventually and weaken your castle and its army of cells, making you vulnerable to the enemy known as disease.

To maintain a healthy kingdom, we must protect our soldiers of cells. For these cells aid and defend our bodies daily. To strengthen our kingdom, to heal our bodies, to create homeostasis, to protect our cells and our knights known as telomeres, we must take care of our cells. The world needs to know that when it comes to health, faster doesn't necessarily mean better. What a change of paradigm. Protect the cell, offset disease, and start to turn back the clock.

Now the "One disease, Two causes, One Cure" theory of health and disease may shock the world of medicine—or do they already know this? Why have doctors made health so complex?

Aging is not a disease

References to "the disease of aging" still make many people uncomfortable. After all, aging is a natural process that has existed forever, so how can it be a disease?

In fact, aging has not existed forever. Approximately 4.5 billion years ago, a cell came into existence on Earth that was the beginning of every living organism that has since existed. This cell had the ability to divide indefinitely. It exhibited no aging process; it could produce a theoretically infinite number of copies of itself, and it would not die until some environmental factor killed it. When the ancestry of any given cell is traced back to this very first living cell, this lineage is called the cell's germ line.

Much later—perhaps three billion years later—some cells of the germ line began to form multicellular organisms: worms, beetles, lobsters, humans. The germ line, however, was still passed on from one generation to the next and remained immortal. Even with the inclusion of multicellular organisms, the germ line itself exhibited no aging process.

As time passed, we began to alter our lifestyle and our environments. We altered the balance of nature. As a result, in some multicellular organisms such as humans, certain cells strayed from the germ line and began to exhibit signs of aging. These cells aged because they became afflicted with a disease: their ability to reproduce themselves indefinitely became broken. The cause of this disease is still speculative, but many scientists are searching for cures. Eventually researchers determined the power of cellular health; most of us were just not aware of it.

The fact that a disease has existed in the genetic code of an animal for a very long time does not mean that it is not a disease. Thousands of diseases, from hemophilia to cystic fibrosis, have lurked in our genes for far longer than recorded history. These diseases should be cured, and aging is no exception.

Health is an inside job. Concern for our health is something we all need to have in common. We all would like to live a high-quality, disease-free life, no matter how long that life may be. But most of us have no idea that a long and healthy disease-free life is just a few chapters away. When people get sick they start to weaken, once that happens their priorities change and we form habits that jeopardize our health. Then we ignore the early signs of ill health and, without knowing it, we lay the groundwork for disaster. Once we realize we add years to our life and life to our years, we are on our way to a new life, a healthier life, and a happier kingdom.

"*If we are creating ourselves all the time, then it is never too late to begin creating the bodies we want instead of the ones we mistakenly assume we are stuck with.*"

—DEEPAK CHOPRA

Chapter 11

CELL CITY

Continually throughout this book, we talk about the importance of the cell and how you must protect the trillions of cells that are working as you read this chapter. Imagine, your cells work 24/7, building, rebuilding, reproducing—never taking one day, one minute, off.

Cells are the essence of life, the building blocks of your bodies. They build your tissues, and these tissues make up your organs and organ systems. Because malfunctioning cells are the one disease, learning to care for our cells is a fundamental key to healthy living.

In order to understand disease, to understand health and prevent aging, you must understand the essence of life—the cell. Cells are the basic building blocks of all living things. They provide structure for the body, take in nutrients from food, convert those nutrients into energy, and carry out specialized functions. Cells also contain the body's hereditary material and can make copies of themselves. This is germane to aging and our knowledge of telomeres and their importance to aging.

Look at yourself in a mirror; what you see are trillions of cells divided into about 200 different cell types. Our muscles are made of muscle cells, our livers of liver cells, and there are even very specialized types of cells that make the enamel for our teeth or the clear lenses in our eyes. Our heart is made of cells, our lungs are made of cells, our skin is made of cells, our brain is made of cells, our bones are made of cells, and so on.

Our body is a community of trillions of individually living cells, and so, our overall state of bodily health is a perfect representation of how healthy, or unhealthy, our individual cells are. Having healthy cells means we have a healthy body, and having stressed out unhealthy dysfunctional cells means the body has disease.

Cells that are constantly subjected to physical, emotional, and energetic stress become dysfunctional, and this dysfunction equates to "dis-ease" because the cells/body is no longer at ease.

If you want to understand how your body works, you need to understand cells. Everything from reproduction to infections to repairing broken bones happens at the cellular level. If you want to understand new frontiers like telomere research through biotechnology and genetic engineering, you need to understand cells.

Cell biology

Cells are the most basic units of life. A cell is much more than a combination of molecules and atoms. A cell represents the miracle of life itself. A single cell is a separate and distinct life form. Where there are living cells, there is life. Each cell is a complex structure that could theoretically survive, grow, reproduce, and die on its own. The cells in our bodies, however, work together with similar cells to form structures called tissues. Tissues make up the different organs and functional material in our bodies.

Each cell is composed of many smaller units called organelles. An organelle in a cell is analogous to an organ in the human body. Important organelles include the plasma membrane, cytoplasm, cytoskeleton, Golgi apparatus, endoplasmic reticulum, mitochondria, lysosomes, ribosomes, and the nucleus. The organelles each perform different functions to keep the cell alive and healthy.

The most important organelle is the nucleus. The nucleus is like the brain of a cell. It controls all actions that the cell undertakes. The nucleus can do this because it contains DNA. DNA is the genetic blueprint for the cell that contains all the necessary information for cells to live, grow, reproduce, and die. It is inherited from the cell's parent and is passed down to the daughter cell when it reproduces. DNA exists as a double-stranded helix made up of four randomly repeating nucleotides, which form a code that tells the cell how to produce all necessary proteins.

Cells grow and divide in a highly regulated system called the cell cycle. During most of the cell cycle, the cell grows at a normal pace and performs its normal functions. However, the key is keeping the cell healthy. When a cell gets too large, it must divide; this is a part of the growth and aging process.

The process by which a cell divides in half to create two identical copies of itself is known as mitosis; it is during this and each process forward that we must preserve our telomeres. Once the two new cells are formed, they are then called daughter cells. For this miracle to occur, the DNA must replicate itself to provide a complete genome for each daughter cell. The organelles must also equally distribute themselves so each daughter cell receives an adequate number to function. The cell must then physically divide, separating the contents of the cytoplasm into the two new cells.

Our body is a self-healing mechanism

In fact, the only thing that our cells do, and what they do 24 hours a day, is protect, heal, repair, regenerate, and rebuild.

The only reason they haven't been able to heal themselves, or stay healthy, thus far, is because of that constant unrelenting cellular stress in our lifestyle.

Throughout the earlier portions of this book, we talked about the importance of the cell. Cells are the building blocks of your bodies. They build your tissues, and these tissues make up your systems. Because malfunctioning cells are the one disease, learning to care for our cells is fundamental to healthy living.

In order to understand disease, understand health, and prevent aging, you must understand the essence of life, the cell. Cells are the basic building blocks of all living things. They provide structure for the body, take in nutrients from food, convert those nutrients into energy, and carry out specialized functions. Cells also contain the body's hereditary material and can make copies of themselves. This is germane to aging and our knowledge of telomeres and their importance to aging.

Telomere shortening

An important property of DNA is that it can replicate, or make copies of itself. Each strand of DNA in the double helix can serve as a pattern for duplicating the sequence of bases. This is critical when cells divide because each new cell needs to have an exact copy of the DNA present in the old cell. It is because of this duplicating process that preserving the length of our telomeres is so important. For every cell division, a chromosome can lose 25–200 base pairs of DNA from its ends.

Fortunately for us, our chromosomes contain protective ends called telomeres. Telomeres are highly repeated sequences that cap both ends of our chromosomes like the plastic tips on shoelaces. My favorite analogy is that telomeres have been compared to the hands of a clock. With each cell division or replication event there is a "click" or movement of the clock's hand that shortens the telomere by loss of a short DNA sequence.

Given enough replication events, telomere shortening is correlated with triggering a natural cell death called senescence. Cellular aging occurs when the cells are no longer able to divide. As our telomeres shorten, we are more prone to disease and aging. If we preserve our cells and maintain our telomeres, we can live longer and better.

Having healthy cells means we have a healthy body, and having stressed out, unhealthy, and dysfunctional cells means the body has disease. With healthy cells, we will protect our telomeres, and we will age more gracefully. Longer telomeres mean longer life.

How do we protect our cells and our telomeres? Our cells are constantly subjected to physical, emotional, and energetic stress. These stresses lead to dysfunction and this dysfunction equates to dis-ease because the cells/body is no longer at ease. This book will teach you how to protect and heal your cells. When you break it down to the most basic level, every single health issue, no matter the name, is about cellular health.

Given enough replication events (named the Hayflick limit), telomere shortening is correlated with triggering a natural cell death called senescence. Cellular aging occurs when the cells are no longer able to divide. What we're learning is how, as our telomeres shorten, we become more prone to disease and aging. If we preserve our cells and maintain our telomeres, we can live longer and better.

There are many theories on what causes aging, and they may all be true—different pieces of the puzzle of why we grow old. These theories can be looked at as multiple sticks of lit dynamite inside our cells, each stick of dynamite representing a different cause of aging. It's only the stick of dynamite with the shortest fuse that will kill us. Which theory of aging has the shortest fuse? No one knows for sure, but given the well-established correlation between telomere length and age, telomere shortening is a good bet.

Scientists around the world are looking for cures for all diseases and how to slow down aging, and the control of telomere length is now often being discussed. The good news is cellular health is making headway in mainstream medicine.

One approach that's receiving a lot of attention is stem cell therapy. Stem cell therapy actually works on a principle similar to telomerase activation; the idea is to periodically infuse the body with young cells to replace cells that have senesced.

Some scientists feel that curing cellular senescence is only a piece of the aging puzzle, and that aging must be addressed on other fronts. An example is Aubrey de Grey's Strategies for Engineered Negligible Senescence. De Grey believes that a cure for aging must include therapies that address not only cellular senescence but also cancer-causing mutations, mitochondrial mutations, intracellular junk, extracellular junk, cell loss, and extracellular crosslinks.

The bottom line is this: As we age, our cells age. The good news is that now we know how to slow down this aging and the key is our telomeres.

Having healthy cells means we have a healthy body, and having stressed out, unhealthy, dysfunctional cells means the body has disease. Having sick cells means disease. With healthy cells, we will protect our telomeres, and we'll age more gracefully. Longer telomeres equal longer life.

Scientists are now convinced that if we could stop our telomeres from shrinking after cell division, we could slow down the aging process and protect ourselves from disease. The good news is there are a number of ways to do just that, and it's my goal to discuss as many of them as I can in this book.

The key to ageless aging is to promote the production of telomerase, the enzyme that makes telomeres in the body that can slow the rate of telomere degradation and even reverse it. In other words, if short telomeres are the problem, then telomerase may be one of the solutions.

In the laboratory, scientists have introduced telomerase into cells in tissue cultures and extended the length of their telomeres. These cells then divided for 250 generations past the time they normally would stop dividing and are continuing to divide normally, giving rise to normal cells with the normal number of chromosomes. By extending the telomeres with telomerase, the mortal cell has the opportunity to become immortal.

This book is not about any one product or solution; it's about cellular healing and cellular repair. Protect the cells and you protect your telomeres.

When the damage to your cells is too extensive, it results in damage to your telomeres.

Cells die every minute

The body continually works to heal, grow stronger, and replicate itself. It has to, as cells die every minute. Scientists estimate that of the 50 to 100 trillion cells in your body, about 300 million cells die every minute. So the obvious question I asked is why do cells die? They die because they are damaged, worn out, finished their lifespan, or destroyed by foreign bodies. The good news is when they die they are replaced with new cells. This is how life is renewed.

We learned earlier in this book that some parts of your body are renewed every week, while some every year. Even your bone cells are renewed regularly; however, when the damage to your cells is too extensive, it will result in damage to your telomeres. In the case of aging diseases like cancer, your body needs assistance to eject the damaged or mutated disease cells (the cancer cells) and boost the abilities of the defensive cells (liver, kidneys, immune system, etc.) and strengthen the normal cells.

When your body is provided with the proper building materials and your cells are being cleansed of the toxic substances, the progressively weaker cells will be replaced by the stronger cells. This is why the duplication process and the protection of your telomeres are so important. Tissue that is damaged and/or dying includes burns and age-related diseases such as atherosclerosis and macular degeneration in the eye. It may eventually be possible to treat these diseases by turning on telomerase. Researchers have already employed telomerase to prolong the lifespan of skin cells, blood vessel cells, and retinal cells.

This concept of cell replacement is known and studied by scientists continually. Cell replacement is accomplished by cell division, which makes more cells to replace cells that have been damaged by wear and tear or senescence (cells growing old and failing to function). The key to ageless aging is to prevent these cells from weakening and dying prematurely. Healthy cells mean a healthy body. Healthy cells have longer telomeres.

The key to maintaining our health is preserving our telomeres as the cells reproduce. In some cases, a single cell of a certain type can divide to give rise to two daughter cells of the same type. This process allows one cell to replace cells of its own type. For example, a liver cell can divide to generate two liver cells.

Much work in sports medicine lately has been done with stem cells. Stem cells are the body's building blocks; they provide a master plan for the growth to come and have the potential to replace any kind of diseased cell in the body. Adult, or somatic stem cells, such as the blood-forming stem cells in bone marrow, currently are the only kind commonly used to treat human disease. A stem cell is a special kind of cell used for cell replacement.

Stem cells also divide into two daughter cells. Some of these daughter cells become stem cells that resemble the mother cell. Other daughter cells become the cell type that needs to be replaced. For instance, our skin contains stem cells called basal cells. These basal cells divide into daughter cells. Some of the daughter cells become basal cells that retain the ability to divide, and other daughter cells become specialized skin cells. That way, some of the cells are used for cell replacement, while other cells retain the ability to divide in the future so that we don't run out of skin cells. Stem cells differ from other kinds of cells in the body and have three general properties: They are capable of dividing and renewing themselves for long periods, they don't have a particular function, and they can give rise to specialized cell types through a process known as differentiation, which is what makes them potentially useful in the treatment of various diseases.

Daily, doctors are utilizing and researching stem cell treatments throughout the world. In the United States, diseases that can be treated with a stem cell transplant are diagnosed in about 30,000 children and adults each year. Perhaps the best known stem cell therapy to date is the bone marrow transplant, which is the replacement of abnormal bone marrow cells with healthy cells.

We still have much to learn about human stem cells. Many of the hoped-for applications of stem cell research are still years away, but we get closer every day. WE have seen great life-changing progress with blood and bone marrow stem cell transplants. Friends, if this is any indication of things to come, stem cell therapies are likely to help many more people in the future. This is important research, but our goal is to keep the cells healthy to begin with. We can do this during the cellular duplication process by protecting our telomeres.

Regardless of the type of cells, the rates at which cells are replaced vary person by person. As we discussed, some cells replace themselves at a faster pace and each person's ability to replace cells is different. Some cells are replaced in a week or less, while other cells may not be replaced for up to a year or more. The key is that cells constantly reproduce.

Sometimes the rate of cell division to replace cells depends on the state or size of the tissue. Liver cells rarely divide, but if there is injury to the liver and the liver is somehow reduced, liver cells will divide to get the liver back to the right size. Similarly, in the skin, the basal cells will divide only to keep the skin at a certain thickness. If the outer layers of dead skin peel away more frequently, the basal cells on the inside will divide more frequently to make up for the lost skin. The body is a self-healing organism, and all disease and healing begins and ends within the cell.

We often resist change as something bad and uncomfortable; however, change is inevitable because it is the essence of life. But often, how we change is up to us. Healing, whether emotionally or physically, is a form of change, from the state of disease and discomfort to the state of health and wholeness. As human beings, we are equipped with powerful healing resources—the mind, body, and spirit—that enable within all of us change, growth, and healing as normal daily tasks.

The facts are simple:

- Doctors do not heal you.
- Drugs do not heal you.
- Machines do not heal you.

They can treat you by helping to remove the infections and assist you in helping your body to heal itself.

The power that created the body heals the body.

Caring for your cells

The health of a person is determined by the health of their cells. This is why caring for your cells is so important. The basics of cell care are as follows:

- Protect and build healthy cell membranes
- Supply cells with all the nutrients they need
- Avoid toxins
- Drink eight 8-ounce glasses of pure water every day
- Provide them with antioxidants
- Exercise
- Maintain your weight
- Meditate
- Avoid stress

Don't ever underestimate the power of your body, or the intelligence of your cells. Our body, through our innate intelligence, is able to identify and eliminate efficiently toxins, germs, and even cancer cells on a daily basis. We have a body so perfect it can produce any medication (painkillers, antibiotics, antidepressants, etc.) manufactured by pharmaceutical companies and administer them in a dosage that is always correct and given on time with no or minimal side effects. And our body can reconstitute damaged cells or replace impaired functions in powerful and creative ways that are still too complex for science to fully understand.

Roger Williams PhD, said, "Cells in the skin, the muscles, the lungs, the liver, the intestines, the kidneys, the blood vessels, the glands, the heart and, crucially, the nerves and brain must be well nourished if we are to lead long and healthy lives. Contrarily, if these cells are undernourished, disabilities and diseases of every description will ensue."

The key to health and ageless aging is to make sure that your cells get what they require on a daily basis. Choosing health and longer telomeres means supplying your cells with what they need while keeping them free of what they don't need. Your body is a fortress under constant assault. You must protect your castle. Infectious diseases, parasites, environmental toxins, food toxins, physical trauma, allergens, and natural disasters are just some of the external enemies our bodies face daily. From the inside, our bodies may be threatened by occasional overzealous allergic, immune, and inflammatory responses. If our cells are healthy, they can ward off these invaders. If the cells are weakened, they are prone to malfunction and allow these invaders to invade and infiltrate the cell. This can be compounded by the cellular mutations as a result of toxins that produce bodily diseases.

The good news is that the body's defenses are remarkably successful, and most of the time we are unaware of the intense drama taking place within our cells and organs. The body is a self-healing organism and will fight the toxins and deficiencies of day to day life. Health is about more than genetics. We are all born healthy, yet we die sick. Sickness and disease are an accumulation of toxins and deficiencies.

Genetics are important, but so are our choices. Life and longevity are about smart choices, healthy choices. Choosing health and longevity means supplying your cells with what they need while keeping them free from what they do not need. Cells are mighty miracles of life. They have super powers, healing powers, they have the power to care for themselves, heal themselves, to stay healthy, and reduce aging, unless they are overwhelmed by toxins, poor eating habits, poor exercise habits, or simply poor lifestyle choices. Your daily choices determine your longevity, your health. Your choices choose whether your cells stay healthy or get sick. Choose to be healthy and make the right choices, the smart choices, every day for the rest of your life. This will surely *Awaken the Wellness Within*.

ONE DISEASE

Cytopathology

TWO CAUSES

Deficiency   Toxicity

ONE CURE

"Each patient carries his own doctor inside him."

—NORMAN COUSINS

Chapter 12

—————=⊙⊙⊙=—————

TO CELL WITH YOU

We have learned if you heal, preserve, and protect the cell, you can literally *Awaken the Wellness Within*.

The fundamental component, of health, life, and aging is the cell. If you were building a house, you wouldn't use a foundation made of sand. If you did, then everything else you built on that house would be in jeopardy. It's the same with your body. Your cellular foundation is the most important aspect of your health. If your cells are not healthy, you will not be healthy and your overall health is definitely at risk. Think of your cells as the foundation of your house of health!

Cellular health means maximized cellular repair and enhanced function of your immune system. A properly functioning immune system keeps your body from being susceptible to disease. The healthier your cells are, the less likely you are to become a victim of disease and the more you can fight and/or heal from disease. Therefore, whether you're 3 or 103, your health strategy must start at the cellular level.

A cell is much more than a combination of molecules and atoms. A cell is the miracle of life, the source of life. Scientist's acknowledge that a single cell is considered a life form. You must daily provide your cells with what they need to be healthy. Choosing health means learning how to supply your cells with what they need to keep them healthy.

139

One of the key ingredients to *Awakening the Wellness Within* is omega-3 fatty acids; they are essential fatty acids necessary for human health.

Now many of us already take these, but please read the labels; not all omegas are the same. There are two families of essential fatty acids: omega-3 fatty acids and omega-6 fatty acids. They are termed "essential" because they cannot be produced by the body and must therefore be obtained from the diet.

Both omega-6 and omega-3 fatty acids are stored in the cell membranes of tissues and have two primary functions. First, they are structural components of cell membranes where they ensure fluidity, stability, and act as gatekeepers in the cell. Second, both omega-6 and omega-3 fatty acids are converted into a number of important, active molecules called prostaglandins.

There are three types of prostaglandins: PG1, PG2, and PG3.

PG1 have many beneficial effects, including reducing inflammation, inhibiting blood clotting, and maintaining various regulatory states in the body. The strong anti-inflammatory properties help the body recover from injury by reducing pain, swelling, and redness.

PG2 have the opposite effects of PG1. They have been found to strongly increase inflammation, constrict blood vessels, and encourage blood clotting. These properties come into play when the body suffers a wound or injury, for without these prostaglandins, a person could bleed to death from the slightest of cuts. However, in excess, these prostaglandins may be harmful.

PG3 have a mixture of functions in the body. In general, they are important in protecting the body from various modes of injury. One of their most important functions, however, is their role in decreasing the rate at which PG2 are formed. Because of their role in reducing inflammation caused by PG2, PG3 are often described as having anti-inflammatory properties.

In people with heart disease, inhibition of PG2 is desirable due to the role of inflammation in the progression of the disease. Studies have found that high omega-3 intake can decrease the production of PG2. To understand how omega-3 inhibits inflammation due to PG2, we need to go over the pathways by which the omega-3 and omega-6 fatty acids are processed in the body.

Alpha-linolenic acid, the primary dietary source of omega-3 fatty acids in the diet, is frequently found in green leaves. The leaves and seeds of the perilla plant (widely eaten in Japan, Korea, and India) are the richest plant source of alpha-linolenic acid, although linseed oil is also a rich source. Fish oil contains very little alpha-linolenic acid, but is rich in the omega-3 derivatives EPA and DHA. Fish are at the top of a food chain based on phytoplankton (algae) that manufacture large amounts of EPA and DHA. Salmon and herring are about 4 or 5 times richer in EPA and DHA than cod.

Your body needs fats to function properly

Nearly half of the dry weight of the brain is fat, and a quarter of this is cholesterol. That is why once cholesterol was the enemy, but now doctors know there is good and bad cholesterol. Cholesterol is an essential part of sex hormones, bile acids, D vitamins, and steroid hormones from the cortex of the adrenal gland—among other important substances. Cholesterol does not need to be eaten, however, because the liver and other tissues can manufacture cholesterol from saturated fats. But too many saturated fats result in excessively high blood levels of cholesterol that can end up being deposited in atherosclerotic plaques on blood vessels, leading to diseases of the cell.

It has been estimated that thousands of years ago the diet of human hunter-gatherers consisted of approximately equal parts of omega-3 and omega-6 essential fatty acids. Since the beginning of agriculture some ten thousand years ago there has been a steady increase in omega-6 at the expense of omega-3 fat in the human diet. This process accelerated about 50 years ago as cattle began to be fed increasingly on grains rather than grass. Recommendations by nutritionists to eat margarine rather than butter (polyunsaturated rather than saturated fats) increased the trend toward pro-inflammatory omega-6 and trans fat consumption. Currently, the ratio of omega-6 to omega-3 fatty acids in the American diet is 7 to 1 or more. There are good reasons to believe that this imbalanced essential fatty acid ratio has led to increased cancer, heart disease, allergies, diabetes, and other afflictions. Much of the reason for this lies in the membranes of our cells.

Your cell factories

Earlier in the book we used the metaphor of your body as a castle. Now let's go deeper into cellular health and utilize the metaphor of a factory to explain in simple terms how a cell works. Imagine a large manufacturing plant, any major factory. This is the most important factory in the world, for without this factory life would cease. This is in essence what your cells are—a manufacturing plant, manufacturing life.

Now a building this important must be protected, right? This building is surrounded by large walls and barbed wire and the most sophisticated security system known to man. Inside this building they manufacture everything needed to sustain life and heal your body. In this factory, every part of your body is built, including your muscles, joints, organs, bones, and blood. Your mission, should you agree to accept it, would be to enter this building.

This manufacturing plant is protected by a security system known as the outer membrane of the cell. This membrane, this outer wall, has one job: to keep out toxins, bacteria, viruses and other toxins, and excrete waste. Like a security team, the outer membrane protects the cell, but it also allows the good material in and allows the waste to leave safely. The security system (the membrane) protects the cell, the same cell we need to sustain life. This outer membrane is made up of fats, preferably omega-3s. Omega-3s protect the cell. If you do not have fats, the cell membrane will utilize whatever fats are in your diet. The worse the fat is in your diet, the worse your security system. You must protect your factory, your kingdom, to obtain maximum health.

A chronic deficiency of essential vitamins, minerals, water, oxygen, or other nutrients causes your cells to malfunction, and cellular malfunction leads to disease. Most often we are not even aware that this malfunction is happening, especially in the early stages of the disease. Any chronic shortage of even one nutrient eventually makes your cells malfunction and ultimately you will become sick. When shortages are chronic, the body stops repairing and self-regulating; cells then deteriorate into a diseased state or die. We must protect our cells and its stars with our security system made up of our cellular membrane.

The fact that our cells house the most powerful manufacturing plants in the world is why the security system is germane. The health and welfare of this security system is so important, in fact, that your very life may depend on its health.

The energy systems inside the factory create energy and assist in manufacturing the products the body needs, such as hormones, antibodies, neurotransmitters, and much more. Your cells have everything they need to sustain life and when they're healthy they have all the energy necessary to keep everything working in balance. Anything that interferes with the cells doing their job interferes with our health.

With every choice you make, you affect your cell's ability to function properly. When you choose to eat fast food, for example, your cellular membrane must arm itself for the invasion of toxins that act as chemical invaders trying to infiltrate your cells. Bad fats put your security system in jeopardy as the cell membrane works as a selective filter that allows only certain things enter the cell. If your cells don't get the omega-3s to make healthy membranes, it will steal other fats from sources such as hydrogenated fats, which weaken your security system.

To be healthy, we must develop healthy cells daily. Each day, our old cells are replaced by new cells. That is why when we are sick we get better, we get new healthy cells that will help fight the invader. The key is to develop new healthy cells.

Now does anyone believe we can build healthy cells by eating unhealthy foods? Will French fries, donuts, or potato chips build healthy cells? Of course not. If we continually deprive our bodies, our cells, of the necessary vitamins, minerals, water, and oxygen we will cause our cells to be weak and malfunction.

Part of the aging process comes from having weak or malformed cell membranes. A diet low in saturated and high in polyunsaturated fatty acids will help protect your cell membranes and help you retain your health.

Protecting the cells

The 21st century is ushering in a new era of nutritional science, demonstrating the unbelievable power of nutrition to benefit human health. It is this new understanding of the cell that proves the search for the Fountain of Youth is no longer a fairytale.

Since before recorded history, people have been searching for ways to live longer. We are all familiar with the story of Ponce de Leon's search for the elusive Fountain of Youth, but even two millennia earlier, emperor Qin Shi Huang of China was sending out ships full of hundreds of men and women in search of an elixir of life that would make him immortal. The desire to live forever is as old as humanity itself.

But it has only been in the last 30 years that science has made any real progress in understanding the fundamental question of why we age and what can be done about it. These discoveries have not yet been widely publicized, so most people are unaware of how close we are to curing the disease of aging once and for all.

Scientific studies now confirm that supplements and proper nutrition may be able to *Awaken the Wellness Within*. Research clearly shows that nutrition can slow your rate of cellular degeneration and biological aging. There is now an emerging body of nutritional science that focuses on helping your cells by improving your telomeres, which we now know is the key to anti-aging. It is so important to protect your cellular factory, your castle, and your knights in shining armor—your telomeres.

When you protect the cell, you protect the telomeres. Each time a cell replicates, the telomere loses some of its length. Eventually, the telomere runs out and the cell can no longer divide and replicate. This triggers a poor state of cell health that contributes to disease risk and eventual cell death. In most cases of aging, scientists now agree that telomeres are the weak link in your DNA. They are readily damaged and must be repaired; yet they lack the repair efficiency of other DNA. This results in an accumulation of partially damaged and poorly functioning telomeres of lower quality, regardless of length. So our goal must be to preserve and protect them.

The cell membrane controls everything that goes in and out of the cell. Cell membranes are made primarily of fatty molecules called phospholipids. Omega-3 fatty acids are used to create the phospholipids of the cell membrane. What makes these oils essential to our diets is that our bodies do not produce them. We must get them through our foods or supplements.

The problem arises when proper materials are not present in our diet. When this occurs, the body makes the cell membrane from whatever it can get its hands on. If your diet is filled with hydrogenated fats, such as margarine, mayonnaise, or saturated cooking oils, this is what your membrane will be made up of. It will not be strong enough to hold the toxins out and cannot regulate waste appropriately. We protect the cell by protecting the membrane.

If the proper materials are not present in our diet, the body will make the membrane from whatever it can get its hands on. This is like hiring terrorists to protect our airports. If your diet is filled with hydrogenated fats, such as margarine, mayonnaise, or saturated cooking oils, this is what your membrane will be made up of. It will not be strong enough to hold the toxins out and or properly regulate waste. We protect the cell by protecting the membrane.

Every day inside this factory, billions of cells are produced. Building a cell will require material—like building a computer, there is hardware and software. If one ingredient is missing, the cell will be defective. If many parts are missing, malfunction is guaranteed.

With every daily choice you make, you affect your cellular manufacturing plant. The security system of this factory cringes when you pull in for fast food. Your cellular membrane now must arm itself for the invasion of toxins and food additives and preservatives that act as chemical invaders trying to infiltrate their cell.

One of the worst invaders are the wrong fats. Bad fats put your security system, your kingdom, in jeopardy. The cell membrane works as a selective filter that allows only certain things to come inside or go outside the cell. It's important in maintaining a homeostatic environment in the cell to keep us healthy and alive.

The first line of defense to protect our telomeres is to protect our cell membranes. Healthy membranes, built from proper materials, protect the cell from harmful invaders. Malfunctioning membranes allow invaders like bacteria, viruses, and other toxins to enter the cell.

Your cell membranes need good omega-3 fats or they will utilize other sources like hydrogenated fats, which will not only weaken your security system but also allow invaders into your kingdom. An overwhelming majority of people in the U.S., some estimate in the range of 90%, may be deficient in the correct assortment of essential fatty acids. When correct raw materials are lacking the body makes cell membranes out of whatever raw materials are available. These include hydrogenated fats found in margarine, mayonnaise, cereals, as well as the trans-fatty acids found in processed fats and cooking oils. Cell membranes built with inappropriate fats and oils cause the membrane and the entire cell to malfunction.

Cell membranes are so fine that they were not discovered and confirmed until modern electron microscopy arrived in the late 1950s. For this reason, it is only recently that scientists have discovered the roles played by membranes in our bodies.

Not only do membranes separate the interior of the cell from the external environment, but something in the membrane itself makes important and correct decisions about which substances can pass in and out of the cell. The membrane treats different molecules in different ways and toxic or unnecessary substances are not permitted to enter.

We now know aging comes from damage to cells and their constituent proteins and DNA. Much of the damage to the cell comes from oxygen-derived reactions generated as the cells utilize oxygen for metabolism.

Scientists sought to determine if extremely old mice had different cell membranes than middle-aged mice. They reasoned that certain individual mice and humans may live very long because their cell membranes were somehow more resistant to oxidative damage. They indeed found that the cell membranes in exceptionally old mice had the highest resistance to oxidative injury, as well as the lowest amount of oxidative damage. They concluded that low lipid oxidation susceptibility and maintenance of adult-like protein lipoxidative damage could be key mechanisms for longevity achievement.

It is not known whether this also occurs in humans of advanced age or what mechanisms may promote this. Therefore, a diet low in saturated fat and high in polyunsaturated fatty acids may help protect your cell membranes and help you retain your health. I start my day with a protein shake, and I take supplements with omega-3s to build my cells, cleanse my cells, and to motivate my cells.

Omega-3s

In human beings, omega-3 fatty acids are important in maintaining the structure of cellular membranes, improving absorption of liposoluble vitamins (A, D, E and K), regulating cholesterol metabolism, and producing eicosanoids, which regulate various cellular processes (vascular and bronchial tone, gastrointestinal and uterine motility, gastric protection, urine output, blood clotting, body temperature, inflammatory and immune processes, etc.).

The improvement of omega-3 fatty acids in endothelial function has been attributed to their ability to augment nitric oxide release by the endothelial cells. Omega-3 fatty acids also show anti-inflammatory properties by reducing C-reactive protein levels.

Omega-3 fatty acids hyperpolarize membrane potential, which increases the ventricular excitability threshold and prolongs the duration of the refractory period, resulting in two of the effects of its anti-arrhythmic properties.

Omega-3 fatty acids are components of the phospholipids that make up cell membranes, which is why they are essential to the growth of nervous system tissue during pregnancy, breastfeeding, and infancy.

Some studies show that omega-3s lower high blood cholesterol and triglyceride levels by as much as 25% and 65%. Omega-3s decrease the probability of a blood clot blocking an artery. They also have been shown to lower blood pressure, reduce inflammation, and lower insulin requirements in diabetics.

UCSF researchers followed 608 outpatients with stable coronary artery disease for 5–8 years. At the start of the study they measured everyone's levels of omega-3s and the length of their leukocyte telomeres, which is a marker of aging. Here's how the lead researcher Dr. Ramin Farzaneh-Far explains the results: "The main result from our study is that patients with high levels of omega-3 fish oil in the blood appear to have a slowing of the biological aging process over five years as measured by the change in telomere length.

"Patients with the highest levels of omega-3 fish oils were found to display the slowest decrease in telomere length, whereas those with the lowest levels of omega-3 fish oils in the blood had the fastest rate of telomere shortening, suggesting that these patients were aging faster than those with the higher fish oil levels in their blood.

"By measuring telomere length at two different times we are able to see the speed at which the telomeres are shortening, and that gives us some indication of how rapidly the biological aging process is taking place in these patients."

Recently, I was on the Dr. Oz show, we spent much time prior to the show talking about health. He is as lovely and polite a man offstage as he is on stage.

As a cardiologist, Dr. Oz understands the importance of healthy fats. Being part Italian, my favorite oil is olive oil. When Dr. Oz was asked about olive oil and anti-aging, he stated, "Olive oil contains monounsaturated fats, which help raise your HDL cholesterol—the "healthy" cholesterol carried through your body by high-density lipoproteins. It actually helps clean out your arteries as it moves through. When it comes to HDL, higher is better—so an HDL level of 60 versus one of 39 will make the average 55-year-old woman four years younger."

In his "You Docs" column, he reported, "Telomeres, in one study, were longest in those eating the most vitamin C-rich foods, such as citrus fruit, strawberries, and red bell peppers, and vitamin E-rich foods, such as whole grains. Add salmon, trout, olive oil, and a cup of tea—or two or three. Researchers in Hong Kong found the longest telomeres in men who drank three cups of green tea or sometimes black tea a day."

Like me, Dr. Oz is a fan of dark chocolate. He says, "A daily dose of dark chocolate revs up power stations called mitochondria in each and every cell in your body. This makes your muscles stronger and increases your endurance. Mega-surveys show that people that eat dark chocolate cut their risk for heart disease by 37%, diabetes by 31%, and stroke by 29%."

Chocolate is packed with flavonoids and flavonoids are essential to ageless aging. Flavonoids are a plant-based chemical that is anti-viral, anti-allergic, anti-inflammatory, anti-tumor, and anti-Alzheimer. I recommend chocolate that contains at least 70% cocoa, and no more than an ounce a day.

We can eat our way to being younger by enjoying chocolate and olive oil. Our diet and supplement habits can help preserve telomere integrity. Once we learn to protect the cells, we have taken our first step to *Awakening the Wellness Within*.

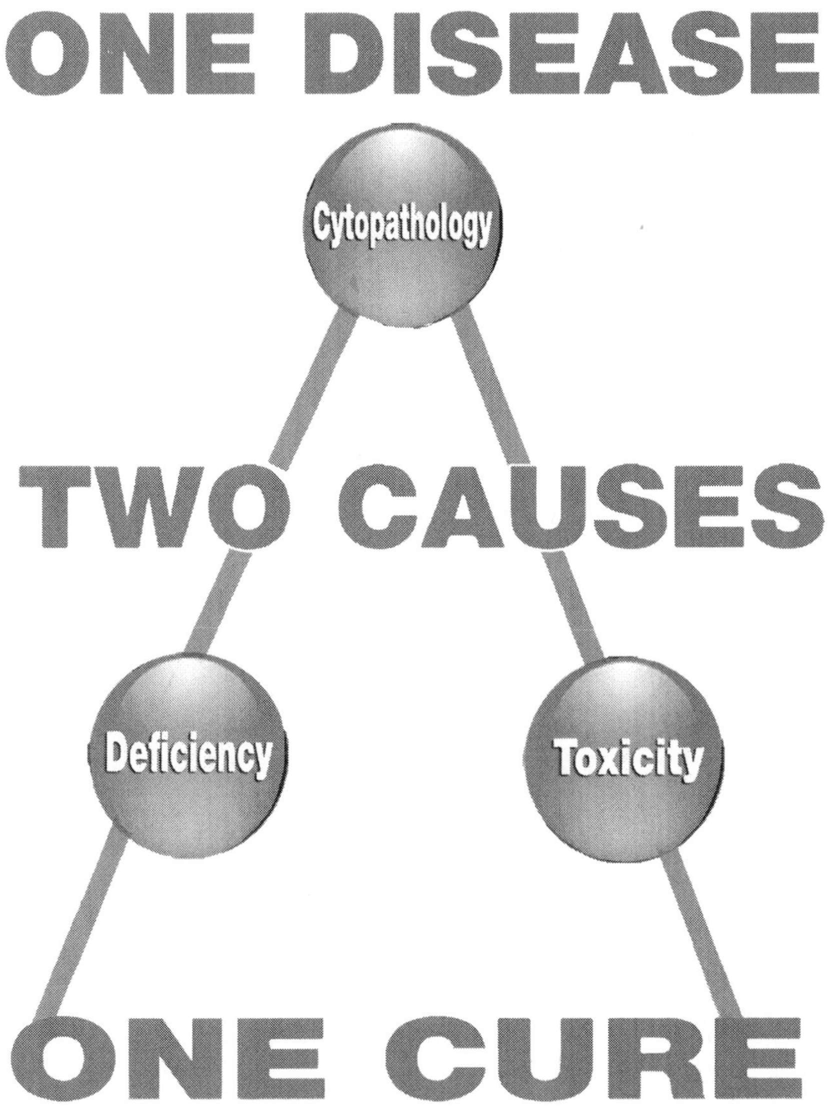
ONE DISEASE
Cytopathology
TWO CAUSES
Deficiency
Toxicity
ONE CURE

"*Healing is a matter of time,*
but it is sometimes also a matter of opportunity."

—HIPPOCRATES

Chapter 13

STRESS AGES OUR CELLS

While everyone experiences stress at times, a prolonged bout of it can affect your health and ability to cope with life. According to the CDC, 90% of illness and disease is caused by stress. Dr. Bruce Lipton of Stanford University Medical School has shown that the real number is closer to 95%. This fact bears repeating: 90% to 95% of all illness and disease is caused by physiological stress, which is an accumulation of situational stress and other factors over time.

These are strong numbers, but remember—we have a strong body. Actually it's not stress itself that causes disease, but how our cells react to stress. When our cells are stressed, they fail to do their job efficiently. If the cells are healthy, free of toxins, and not deficient, they can handle stress.

Stress is a major factor that contributes to disease, but that is because the cells malfunction when under stress. Chronic stress results in an excessive buildup of natural chemicals in the body, which at higher levels become toxic. In addition, stress depletes the body of certain nutrients, resulting in deficiency. Stress is a contributor to disease, but only by expressing itself through the common denominators of all disease: deficiency and toxicity. Deficiency and toxicity, regardless of their cause, increasingly compromise the functioning of cells, making a person steadily more vulnerable to developing a diagnosable disease and aging prematurely.

Stress can hit you when you least expect it—before a test, after an accident, or during conflict in a relationship. While everyone experiences stress at times, a prolonged bout of it can affect your health and ability to cope with life. That's why social support and self-care are important. They can help you see your problems in perspective, and the stressful feelings ease up.

Sometimes stress can be good. For instance, it can help you develop skills needed to manage potentially threatening situations in life. However, stress can be harmful when it is severe enough to make you feel overwhelmed and out of control. When this happens, the cells become negatively affected.

Strong emotions like fear, sadness, or other symptoms of depression are normal as long as they are temporary and don't interfere with daily activities. If these emotions last too long or cause other problems, it's a different story.

Symptoms of Stress

Common reactions to a stressful event include:

- Disbelief and shock
- Tension and irritability
- Fear and anxiety about the future
- Difficulty making decisions Being numb to one's feelings
- Loss of interest in normal activities
- Loss of appetite
- Nightmares and recurring thoughts about the event
- Anger
- Increased use of alcohol and drugs
- Sadness and other symptoms of depression
- Feeling powerless
- Crying
- Sleep problems

- Headaches, back pains, and stomach problems
- Trouble concentrating

The response to stress evolved as a vital defense system that primes the body for fighting or fleeing dangers. But when ongoing daily stresses provoke the defense system into prolonged action, inflammation and other side effects can cause widespread damage to cells and organs.

Stress can have effects on other hormones, brain neurotransmitters, additional small chemical messengers elsewhere, prostaglandins, as well as crucial enzyme systems, and metabolic activities that are still unknown.

Research in these areas may help to explain how stress can contribute to depression, anxiety, and its diverse effects on the gastrointestinal tract, skin, and other cells and organs.

According to the CDC, the following diseases and health issues are the leading causes of death in the U.S. They have a huge economic impact on the nation's healthcare system and all are affected or caused in some manner by stress. Stress to the body or stress to the cell. An overworked, toxic or deficient cell, is a cell under stress.

Heart disease is the leading cause of death in the U.S. It's a major cause of disability for Americans. The most common heart disease is coronary heart disease; this often appears as a heart attack. An estimated 785,000 Americans were projected to have a new heart attack in 2009 and about 470,000 will have a recurrent attack. About every minute, one American will die from a heart attack.

Cancer is the second leading cause of U.S. deaths. More than 559,000 Americans died of cancer in 2005; this is the most recent year for which incidence data is available. More than 1.3 million people in the U.S. are diagnosed with cancer each year. The overall cost for cancer in 2008 was estimated by the National Institutes of Health to be $228 billion.

Stroke is the third leading cause of U.S. deaths. Heart disease and stroke account for more than one-third of all U.S. deaths. More than 80 million Americans currently live with a cardiovascular disease. In 2009, the cost of heart disease and stroke was projected to be more than $475 billion in the U.S.

Diabetes is the seventh leading cause of U.S. deaths. Diabetes-related complications cause over 200,000 deaths each year. More than 23.6 million Americans have diabetes—and about 5.7 million don't know that they have the disease. The estimated cost of diabetes in 2007 was $174 billion.

Common Stress-Related Diseases

- Acid Peptic Disease
- Alcoholism
- Asthma
- Fatigue
- Tension Headache
- Hypertension
- Insomnia
- Irritable Bowel Syndrome
- Ischemic Heart Disease
- Psychoneuroses
- Sexual Dysfunction
- Skin diseases like Psoriasis and Neurodermatitis

Stress Facts

- 75% of the general population experiences at least some stress every two weeks (National Health Interview Survey).
- Half of those experience moderate or high levels of stress during the same two-week period.
- Millions of Americans suffer from unhealthy levels of stress at work.

- Worker's compensation claims for mental stress in California rose 200–700% in the 1980s, whereas all other causes remained stable or declined.
- Stress contributes to heart disease, high blood pressure, strokes, and other illnesses in many individuals.
- Stress also affects the immune system, which protects us from many serious diseases.
- Tranquilizers, antidepressants, and anti-anxiety medications account for one fourth of all prescriptions written in the U.S. each year.
- Stress also contributes to the development of alcoholism, obesity, suicide, drug addiction, cigarette addiction, and other harmful behaviors.
- The U.S. Public Health Service has made reducing stress by the year 2000 one of its major health promotion goals.

Stress has a double effect on your body. Stress is toxic and this toxicity will create a deficiency. In other words, stress shortens our life by shortening your telomeres. There's a way to reduce the stress on your telomere. First, we must understand stress and then we can treat it.

The time and place in which we live offers us more opportunity than has been enjoyed by any culture in history. But one of the byproducts of modern living is stress. As a chiropractor, one of my functions is to help people reduce the effects of stress, for it can cause significant health problems. We can't completely avoid stress, but we can minimize it—in fact, we *must* minimize it.

There are two types of stress: internal and external. Within these two categories, there are various degrees of mental, emotional, and physical stress. More important than the stress itself is the ability of the body to adapt to it. The body can react favorably to stress, in which case no harm is done. Conversely, an adverse reaction will produce adverse consequences. The degree to which a person reacts to stress is subjective, and some people have a higher tolerance than others.

While some people thrive on stress, my opinion as a physician is that these sturdy souls are in the minority. I have found that most people suffer from numerous ailments when their stress tolerance is exceeded. I am one of them. Stress may lead to diseases such as hypertension, atherosclerosis, and heart disease. It can cause irritability, insomnia, anxiety, anger, frustration, and a variety of other unpleasant emotions. Stress can decrease the quality of life, cause premature aging, and even hasten death.

There is no such thing as good stress, yet stress is a part of our everyday life. Let us start with the basics. Any type of stress will affect your telomeres. Oxidative stress, for example, will shorten telomere length and cause aging in cellular tissue. Substantial evidence has led to findings that premature aging and its core cellular mechanisms are governed by the onset of chronic oxidative stress and resulting in telomere attrition. Research on telomeres and cells also indicated that chronic oxidative stress not only causes progressive damage to cellular membranes, proteins, and molecules, but also induces an arrest of existing telomerase activity and accelerates telomere attrition.

Stress does not only affect older people; children are also vulnerable. "A long-term study of children from Romanian orphanages suggests that the effects of childhood stress could be visible in their DNA as they grow up. Children who spent their early years in state-run Romanian orphanages have shorter telomeres than children who grew up in foster care, according to a study published in *Molecular Psychiatry*. The study focused on 136 orphanage children aged between 6 and 30 months, half of whom were randomly assigned to foster families. The other half remained in orphanages. "It shows that being in institutional care affects children right down to the molecular level," says clinical psychiatrist Stacy Drury of Tulane University in New Orleans, Louisiana, one of the lead authors on the study.

The researchers obtained DNA samples from the children when they were between 6 and 10 years old, and measured the length of their telomeres. They found that the longer the children had spent in the orphanage in early childhood—before the age of four and a half—the shorter their telomeres. Other studies have found short telomeres in adults who said they had experienced childhood psychological stress.

The good news is we can change and reverse this dilemma

Iiris Hovatta of the Molecular Neurology Research Program at the University of Helsinki, who was not involved in the Romanian study, suggests that shortened telomeres might not be permanent. "Studies in adults have shown that telomere length in some individuals increases over time, and this tends to occur in those people who have shorter telomeres to begin with," says Hovatta.

This is also true for adults. Edward Nelson, MD, division chief of hematology/oncology at the University of California-Irvine said, "We are trying to understand the interconnections between the mind and the body; that is, how does the diagnosis and treatment of cancer impact patients not only psychologically, but also physiologically and how can we improve their outcome. Cancer drives a chronic stress response in some patients' improved quality of life and reduced stress response was associated with changes in telomere length."

Obesity is an especially dangerous form of physical stress. When we overeat, the digestive system is burdened by the need to break down the excess food we consume. Obesity also leads to numerous diseases, as the immune system of the body becomes fatigued and sluggish. Proper diet, exercise, and nutritional supplements are important because stress will take its toll on the body as well as the emotions. Two other items that can help reduce stress are the herbs valerian root and kava kava. As I said before, a body not at ease is in a state of dis-ease, which can eventually lead to disease. One of my goals is to teach you to listen to your body and to use your emotional reactions as a stress barometer.

So what do we do? As with any disease, we find and remove the cause. Here's how:

4 Steps to Stress Reduction

1. Learn what causes your stress. Stress triggers are different for all of us. Some are work related, others diet related. Both deficiency and toxicity puts stress on the body. Know what causes your stress, such as overeating, working too long, relationships, etc. Notice every time you find your stomach in knots. Pay attention to where it came from. Keep a list.

2. Exercise. One of the greatest natural stress reducers is exercise. Plus, exercise helps your cells and your telomeres. The mood-elevating effects of exercise have been widely documented. Various theories have been proposed to explain this effect. Some experts believe exercise increases the level of certain hormones in the brain, thus producing a feeling of well-being. Others claim that the beneficial effects of exercise are due to increased blood supply, which in turn increases the oxygen level throughout the circulatory system and brain. Whatever the reason, the message is clear— you can exercise a good deal of your stress away. The over-prescription of valium and other drugs might stop if more people used the natural and beneficial tranquilizer they have available to them through exercise.

3. Take supplements. If your body is deficient, you will need to supplement your diet to assist the cells. Cells that are toxic or deficient from oxidative stress, work stress, etc., can be helped by certain antioxidants and supplements.

4. Do everything you can to avoid stress in your life.

Meditation, supplements, and especially antioxidant supplements can potentially reduce oxidative stress very effectively in addition to exercise, which will ultimately improve oxidative defenses, mitochondrial function, reduce inflammation and slow vascular aging. Targeted supplementation is key to good health. Increasing antioxidant capacity at the cellular level is critical to maintaining telomere length.

Stress and diet

The interaction of improper diet and stress contributes to the plight of many ulcer patients. It is commonly believed that ulcers are caused solely by emotional conditions. I disagree. Webster's Dictionary defines an ulcer as a necrotic or eroded sore that often discharges pus. Ulcers are often caused by dietary stress and the two substances most often responsible are sugar and dairy products.

Sugar creates excess stomach acid and dairy products are hard to digest; both of them will act as an irritant. Yet dairy products—which include sugar-laden ice cream—are regularly prescribed to help heal ulcers. For years, ulcer sufferers were advised to consume milk to ease the pain. Natural hygienists voiced their disbelief of such absurd advice from the beginning, knowing that acid-forming foods are the worst thing for an ulcer sufferer, and all the dairy products, except butter, are acid forming. The natural hygienists were first scoffed at by the elite credentialed health experts. But check with medical professionals or dietitians today and they will now agree with the very hygienists they used to attack. Dairy products aggravate ulcers.

Ulcerative colitis is another extremely painful and uncomfortable ailment. Frequently it is a precursor to colon cancer. Dairy products not only contribute to colitis, but removal of dairy products results in a dramatic improvement of colitis.

All too often, we worsen dietary stress by the remedies we use to relieve it. We get upset about something, which causes our blood sugar levels to jump, and eat the wrong foods (sugar) to console ourselves. Our stomachs, in response to this external and internal stress, produce excess acid. So we run to the medicine cabinet, forgetting to treat the cause. A diet high in refined sugar, dairy products, or alcohol are all acid producers. This puts stress on the cells and shortens our telomeres.

For more information on diet, vitamins, and stress, read my first book *Lifestyle of the Fit & Famous*. Go to www.5minutemotivator.com to order a copy.

Cigarette smoking

Cigarette smoking is one of the key toxic products we can put in our diet. It will stress your body and make your body deficient at the same time. Cigarettes killed my mother (she died of pneumonia), my brother (lung cancer), and my father (heart disease). Are you getting the picture?

Ever since the 1960s, federal law has required that tobacco companies place warnings from the Surgeon General on all cigarette packs. The studies done on cigarette smoking over the years have produced astonishing findings. Smoking has been associated with lung cancer, emphysema, bronchitis, cardiovascular disease, arteriosclerosis, vascular disease, gastrointestinal distress, urinary tract disease, nerve-related disease, and many other maladies. Yet people continue to smoke. Smoking is a toxin that will shorten telomeres and your life.

Dr. Perry Bard and I founded Smoke Arrest Centers, a doctors' program working with lasers and acupuncture points to aid anyone in quitting smoking. Smoking will age you and lower your immunity system. The toxins in cigarettes create accelerated telomere shortening, which research has shown to increase mortality, not from any one disease in particular, but from a wide variety of age-related diseases. It seems intuitive that cigarette smoking would increase the risk of lung cancer (toxic to the lung cells)—you're putting poison in your lungs, so it is expected that they would be affected. But has it ever struck you as a little odd that cigarette smoking also increases the risk of dozens of other diseases, including osteoporosis and osteoarthritis (in your bones, where cigarette smoke would presumably never reach), and that smoking cigarettes has even been shown to slow down wound healing? Telomere shortening is the common factor.

When public service announcements informed people that cigarettes made you "look older," the explanation was usually that the toxins in smoke affected capillaries under the skin in a way that led to wrinkling of the skin. Now we're finding out that these warnings actually understated the case. Cigarettes don't just make you look older, they actually make you older.

Numerous studies have shown that cigarette smoking is associated with short telomeres. The free radicals in cigarettes actually attack DNA directly, and since telomeres are the exposed sections of DNA, they have been shown to cleave sections of the telomere directly from the chromosome. But it gets worse. When telomeres get short, they actually induce mitochondrial dysfunction, which causes the mitochondria to start pumping out free radicals. It is a terrible, vicious cycle: Cigarettes not only age us and damage our tissues, but they reinforce a feedback loop that inspires our body to further age us and further damage our cells and tissues.

Could lengthening telomeres by inducing telomerase help alleviate this process? Absolutely. Could it actually erase all the damage done by smoking and allow a smoker to return to the same health and the same biological age he or she enjoyed before starting the habit? A cautious "maybe." It is too soon to give a definitive "yes," but there is no research that suggests that such a thing is impossible, and plenty to suggest that it is possible.

So what do we do to help our telomeres, remove stress, and live longer? Recent evidence suggests that a high-quality and balanced multivitamin, along with avoiding toxins and getting plenty of exercise, will help maintain telomere length. Specifically, studies have linked longer telomeres with levels of vitamin E, vitamin C, vitamin D, omega-3 fatty acids, and the antioxidant resveratrol. In addition, homocysteine levels have been inversely associated with telomere length, suggesting that reducing homocysteine levels via folate and vitamin B supplementation may decrease the rate of telomere loss.

Together, after 28 years, Dr. Bard and I worked to develop a program that would be specific to smoking cessation and help doctors create one more non-smoker at a time naturally.

What makes the Smoke Arrest program unique is that it is "doctor supervised" and utilizes a comprehensive approach by providing the latest natural techniques for smoking cessation. This course combines patient assessment, laser therapy, nutrition, doctor support, and proprietary combined methods of providing back-up support to patients. The program centers on empowering and enabling individuals who require a smoking cessation intervention.

Smoke Arrest Proprietary Five-Step Approach

- Physician Evaluation and Assessment
- Specific Laser Therapy
- Strategic Auricular Energy Magnets and Specific Sprays, and other Nutraceuticals
- Behavior Modification and Counseling
- Physician Supervision

Any smoker knows the feeling that they get when they are under stress or find themselves in a situation where they have become accustomed, for one reason or another, to lighting up a cigarette. Also, when a smoker has a meal or a cup of coffee or a soft drink, they have a strong desire for a cigarette.

For simplicity, we have broken the many aspects of smoking down into three main categories:

1. Physical
2. Psychological
3. Habitual (or Sociological)

Yes, solving the smoking problem is much like solving a complex puzzle. There are many pieces of the puzzle, and to solve it, you need to address all of these factors.

The benefits of quitting smoking are many fold. A smoker's entire life will begin to change from the first minute that he or she quits smoking for good. Many aspects of their lives will be improved in countless ways. While the physical health benefits are certainly among the most important ones, the self-esteem and mental health of the ex-smoker, and the effects that these things have on so many other people, is of paramount importance.

The key to Smoke Arrest Centers is their "doctor supervised" Low-Level, Cold-Laser program.

A clinically validated and scientifically specific laser is a key to their system, which makes their program unique.

Low-level laser therapy (LLLT) aims to bio-stimulate the body. Because of the low-power nature of the low-level laser, the effects are biochemical and not thermal and cannot cause heating and thereby damage to living tissue. Four distinct effects are known to occur when using low-level laser therapy:

1. Growth factor response within cells and tissue as a result of increased ATP and protein synthesis; Improved cell proliferation; Change in cell membrane permeability to calcium up-take.
2. Pain relief as a result of increased endorphin release; increased serotonin; Suppression of nociceptor action.

3. Strengthening the immune system response via increasing levels of lymphocyte activity and through a newly researched mechanism termed Photomodulation of blood.
4. Acupuncture point stimulation.

LASER

Laser is an acronym for Light Amplification by Stimulated Emission of Radiation.

Low level laser therapy (LLLT) has proven to be very effective for many conditions that have not responded well to other forms of treatment. LLLT has been thoroughly tested and proven effective in most countries of the world. It is a well-accepted and recommended form of treatment in England, Italy, Ireland, the Netherlands, Russia, Israel, Japan, Canada, India, Venezuela, and many other countries in Europe, South America, and the Far East

The treatment material is based on our clinical experience, including scientific works as well as the experience of specialists in the field of laser therapy.

Smoking Cessation Patient Facts

In 20 minutes of not smoking, your blood pressure drops to a level close to that of before you had your last cigarette. The temperature of your hands and feet may increase to normal.

In 8 hours of not smoking the carbon monoxide level in your blood drops to normal.

In 24 hours of not smoking your chance of a heart attack decreases.

In 2 weeks to 3 months of not smoking circulation improves and your lung function has the potential to increase up to 30%.

In 1 to 9 months of not smoking coughing, sinus congestion, fatigue, and shortness of breath decrease; cilia regain normal function in your lungs, increasing your ability to handle mucus, clean your lungs, and reduce infection.

In 1 year of not smoking your chance of having a heart attack is cut in half.

In 5 years of not smoking your risk of stroke is reduced to that of a non-smoker.

In 10 years of not smoking your risk of dying from lung cancer is about half that of a continuing smoker; risks of cancer of the mouth, throat, esophagus, bladder, kidney, and pancreas decrease.

In 15 years of not smoking your risk of coronary heart disease may become that of a non-smoker.

Go to www.smokearrest.com for more information.
844-NO2-SMOKE (844-662-7665)
Email: info@smokearrestcenters.com

Alcohol

Alcohol, the great social lubricant, is often used to combat stress; it relaxes muscles and decreases anxiety. But alcohol used to excess can be a source of stress, and it is one of the major drug problems in the United States. Listen, most people enjoy a drink every now and then; personally, I enjoy a good glass of wine. More on wine later. The fact remains that, as with anything, the key is moderation and too much alcohol will have an effect on your telomeres. Yet, you will learn later that a little wine can benefit your cells and telomeres.

The problem with any substance is abuse and alcohol, like drugs, is often abused. According to the National Council on Alcoholism, "There are 3.3 million alcoholics and problem drinkers age 14–17,

10 million aged 18–65, and 1.6 million over 65—a total of nearly 5 million alcoholics. Approximately 5 million Americans have alcohol-related health problems. As a central nervous system depressant, alcohol does not increase either physical or mental ability, nor does it dilate the cornea vessels as some believe. Studies show that even in low or moderate amounts, alcohol actually increases the workload of the heart. Moderate amounts significantly impair visual and motor coordination in the ability to estimate speed and distance of objects and motor coordination in the ability to estimate speed and distance of objects and judgments of passage of time. Sexual function is diminished by even a moderate amount of alcohol. Addiction to alcohol is characterized by tolerance and physical dependence. Illnesses associated with alcohol abuse include cirrhosis, gastritis, pancreatitis, nutritional disorders, organic brain disease, coronary artery disease, and hypertension. Over 50% of all highway fatalities are directly related to alcohol abuse."

Alcohol and nicotine are drugs; they're products that have the capacity to alter the natural chemistry of the body. *Newsweek* recently reported that drug abuse has become America's number one problem in business. Drugs in today's society have moved into the corporate board rooms, courtrooms, airline hangars, nuclear plants, factories, construction sites, and even our schools. Drugs and alcohol are byproducts of stress. People utilize these substances to alleviate their problems, not realizing that they are actually feeding them. Stress can be reduced by proper diet, proper exercise, and proper health habits. Any dependency is an addiction, and addiction is a problem, and problems are a major source of stress.

Alcohol creates biochemical stress within the body. When it enters the blood it stimulates an increased production of our stress hormone norepinephrine. This hormone mobilizes all our resources to fight stress. The fact that alcohol stimulates norepinephrine production suggests that regular drinking takes its toll on the body's capacity to cope with stressful life situations.

Andrea Baccarelli, the lead researcher at the University of Milan in Italy, said, "Heavy alcohol users tend to look haggard, and it is commonly thought heavy drinking leads to premature aging and earlier onset of diseases of aging."

The researchers looked at more than 250 volunteers, some of whom drank more than 4 alcoholic drinks per day.

They were similar in age and other factors that might affect telomere length, such as diet, physical exercise, work-related stress, and environmental exposures.

Results showed that telomere length was dramatically shortened in those who consumed heavy amounts of alcohol. In some, telomere length was nearly half as long as telomere length in the non-abusers.

Stress telomeres and DHEA

I am always on the lookout for supplements to keep me young and my cells fit. One way to counteract aging and make your body feel like it did years ago is with Dehydroepiandrosterone (DHEA). Although many people have heard of DHEA, hardly anyone can pronounce its full name and few know anything about it. DHEA is the most abundant product of your adrenal glands.

Throughout the rest of this book we will continue to discuss and explore many supplements that will help you turn back the clock, but it is important that you have a guide, a coach, along your journey through time. A qualified doctor, health coach, or nutritionist should be the leader of your expedition. DHEA is one supplement I recommend taking under a doctor's guidance. Your doctor can check your DHEA levels and guide you through this process. No supplement should be taken randomly without your doctor's or nutritionist's guidance. This is especially true for DHEA. DHEA is one that definitely should be taken under a doctor's guidance.

We call DHEA the "anti-stress hormone." It is the precursor used by your body in producing sex hormones like testosterone, estrogen, and progesterone. You secrete DHEA when times are good—when you are well-fed, secure, and free of stressors. The more DHEA in your body, the less effect stress will have on you. That's because DHEA is the counter to another hormone called cortisol. When you are under stress, cortisol tells your body "just get through the moment, don't worry about tomorrow." Where there is stress, there is cortisol. Since it inhibits maintenance and repair, cortisol accelerates aging. Most hormones decline with age, but cortisol, the stress hormone, actually increases with age. Cortisol plays havoc with your body because it's like burning your candles at both ends. People with DHEA deficiency have been documented to experience cognitive decline, an aged appearance, and a shortened lifespan.

A study in the *Journal of the American Geriatric Society* showed people between 60 and 80 with the highest levels of DHEA performed better on both cognitive and physical tests. Study authors even noted that those with higher levels of DHEA seemed younger. If you want to turn back the effects of our stressful modern environment, you can supplement with DHEA. DHEA therapy has successfully treated many patients who suffer from lack of energy, depression, and chronic fatigue syndrome. It's important for you to get your DHEA levels checked. Your doctor can perform the simple test. After your levels have been checked, you can determine optimal dosing. DHEA is absorbed well and can be taken at any time but best mimics the natural daily levels when taken first thing in the morning.

Inflammation and infection drive telomere loss

At this time in our scientific understanding of telomeres, the most realistic expectation is to be able to slow the rate of telomere loss, which will hopefully enable you to fulfill your Hayflick obligation of 120 years of healthy life—or even longer. This means you must manage wear and tear effectively. High stress and infection are two examples of wear and tear that will shorten your telomeres. Both situations are highly inflammatory, causing significant cell damage. As inflammation rises, so does free radical damage. For example, patients with periodontal inflammation, which is typically accompanied by low-grade mouth infections, have higher levels of inflammatory markers, higher amounts of free radical damage, and shorter telomeres.

Under conditions of higher inflammatory stress, cells increase their rate of replicating and dividing in order to restore themselves. This need to recover from cellular damage actually speeds up the loss of telomeres due to significantly increased cell turnover. Additionally, the free radicals generated during the inflammatory situation also damage existing telomeres. Thus, we want to do everything we can to reduce inflammation (especially traumatic injury, physical or emotional) and prevent infectious illness. In addition to the more obvious acute and intense issues we also need to manage the low-grade chronic issues, such as infections in our sinuses, mouth, or digestive tract.

It is simply not realistic or even desirable to avoid all stress or inflammation. However, it is important to manage your life effectively so as to prevent your telomeres from shortening too quickly. And in the unfortunate event of trauma or a nasty infection, it is a good idea to boost and support nutrition until there is a full recovery. The most basic supplements to address the inflammatory issue are vitamin D and DHA, an essential omega-3 fatty acid integral to the health of cell membranes, nerve, and brain function. It must be received in the diet via cold water oceanic fish, although some plant sources are available.

Conquering inflammation is a pillar of anti-aging medicine. By defeating the chronic diseases that threaten to cut short your life, you set yourself on the path of "healthy aging."

Oxygen that kills inflammation

Former NFL great and friend, Duane Clemons, former captain of the Cincinnati Bengals and Kansas City Chiefs first told me about barometric chambers. This was later shared with me by my special friend Joe Jillson. So hearing about oxygen from these two special men made me do my research.

Researchers and forward-thinking doctors have been putting patients into hyperbaric chambers to breathe oxygen at 1.5 times normal atmospheric pressure for all kinds of problems for more than 30 years. And it's worked on patients from children with cerebral palsy and athletes with sports injuries to victims of chronic and slow-healing medical conditions.

But only recently has science discovered why it works so well on inflammation.

In 2002, Professor Jürg Tschopp and his team at the University of Lausanne in Switzerland discovered a multiprotein group he called "inflammasomes." The job of inflammasomes, Prof. Tschopp revealed, is to produce inflammation as part of your body's immune system response.

Of course, all inflammation isn't bad. You need it when you have a cut or a broken bone. Without this "acute" inflammation, your body wouldn't heal because no white blood cells from your immune system could ride to the rescue and fight off the foreign bodies attacking you.

But inflammasomes also cause the low-level inflammatory responses you can't see—those that go on for years and slowly kill you with cancer and the other chronic diseases. Inflammasome triggers are all around us. In fact, they attack every day and are one of the two causes of disease. These include:

Environmental toxins and pollutants
Stress
Poor diet

Excess weight

Cigarette smoke

Inflammasomes can also be activated by live bacteria, as well as xeno-compounds and hormone-disrupting chemicals,1 like Bisphenol A (BPA).

But recent research reveals the power of HBOT in the battle against inflammasomes. A study published earlier this year tested the impact of HBOT on lab mice with spinal cord injuries.

Inflammation was running rampant in the mice. But after a series of HBOT sessions, it became clear that the pressurized oxygen had "inactivated" inflammasomes.

The explanation is simple. Breathing pressurized oxygen raises the concentration of oxygen in the blood, thereby increasing the number of oxygen molecules getting through without having to increase the flow of blood to the area.

The oxygen jolt wakes the cells and gets them working again, allowing their repair mechanisms to go into action. That repair mechanism begins by inactivating inflammasomes.

We only have one body; let's give it what it wants, what it needs, and get ourselves on the road to health.

I believe that with some guidance, a certain amount of discipline, and a lot of education, we can achieve a happier, healthier existence. Stress, like disease, will always be with us, but we can reduce it and learn not to let it run us. Befriend yourself, learn from your failures, and acknowledge your successes. Accept that plans do not always work out and that worrying will not improve matters. Most of all, be willing to accept that the life you deserve is available to you. *Awakening the Wellness Within* is about developing the right habits, habits that will help your cells stay healthy and assist your telomeres in remaining longer so you can live a longer, more fulfilled life.

"The doctor of the future will be oneself."

—ALBERT SCHWEITZER

Chapter 14

TOXINS AND DISEASE

We now know how caring for our cells cares for our telomeres, which prolongs our lives. To defeat the enemy, in this case toxins, we must know the enemy.

With only two causes of disease we must look at each cause closely. Toxins come in different forms and have many disguises. The upcoming chapters will help you identify the toxins in the environment you live in.

Let's begin to look at our enemy. Toxins in the form of synthetic pollutants have increased as a result of the technological leap made since the industrial revolution. The toxins we use on a daily basis are finding their way into our cells and creating a health crisis of pandemic proportions. Just look at the ingredients in the foods you eat.

We live in a world where many new hazards pose a danger to human health in this modern age where synthetic and potent toxic chemicals run abundant in the products used on a daily basis. Toxins shut our systems down and are the cause of many chronic diseases today. Like grains of sand, toxins can jam the cellular machinery and cause the entire cell to shut down.

Countless toxins enter our bodies on a daily basis, whether it's from driving in a brand new car for a few hours, using conventional cosmetics and skin care products, or eating certain foods. Even for those of us who carefully avoid pesticides, parabens, and phthalates whenever possible, we can't help but come into contact with them because of their ubiquitous presence in the world.

Canadian authors and environmentalists Bruce Lourie and Rick Smith alerted much of the world to the toxicity of everyday household items in their first best seller *Slow Death by Rubber Duck.* While that book did a great job of educating people, it didn't answer the next, logical question: How do I get this stuff OUT of my body?

Imagine, in modern societies we must combat the risk of radiation from nuclear waste, as well as contamination from polluted air and water. Our world today has been reshaped by humans, leading to the production of many new health hazards that were absent just two centuries ago. The many synthetic chemicals and drugs we use on an increasing basis find their way into the food chain, threatening not only our cells but our health and natural environment as well.

It all begins with the chemicals in our water and the chemicals sprayed over our neighborhoods to maintain our lawns, to the poisons killing our insects and making our food toxic "medicine." The fact is, we need a way to purge the deadly elixirs of a greedy government, owned and run by corporate interests. For the sake of keeping your attention, I won't go on *ad nauseum* about fluoridated water, oil spills, and contaminated air and water due to fracking and mining. However, isn't it amazing that we spend money weekly for water, the same water that flows freely through our homes?

Toxins are enemies to our cells and infiltrate our homes even in the form of water. Research since the early 1900s suggests our bodies simply cannot handle the level of toxicity in our environment without some help, though it was originally designed to cure itself from every conceivable toxin—from heavy metals to the common cold. We have simply burdened the mechanism so profoundly that the intelligence of the human form is being strained to its acme. We either learn to adapt to the toxic environment that our governments so blatantly support or we die. We can't wait for congress or the senate to do the right thing. It's time to get radical. It's time to tell your friends about this, even if it is absolutely rabble-rousing.

We are a toxic world. Our blood and bones now contain over 50,000 different chemical pollutants. There are too many other toxins to name here. Their names and devastating health effects could fill books. These toxins have seeped into our cells, causing cancer, depression, and even insanity.

These pollutants are making our children less intelligent and slowly breaking down our immune systems until they can't even fight a simple virus. Our hormonal systems are so out of whack from these toxins that both boys and girls are starting puberty way too soon, and fetuses are not developing properly. ADHD, ADD, and autism are on the rise like never before. Our bodies are fat and tired because a toxic body can't metabolize fats and proteins properly.

The average man or woman in the 21st century consumes artificially refined foods in sugar, salt, and carbohydrate-rich diets in alarming quantities. Daily, the consumers of the world weaken his or her body by consuming artificial stimulants and sedatives, as well as the industrial cleaners utilized in our homes. Combine this with the pesticides in our food and contaminants in our water, as well as the millions of synthetic products we come in contact with on a daily basis. Is it surprising then that the number of people suffering from cancer and cardiovascular disease is sky-rocketing? Every imaginable disease, including allergies, arthritis, obesity, acne, basal cell cancers and other disorders of the skin are increasingly becoming major health issues across the world. In many countries, the number of people who complain of a variety of physical symptoms like constant weakness, fatigue, persistent headaches, vague pains, chronic coughs, disorders of the gastrointestinal tract, immune impairment, sexual impairment, as well as psychological disorders are all showing a steep increase.

Toxins, meaning substances that at high enough levels are poisonous to our bodies, exist in many everyday foods and products.

Take your breakfast meal, for example. If you eat a simple breakfast of cereal with milk and fruit, some researchers suggest you are likely to be exposed to more than 25 toxins. If you eat a breakfast of bacon or sausage and eggs, you are likely to be exposed to more than 57 toxins. What about coffee and a pastry—no toxins, right? Wrong. Even that simple breakfast can expose you to more than 10 toxins. This is why I start my day with a protein shake.

It is estimated by some journals that if we follow you through a normal day in the U.S. and you do nothing more than simply eat 3 meals and get to work and back, you are likely to have been exposed to over 450 toxins. Many of these toxins are even present in newborns. One study in 2004 randomly tested the discarded umbilical cords of newborn infants in the U.S. found 187 known carcinogens, 217 known neurotoxins, and 208 substances known to cause birth defects.

Because toxins and contaminants can be either water-soluble or fat-soluble, these toxins can hide in the fat tissues of the body for a lifetime. Over a lifetime, the bioaccumulation of toxins has been lifetime can reach or exceed recommended levels for safety established by the Centers for Disease Control.

Toxins have an adverse affect on the cell; they weaken and stress the cell. Toxins may be defined as substances that produce physical, emotional, and psychological imbalances in an individual. We are consistently exposed to toxins every day.

I mentioned the two types of types of toxins in Chapter 4: exogenous and endogenous. Remember, exogenous toxins are present in the outside environment, whereas endogenous toxins are produced as a result of imbalances in our metabolism. Remove the cause and you are on your way to health and well-being. So let's start reviewing the cause of how toxins get into our bodies and figure out how to eliminate toxins from our cells.

1. **Endogenous Toxins** are toxins that are produced inside of your body. This becomes a problem when the cells become weak,

especially the cell membrane that has to regulate the outflow of toxins. Toxins are waste products from normal metabolic activities. Carbon dioxide, urea, and lactic acid are examples of endogenous toxins that your body churns out by the second. Unless your cells are severely compromised, your body is well equipped to eliminate these endogenous toxins from your system. An often overlooked source of endogenous toxins is an unhealthy gut. Over time, a diet that's rich in highly refined foods, poor eating habits, and emotional stress can lead to an unhealthy balance of microorganisms in your gastrointestinal tract. This can be diagnosed as intestinal dysbiosis, but it's a state of cytopathology. Intestinal dysbiosis is accompanied by a steady production of endogenous toxins by undesirable yeasts, fungi, bacteria, and in rare cases even parasites. These toxins include various aldehydes, alcohols, indols, phenols, and skatols—to name just a few. While some of these endogenous toxins are eliminated as gas, some make their way into your bloodstream by traveling through your intestinal walls, and once they make it into your bloodstream, they can get into your cells. Once this happens, the cells become weakened and disease sets in. This is why the cell membrane is so important as it filters and protects our cells.

2. **Exogenous Toxins** are chemicals that are made outside of your body and can harm your cells if they are ingested, inhaled, or absorbed into your bloodstream through some other channel. While it's unrealistic to live and work in an environment that's free of exogenous toxins, you should strive to minimize your exposure to the following most common exogenous toxins:

- MSG and aspartame, both are especially toxic to your nerve cells
- Drugs (medical and recreational)
- Water

- Plastic
- Anything not natural will probably be toxic to your body
- Any over-the-counter or prescription drug that comes with a warning that use of the drug in question may lead to liver damage. Tylenol, for example.
- Many household and hygiene products, especially cosmetics that are applied around the mouth, which are easily swallowed in small but significant amounts

Vaccines—the toxic truth

Imagine injecting a child with toxins soon after their birth, before their immunity system is fully formed This puts cellular stress on the child from the beginning which clearly affects 13% of parents are now using an alternative vaccination schedule, and 2% refuse all vaccines for their children. Still, 28% of parents following the childhood vaccination schedule think it would be safer to delay the use of vaccines.

The CDC vaccination schedule for children aged six and younger includes vaccines for measles, mumps, rubella, whooping cough, chicken pox, hepatitis, seasonal flu, and others. All in all, U.S. children are expected to get 48 doses of 14 vaccines by the time they're 6 years old. By age 18, federal public health officials say they should have gotten a total of 69 doses of 16 vaccines.

Is this safe and beneficial in the short- or long-term? No one really knows, primarily because large studies comparing the health outcomes of vaccinated versus unvaccinated children have not been a priority for vaccine researchers. Most vaccine studies are about developing more vaccines for children and adults to use.

Some claim studies comparing the health of highly vaccinated and unvaccinated children cannot be done because it would be "unethical" to leave children participating in the study unvaccinated in order to do the comparison.

But since there are a number of American parents who are already delaying or avoiding vaccinating their children altogether, this hardly seems like a reasonable excuse. It seems more likely that comparing the health of vaccinated and unvaccinated children in appropriately designed studies are avoided because the results might upset the proverbial apple cart.

In German children, 11% of those vaccinated reported having ear infections, compared to less than 0.5% of unvaccinated children. Similarly, sinusitis was reported in over 32% of vaccinated children, while the prevalence in unvaccinated children was less than 1%.

There are basic differences between naturally acquired immunity and temporary vaccine-induced antibody production. But few are willing to look at this issue—least of all conventional medicine, which is so dominated by pharmaceutical companies seeking bigger markets and more profits from the investment they make in developing new vaccines. As a parent, you need to educate yourself on each individual disease and corresponding vaccine in order to make an informed decision about the risks and benefits of the choices you make.

An important vaccine safety review was issued by the Institute of Medicine (IOM) in August. According to this review of over 1,000 independent studies on vaccines, they were unable to determine whether or not vaccines are a causative factor in over 100 serious adverse health outcomes. In short, the research available is insufficient and cannot be used to confirm nor deny causation for many poor health outcomes and vaccinations.

In the United States, people get in line yearly for their flu shots and all kinds of other vaccines with complete trust that they will be protected from illness. In all actuality, some vaccines may be riskier than the diseases themselves. In the '70s, the last time there was a true mass epidemic of the swine flu, the vaccination caused more deaths than the flu itself.

Sure, the rates of serious illnesses that we are vaccinated for can be clearly shown to have decreased over 90% since vaccinations have been used. While this number is remarkable, we don't live in a country where these diseases are prevalent. We don't even hear of most of these diseases anymore, and the risks are lower than ever.

Current studies show that approximately 50% of Americans are fearful of vaccinations. Naturally, parents are hesitant before vaccinating their babies without fully understanding the risks, but they are often not given the facts or a choice in the matter by their doctors.

Many doctors, parents, and others in the medical community feel strongly that there is a clear link between vaccines and autism. Just think, 30 years ago most people had never heard of autism, but now approximately 1–2% of children will be diagnosed with autism in their lives. There has to be something to this.

So while some people say this is just coincidence, the real shock is when you look at entire communities that do not use vaccines at all, like the Amish community, where there are actually no cases of autism at all. While some believe they are just not diagnosed, many others think it is because they stay away from vaccinations and the dangerous mercury that vaccinations include.

Many vaccines actually have viruses in them. So in reality you are injecting yourself with a live virus to try to avoid catching an alternative disease, which you may not have any chance of catching in the first place. Does this sound crazy to you too?

Flu shots, which include mercury, are toxic. The National Institute of Health (NIH) admits that mercury is toxic, even in very small amounts, but it remains in vaccinations. Just the flu shot contains ingredients that cause symptoms like allergic reactions, death, neurological problems, dementia, convulsions, speech problems, respiratory problems, issues with intestines or liver, skin disorders, cancer cells, and more.

There are numerous cases where children were developing normally until they received these vaccinations, when their behavior almost immediately changed. These children went from being engaged, happy 12 to 16-month-old children, and then after receiving vaccinations, their speech and other abilities declined, eventually leading to autism. There are thousands of reports of this happening, so it is far from a standalone case.

Many parents who have sworn off vaccinations are also reporting that their kids are healthier than other kids who have been vaccinated, overall, lessening chances of regular day to day illness.

So why on earth would anyone intentionally put these chemicals into their children when the risks are not there? Don't just listen to your doctor and do what everyone else does because it is the recommended procedure. Do the proper research and understand the risks of all vaccinations and the chances that your child may wind up with autism.

For example, there have been absolutely zero cases of polio in the United States since 1979. Are you worried that your child will become the first to catch polio in over 20 years? Worried enough to get a potentially harmful vaccine to prevent it, when there are such low risks to be worried about?

While autism and other diseases have not been directly tied back to vaccinations as the 100% solidified cause, vaccinations and the prevalence of mercury are so apparent, and obvious lines have been drawn to show that vaccinations should be avoided. Every parent and person needs to make their own decision, but before trusting your doctor that vaccinations are the way to go, get multiple opinions and truly consider your risk before doing so. You do this by speaking with your doctor and doing your homework.

Toxic city

The key to cellular health is avoiding toxins that we come in contact with daily and can remove from our homes and lives. According to Dr. Joseph Mercola, toxins are abundant in our homes.

"Household consumer products injure 33.1 million people in the United States every year. These incidents cost $800 billion in related expenses from death, injury, or property damages. And many scientists are starting to believe that, in particular, the chemicals found in a wide variety of the goods you use every day may be more toxic than previously thought." Here are his top 10 of the most common products that may be hazardous to your health.

10. Mothballs

Since moths chew holes through clothing and other textiles, people pack away these stinky repellents to kill them. But studies on one active ingredient in some repellents, paradichlorobenzene, found that it can cause cancer in animals. Other types of moth balls use naphthalene, which after prolonged exposure can damage or destroy red blood cells and can also stimulate nausea, vomiting, and diarrhea.

9. Pesticides

99% of households in the United States use some form of pesticide, a broad term that encompasses a variety of chemical formulas that kill everything from tiny microorganisms up to rodents. In 2006, the American Association of Poison Control Centers received nearly 46,000 calls regarding children under 5 years old who had been exposed to potentially toxic levels of pesticides.

8. Pressed Wood Products

This faux wood takes bits and pieces of logs and wood leftovers and combines them together. Pressed wood products include paneling, particle board, fiberboard, and insulation, all of which were particularly popular for home construction in the 1970s. However, the glue that holds the wood particles in place may use urea-formaldehyde as a resin. The U.S. EPA estimates that this is the largest source of formaldehyde emissions indoors. Formaldehyde exposure can set off watery eyes, burning eyes and throat, difficulty breathing, and asthma attacks. Scientists also know that it can cause cancer in animals. The risk is greater with older pressed wood products, since newer ones are better regulated.

7. Chemicals in Carpets

Indoor carpeting has recently come under greater scrutiny because of the volatile organic compounds (VOCs) associated with new carpet installation. The glue and dyes used with carpeting are known to emit VOCs, which can be harmful to your health in high concentrations. However, the initial VOC emissions will often subside after the first few days following.

6. Laser Printers Chemicals

A 2007 study found that some laser printers give off ultra-fine particles that can cause serious health problems. Another study confirmed that laser and ink-jet printers can release volatile organic compounds (VOCs) and ozone particulates. All of these have been linked with heart and lung disease.

5. Lead Paint

In 1991, the U.S. government declared lead to be the greatest environmental threat to children. Even low concentrations can cause problems with your central nervous system, brain, blood cells, and kidneys. It's particularly threatening for fetuses, babies, and children because of potential developmental disorders. Many houses built before 1978 contain lead paint. Once the paint begins to peel away, it will release the harmful lead particles that you can inhale.

4. Air Fresheners and Cleaning Solutions

Air fresheners and cleaning solutions, when used excessively or in a small, unventilated area, can release toxic levels of pollutants. This comes from two main chemicals called ethylene-based glycol ethers and terpenes. While the EPA regards the ethers as toxic by themselves, the non-toxic terpenes can react with ozone in the air to form a poisonous combination. Air fresheners in particular are linked to many volatile organic compounds, such as nitrogen dioxide, and some fresheners also contain paradichlorobenzene, the same chemical emitted by mothballs.

3. Baby Bottles and BPA

Canada has taken the first steps to outlaw the sale of baby bottles made from polycarbonate plastics, which are the most common type on the market. It has done so because the plastics are made with a chemical called bisphenol-A (BPA). BPA has a structure very similar to estrogen and for that reason is referred to as a "hormone disruptor." Hormone disruptors can interfere with the natural human hormones, especially for young children.

2. Flame Retardants

Commonly used in mattresses, upholstery, television, and computer casings and circuit boards, flame retardants use polybrominated diphenyl ethers (PBDEs). Two forms of PBDEs were phased out of use in manufacturing in the United States in 2004 because of related health threats, but the products containing them linger on. Studies have linked PBDEs to learning and memory problems, lowered sperm counts, and poor thyroid functioning in rats and mice. Other animal studies have indicated that PBDEs could be carcinogenic in humans, although that has not yet been confirmed.

1. Cosmetic Phthalates

Phthalates, also called plasticizers, go into many products including hair spray, shampoos, fragrances, and deodorants. Phthalates bind the color and fragrance in cosmetic products, and are also used to increase the durability and flexibility of plastics. Like BPA, these hormone-like chemicals are linked to reproductive and developmental problems in animals. Because of these findings, California and Washington State have banned the use of phthalates in toys for younger children.

Toxic talk

Is there a link between the toxins we live with daily and the increases in disease like cancer, Alzheimer's, etc.? Only recently have researchers and health practitioners begun to understand the long-term effects of the thousands of chemicals we now encounter in our daily lives. At the time of my birth, the majority of these chemicals did not exist, or at least we didn't know about them as we do today. Now they are all-pervasive and attack our cells on a daily basis.

A growing body of scientific evidence links toxins to a wide variety of symptoms and syndromes, such as mental and behavioral disorders, learning disabilities, fatigue, migraines, allergies, rashes, and gastrointestinal disorders.

Frightening new evidence suggests that low-level exposures to certain dietary and environmental chemicals are causing hormone disruptions, resulting in serious problems that range from birth defects to cancer.

Many of the diseases that confuse doctors today (often misdiagnosed as "diseases of aging" or "diseases of civilization") are the results of the toxic overload caused by modern industrialized society. These diseases are difficult to diagnose and impossible to cure using conventional medical approaches that just treat symptoms, rather than minimizing toxic exposure and optimizing detoxification. This is a major reason why my disease approach makes so much sense. With new toxins will come more diseases and more new names.

Chemicals posing little cancer risk can trigger cancer when combined together with other toxins on a daily basis; it is the combination that causes a severe toxic chemical reaction, like the makings of a bomb. It is a group of ingredients together that creates combustion.

Many chemicals and metals are toxic in any amount; others are beneficial or even essential in small amounts— such as vitamin A— but toxic in large amounts.

It is scary to know that every day we're exposed to hundreds of toxins—from the food we eat, to the air we breathe, to the water we drink, to the items we touch. Without proper cleansing of impurities, the body struggles to maintain good health. Cleansed and revitalized cells makes the body stronger, resist illness better, is more efficient, and performs at a higher level than one that is filled with impurities.

"The human body has approximately 5 liters of blood circulating at any given time, consisting of cells and plasma," notes the Franklin Institute. Keeping the blood cleansed attributes to increased health and life expectancy. We will talk more about cleansing the cells in the next chapters. Cleansing will help you *Awaken the Wellness Within*, by empowering your cells and allowing your body to heal.

ONE DISEASE

Cytopathology

TWO CAUSES

Deficiency

Toxicity

ONE CURE

"No disease that can be treated by diet should be treated with any other means."

—Maimonides

Chapter 15

———◦◦◦———

TOXIC FOOD FACTS

The toxic truth is that one of the main ways toxins enter our bodies is through the foods we eat. Our foods are so toxic, so full of additives and preservatives, that I had to write an additional chapter on the toxins in the foods we eat. Friends, if we are what we eat, remember, we eat what we buy. Various shelves throughout every aisle of your grocery store are stocked with wolves in sheep's clothing. Colorful packaging, appetizing pictures, and nutrition claims hide the truth: Unhealthy chemicals are lurking in many of these seemingly harmless foods.

We are now adroit in understanding how toxins affect our cells. Did you know that more than 6,000 additives and chemicals are used by food manufacturers to process and produce our food? I didn't know this and was alarmed when I found out. Today's conventional food system is heavily dependent on toxic chemicals and synthetic inputs that pose threats to our health—especially children's. Just look at their cereal box, and it only gets worse from there. Forget about the soda they drink, the candy they eat, the snacks they snack on. The food industry and its marketing prey upon children and the foods they eat.

Imagine a world where

Wouldn't it be great if we didn't have to read labels? But we do. Imagine a world where:

- Diabetes, heart diseases, autoimmunity and other modern diseases are rare or don't exist at all
- We are naturally lean and fit
- We are fertile throughout our childbearing years
- We sleep peacefully and deeply
- We age gracefully without degenerative diseases like Alzheimer's and osteoporosis

While this might sound like pure fantasy today, anthropological evidence suggests that this is exactly how human beings lived for the vast majority of our evolutionary history. Let's face the facts, our grandparents ate healthier foods, more nutritious foods than our generation. I only see it getting worse; we must stand up for our health rights.

Today, most people accept diseases like obesity, diabetes, infertility, and Alzheimer's as "normal." But while these diseases may now be common, they're anything but normal. One of my best friends, a "brother," Joe Jillson, is 72 and the picture of good health; however, it was not just a genetic gift. He is one of the most dedicated men I know, a true inspiration. Joe awakes every morning at 5:00 am to exercise. He knows you must pay a price for health, and he pays it tenfold.

It is time for us to remember that humans evolved roughly 2.5 million years ago, and for roughly 84,000 generations we were naturally free of the modern diseases that kill millions of people each year and make countless others miserable. In fact, the world I asked you to imagine above—which may seem preposterous and unattainable today—was the natural human state for our entire history on this planet up until a couple hundred years ago.

What was responsible for the change? What transformed us from naturally healthy and vital people free of degenerative disease into a world of sick, fat, infertile, and unhappy people?

Though there are several aspects of our current lifestyle that contribute to disease, the widespread consumption of food toxins is by far the greatest offender. Specifically, the following dietary toxins are to blame:

- Cereal grains
- Refined flour, gluten products)
- Omega-6 industrial seed oils (corn, cottonseed, safflower, soybean, etc.)
- Sugar (especially high-fructose corn syrup)
- Milk
- Margarine
- Salt
- Processed soy (soy milk, soy protein, soy flour, etc.)

The role of dietary toxins in contributing to modern disease

Before you get worried, relax, sit back, and continue to learn. Your body is perfect; it is a self-cleaning, healing machine. As a result of this great machine and the knowledge we now possess, most of us won't get sick from eating a small amount of any food. However, in quantity, foods like sugar, cereal grain, soy, and industrial seed oil are harmful to our cells. When we eat these nutrients (or rather anti-nutrients) in excessive quantities, our risk of developing cellular malfunction and modern diseases rises significantly.

That's exactly what's happening today. These four food toxins—refined cereal grains, industrial seed oils, sugar, and processed soy—comprise the bulk of the modern diet. Bread, pastries, muffins, crackers, cookies, soda, fruit juice, fast food, and other convenience foods are all loaded with these toxins. And when the majority of what most people eat on a daily basis is toxic, it's not hard to understand why our health is failing.

Let's look at each of these food toxins in more detail.

Cereal grains: one of the unhealthiest "health foods" on the planet?

The major cereal grains—wheat, corn, rice, barley, sorghum, oats, rye, and millet—have become the staple crops of the modern human diet. They've also become the "poster children" of the low-fat, high-carbohydrate diet promoted by organizations like the American Heart Association (AHA) and American Diabetes Association (ADA). If you say the phrase "whole grains" to most people, the first word that probably comes to their mind is "healthy."

But the fact is that most animals, including our closest relative, the chimpanzee, aren't adapted to eating cereal grains and don't eat them in large quantities. And humans have only been eating them for the past 10,000 years. So I ask you, Why?

Grains are not made the way they once were. Cereal is basically manufactured candy. Most cereals are cooked and come from refined flour, which can irritate our stomach in many different possible ways, such as:

- Producing toxins that irritate or damage the lining of the gut
- Producing toxins that bind essential minerals, making them unavailable to the body
- Producing toxins that inhibit digestion and absorption of other essential nutrients, including protein

One of these toxic compounds is the protein gluten, which is present in wheat and many of the other most commonly eaten cereal grains. In short, gluten damages the intestine and makes it leaky. And researchers now believe that a leaky gut is one of the major predisposing factors for conditions like obesity, diabetes, and autoimmune disease.

Celiac disease (CD)—a condition of severe gluten intolerance—has been well known for decades. Celiacs have a dramatic and, in some cases, potentially fatal immune response to even the smallest amounts of gluten. I didn't know I was gluten intolerant until recently. Having stomach issues, I went to doctor after doctor and took Prevacid daily for acid. Once I cut my sugars, my carbohydrates, and my glutens my stomach issues resolved. I am 25 pounds lighter and drug-free as well as symptom-free. I eat more and weigh less.

The understanding of cytopathology of the stomach cells, or celiac disease, is just the tip of the iceberg when it comes to intolerance to wheat and other gluten-containing grains. Celiac disease is characterized by antibodies to two components of the gluten compound: alpha-gliadin and transglutaminase. But we now know that people can and do react to several other components of wheat and gluten.

Current laboratory testing for gluten intolerance only tests for alpha-gliadin and transglutaminase, the two components of gluten implicated in celiac disease. Fact is, wheat contains several other components including lectins like wheat germ agglutinin, other epitopes of the gliadin protein like beta-gliadin, gamma-gliadin and omega-gliadin, another protein called glutenin, an opioid peptide called gluteomorphin, and a compound called deamidated gliadin produced by the industrial processing or digestion of gluten. I could hardly spell these words so you can imagine how hard they are to digest.

Studies now clearly show that people can react negatively to all of these components of wheat—not just the alpha-gliadin and transglutaminase that celiacs react to. And the worst part of this is that up until recently, no commercial labs were testing for sensitivity to these other subfractions of wheat.

This means, of course, that it's extremely likely that far more people are intolerant to wheat and gluten than conventional wisdom would tell us. In fact, that's exactly what the latest research shows. Dr. Kenneth Fine, a pioneer in gluten intolerance research, has demonstrated that 1 in 3 Americans are gluten intolerant, and that 8 in 10 have the genes that predispose them to developing gluten intolerance.

This is nothing short of a public health catastrophe in a nation where the #1 source of calories is refined flour. But while most are at least aware of the dangers of sugar, trans fat, and other unhealthy foods, fewer than 1 in 8 people with celiac disease are aware of their condition. A 1999 paper in the *British Medical Journal* illustrated this well:

Patients with clinically obvious celiac disease (observable inflammation and destruction of the gut tissue) comprise only 12.5% of the total population of people with CD. And 87.5% of those with celiac have no obvious gut symptoms. For every symptomatic patient with CD, there are 8 patients with CD and no gastrointestinal symptoms. We will discuss gluten more later in this chapter.

Know your oils

Most cooking oils are already oxidized (rancid) before they are even bottled because of the processing. Even otherwise healthy oils become slightly toxic and carcinogenic when they are rancid. It is vital to get cold-pressed oils for this reason. Chemical deodorizers are sometimes added to hide the unpleasant scent of rancidity. Rancid (oxidized) fats are chemically unstable and provide damaging free radicals. Trans fats cause inflammation that may induce arterial patching. Beware of both trans fats and healthy oils that have been made rancid. Use cold-pressed, extra-virgin olive oil for most cooking, and peanut oil for high-heat applications. Cold-pressed, extra-virgin coconut oil is easily the healthiest oil of all for cold recipes, but it breaks down rapidly in heat to become rancid. Pristine coconut oil is an extremely healthy dietary supplement that will help to protect the arteries, like other healthy saturated fats will. Trans fats are industrially produced artificial foods. They commonly contain aluminum, lead, and cobalt residues as a result of their manufacturing processes.

Did you know that soy and canola oils are used as pesticides? When I learned this I was flabbergasted. Remember, anything toxic to the cells will cause cellular malfunction. We must remove toxins daily.

Soy is toxic even in its organic state, and it has to undergo a fermentation process just to make it safe for human consumption—with very mixed results. Soy causes drastic hormone imbalances, which has resulted in the epidemics of hypothyroidism and endometriosis.

The canola plant has no organic variety because the first canola plant was born in a test tube in the 1970s. The nuclear industry assisted in genetically engineering it. It is time we take our lives back and know what we are eating and better yet, where it comes from. Canola oil is considered, in my opinion, the Frankenstein of oils. It is the child of the deadly rapeseed plant. Rapeseed oil was banned in foods for causing heart tumors. Rapeseed's unwanted child, canola, is being deceptively marketed as being free of trans fats. The lie is based upon the fact that they only use the test results from before the oil is heated, and flagrantly ignore the test results of heated canola oil. Then, they market canola as the healthiest cooking oil, using cherry-picked test results from only uncooked oil. The biotechnology companies forget to mention that canola oil becomes a trans fat as soon as it is heated. However, they never forget to place the FDA-approved "heart healthy" label on every bottle of canola oil. Canola oil is also marketed as being high in omega-3, but all of the omega-3 becomes rancid and carcinogenic as soon as it is heated. Studies have shown that canola oil can produce heart lesions, particularly when accompanied by a diet that is low in protective saturated fats. It also produces high levels of benzene and formaldehyde when it is heated. The biotech industry brought us trans fats to ironically save us from heart disease, and it is now bringing us genetically engineered canola and soy, whilst promoting the very same con-job.

Margarine madness

In my first book, *Lifestyle of the Fit & Famous*, I talked about the difference between margarine and butter. Many of us were raised with the belief that margarine is better for you than butter and that margarine promotes heart health. This is simply not true. Our body needs good fats to protect our cells and margarine is a bad fat.

Today, it is estimated that margarine users outnumber butter users by more than 2 to 1. This is hardly surprising, for most of us were hearing of the virtues of the margarine (courtesy of television) before we knew the difference between a polyunsaturated fat and a polysyllable.

We have been led to believe that polyunsaturated fats, especially linoleic acid, can lower body fats and break down saturated fats. So in theory, it seems logical that if we switch to a polyunsaturated oil or margarine, we will be helping to lower the body's serum cholesterol level.

But the facts may not fit this appealing hypothesis. In his book, *Super Nutrition*, Richard A. Passwater, PhD, explains that, "The danger of polyunsaturated fats began to be noticed when Dr. Fred A. Kummerow and his colleagues from the University of Illinois at Urbana reported their studies at the 1974 Federation of American Societies for experimental biology meeting of nutritionists and related science. Newspapers carry the story of such titles as 'Margarine Found Health Hazard.' It is a shame that the story didn't make the front sections but that findings showed that fat present in margarine may present a greater health risk than cholesterol-rich foods such as beef fat, butter fat, and powdered eggs."

It's been around for over 100 years and was originally manufactured to fatten turkeys. It used to be white and tasted something like lard. Not very palatable. Eventually, margarine manufacturers won the right to color the stuff, but not without a fight because the dairy board tried to stop them in the U.S. The dairy board lost, and it was colored, flavored, and made to look and taste like butter.

Once the marketing campaign started, they did a great job of convincing the consumer, including the medical profession, that margarine was the superior product. Saturated fats were given the big thumbs down and we were told that butter, along with eggs, was bad and unhealthy.

Eventually research showed that although margarine consumption has gone up over the years, heart disease hasn't gone down. Neither has obesity. In fact, chronic disease in all its forms has gone up.

Margarine is unhealthy because it's made from cheap oils that are heat-extracted using petrochemical solvents—toxins, in other words. It's then hydrogenated to make it solid, which generally creates trans fats, which will give you heart disease as well as other health issues, before having colorings, flavorings and who knows what else added to it.

Recently, a study reported in the *Associated Press* claimed that men and women who ate the most margarine and certain processed foods had more than twice the heart attack risk. This study, which was presented at the annual American Heart Association Epidemiology Meeting, is one of the first to link margarine directly to heart disease. The problem occurs when polyunsaturated oils (which do not pose a heart risk) are modified to make them solid or semisolid in a process known as hydrogenation. Hydrogenated or partially hydrogenated vegetable oils are used to make margarine, a variety of cookies, potato chips, crackers, and other processed foods. Dr. Alberto Asherio of the Harvard School of Public Health in Boston analyzed the diets of both heart attack and non-heart attack victims. He found those highest in trans fatty acids (margarine) had 2.44 times the heart risk of those whose diets were lowest in trans fatty acids.

I suggest to my patients that they conduct a simple experiment. It involves taking a pat of margarine in one hand and a pat of butter in the other, then rubbing the fingers back and forth. The butter will dissolve, practically liquefy, in your hand. The margarine, on the other hand (pun intentional), maintains a thick, course texture that is not broken down by the heat given off by the body. If we are not able to break down this viscous, gelatinous substance in our hands, how can the body break it down in the circulatory system?

Our bodies don't know what to do with it because it's not a real food. Butter is a real food; the cells in our bodies know how to use it. When it comes to food, it's just common sense. Eat what we've always eaten, not for the last 50 or 100 years, but for the last 1,000 years or more.

Margarine Facts

- Very high in trans fatty acids
- Triples risk of coronary heart disease
- Increases total cholesterol and LDL (the bad cholesterol)
- Lowers HDL cholesterol, (the good cholesterol)
- Increases the risk of cancers up to five times
- Lowers quality of breast milk
- Decreases immune response
- Decreases insulin response

Margarine is only one molecule away from being plastic and shares 27 ingredients with paint.

Butter is better

Butter has been eaten for centuries, while margarine has only been on the market for 30 to 40 years. Butter is a natural food, while margarine is a chemical concoction. The widespread fear of dietary fats makes margarine an advertiser's dream, but it is a consumer's nightmare.

Butter contains no carbohydrates, which is why it is allowed on my diet. I'm not suggesting you gorge on it, but by all means use it, as long as it is not combined with a refined carbohydrate. That means no bread and butter because this mixture can go straight to your waistline.

Fats are essential to the body. Remember our prior learning about cholesterol and fats? Fats form the outer wall of our cell membrane and omega-3s are our # 1 choice. The fact remains: Our bodies need fats, just good fats. Fats keep your skin and your vital mucous membranes smooth and lubricated. Most importantly, they transport the fat-soluble vitamins (A, D, E, K) to the sites where they are needed. Following digestion, fats are absorbed and then oxidized to produce energy, carbon dioxide, and water.

Fats are a reserve of fuel, which is why my dietary principles work. When we cut down on carbohydrates, the fat mobilizing hormone is released and turns fat into energy—the purpose for which nature intended it.

Fats are also important in my program because they ward off boredom, which has been the downfall of many a diet. A little butter goes a long way toward adding zest to vegetables. In addition, fats help stabilize blood sugar, and when our blood sugar is under control, our appetite is reduced, so our overall consumption of food—including fat—is reduced naturally.

I find it amazing, day after day, to find that the same people who won't eat eggs for fear of their cholesterol levels will gorge themselves on sweets, starches, and refined carbohydrates. They compound insult to injury by consuming gobs of margarine (they have no fear of margarine's side effects) on their foods. They wash this all down with a glass of milk. The facts are the facts: Our country is not the healthiest in the world. It appears to me that chemical nutrition has kept up with medical technology—the result being no major increase in life expectancy over the past 15 to 20 years. Eat wisely and be an educated consumer.

Furthermore, a certain amount of cholesterol is not only acceptable, but vital. Cholesterol is a complex chemical that is absolutely essential to life. It is the basic molecular building block, from which adrenal hormones, sex hormones, vitamin D, and the bile acids necessary to digestion are formed. Cholesterol forms part of the membranes that surround every cell in our body. It is part of the protective covering of nerve fibers; it makes up a large part of the brain, it combines with various proteins to form lipoproteins needed to transport fats used as energy. Recent findings indicate that cholesterol may be essential to normal growth, longevity, and resistance to infection and toxicity.

Butter Facts

- Eating margarine can increase heart disease in women by 53% over eating the same amount of butter, according to a recent Harvard medical study.
- Butter has many nutritional benefits where margarine has a few and only because they are added!
- Butter tastes much better than margarine and it can enhance the flavors of other foods.
- Butter has been around for centuries where margarine has been around for less than 100 years.

Milk ain't what it used to be

As stated, there are good fats and bad fats. Milk is considered a bad fat. No longer is milk the beverage of choice. Cow's milk is ideal—for calves. That is the animal for which nature designed this product, and its components are proof of this. For example, all milk products contain a vital substance called casein. But, as I'll explain, there is far more casein in cow milk than a human can comfortably handle.

Before making a decision, know the facts. Don't be afraid to ask your doctor questions. You can be misled if you only have part of the information you need, as the following story illustrates.

Two men were thrown into the army guardhouse. One prisoner asked his cellmate, "How long are you in for?"

The other prisoner replied, "Twenty-four hours."

The first prisoner asked what offense he had committed.

"I killed the general," he said.

Confused, the first prisoner asked, "How come I got 30 days for going AWOL and you only get 24 hours for murdering the general."

He replied, "Because they're hanging me tomorrow."

Listen, like most Americans my age, milk and dairy were abundant in my diet. It was only later that I learned I was lactose intolerant. No wonder I had severe acne. Humans are the only species that continue to drink milk after they are weaned. If you put a bowl of milk in front of an adult cow, she would probably ignore it and munch on grass. Domesticated animals, such as cats, are different—they will drink milk because humans have tampered with their tastes. The enzymes necessary to break down and digest milk are rennin and lactase. Is it coincidence that most people no longer produce these enzymes after age three?

There is 300% more casein in cow milk than in human milk. Cow milk does indeed make cows strong. This drink is intended by nature for a huge, big-boned animal with four stomachs. A calf weighs about 90 pounds at birth and may attain a weight of 2,000 pounds in approximately two years. Humans, on the other hand, enter the world weighing about 5 to 10 pounds, and on the average weigh 100 to 200 pounds at maturity. We simply don't need the extra casein that a growing cow requires.

Casein coagulates in the stomach and forms large, tough, dense, difficult-to-digest curds that are adapted to the four stomachs and digestive apparatus of a cow. Once inside the human system, this thick mass of goo puts a tremendous burden on the body to somehow get rid of it. In other words, a huge amount of energy must be spent dealing with it. Unfortunately, some of this gooey substance hardens and adheres to the linings of the intestines and prevents the absorption of nutrients into the body. Resulting in lethargy. Also, the byproducts of milk digestion leave a great deal of toxic mucous in the body. It is very acidic, and some of it is stored in the body until it can be dealt with at a later time. The next time you are going to dust your home, smear some paste all over everything and see how easy it is to dust. Dairy products do the same to the inside of your body. That translates into more weight instead of weight loss. Casein, by the way, is the base of one of the strongest glues used in woodwork.

This is not to say that you cannot consume milk products, but it is important to exercise moderation. And dairy products should not be combined with other animal products or with carbohydrates.

Earlier, I referred to white flour, sugar, and salt as the "three whites." Milk is the fourth white. While it is less harmful than the other three, it does present health risks. And it is impossible to consume the four whites in large quantities and remain thin.

Homogenized milk is one reason why heart disease is the number one killer in America, and we suspect that it could actually be the main culprit. Homogenization causes the fat in milk to be broken into such tiny particles that milk does not separate from its cream. These fat particles are so unnaturally small that they are absorbed directly into the bloodstream without proper digestion. These undigested fat particles stress the immune system greatly and cause extreme inflammation. There is an enzyme in cow milk that becomes dangerous whenever milk is homogenized. It is called xanthine oxidase or simply XO. This enzyme is used by young calves to aid with digestion, but it causes cardiovascular disease in humans whenever it is unbound from the fat by homogenization. With raw, or even pasteurized milk (creamlike milk), this toxic substance is not absorbed into the blood. Prior to homogenization, this offensive enzyme was always chemically bound inside milk fats, which were too large to enter into the human bloodstream undigested. The natural particle size of fat inside unadulterated cow milk acts as a shield to protect humans from the milk's xanthine oxidase. Homogenized milk should always be avoided, but if complete avoidance is not an option, then some of its negative effects can be neutralized with folate or folic acid supplements combined with vitamin C. Folic acid is inferior to folate for supplementation purposes. Be advised that the homogenized fats will still be damaging to the heart, even if the arteries are somewhat shielded from the xanthine oxidase. I recommend whole cream (non-homogenized) milk, which can be found at many health food stores. There is no significant benefit to using raw milk over pasteurized milk, so my recommendation is to simply stay with sterile milk.

> "Bovine milk xanthine oxidase (BMXO) may be absorbed and may enter the cardiovascular system. People with clinical signs of atherosclerosis have greater quantities of BMXO antibodies. BMXO antibodies are found in greater quantities in those patients who consume the largest volumes of homogenized milk and milk products."
> — The XO Factor by Kurt Oster, MD,
> and Donald Ross, PhD

Most soft dairy products are made with homogenized milk. Although they are rarely labeled as being so. Some people eat yogurt in an attempt to become healthier, and it is something that we have recommended many times in the past. Overall, yogurt usually helps more than it harms, but due to homogenization it is not as healthy as most people believe. Most soft dairy products will cause inflammation and arterial damage because of homogenization. Those who eat homogenized products should compensate somewhat with vitamin

C and folate (or folic acid) in order to shield the body. Hard cheeses and butter are currently not being made with homogenized milk, so they are safe. Goat milk and products made from it are safe because goat milk is never homogenized.

Salt

To be healthy, the nutrients in our bodies must be in proper balance. Upsetting the natural balance of chemicals inside the cell may cause the cell to malfunction. This is what is happening to the balance of sodium and potassium in our cells if we consume too much of the wrong salts. For our body to stay healthy, it's fundamental to have a constant balance of the water inside and outside the cells, and salt provides this balance through the process of osmosis. Each and every cell in our body absorbs nutrients and energy from the salt carried through the body by water.

Unfortunately, the "table salt" that we know and use every day has undergone a great amount of processing, filtering, and bleaching to eliminate each and every trace of the 84 minerals that are normally found in sea salt and rock salt. After all this processing, the product that reaches our tables is no longer salt but is reduced to no more than just sodium and chloride (NaCl).

The problem is that sodium and chloride, in order to be available to our body, need other minerals like potassium, calcium, magnesium, and zinc, just to name a few. Since common table salt is only made of sodium and chloride, our body has to provide all the other minerals needed, sourcing them from the cells.

Therefore, when we consume regular table salt (not sea salt or rock salt), instead of giving our body the fundamental nutrients needed by the cells to work and keep us healthy, we are actually introducing in our system a substance that robs the cells of precious minerals and energy. Our body reacts to this attack with a domino effect of physiological responses like high blood pressure, cellulite, fluid retention, heart enlargement, and osteoporosis (due to the extraction of calcium from the bones in order to process the sodium chloride). An excess of sodium chloride in our body also causes airway restriction and consequently increases the number of attacks in asthma sufferers.

Sodium is also used by the food industry as a preservative. Pick up any jar from your pantry, even jam, and you will find that it contains some amount of sodium, which increases by many times our total amount of sodium and chloride intake, creating an increased burden on our body.

Salt and your cells

To be healthy, the nutrients in cells must be in proper balance. Upsetting the natural balance of chemicals inside a cell causes the cell to malfunction, which is what is happening to the balance of sodium and potassium in our cells. Over the past 100 years, our diets have changed dramatically, increasing the amount of sodium and decreasing the amount of potassium in our diet, thus reversing the natural balance. Modern food manufacturers add lots of salt (sodium chloride) to their products, while modern diets do not include enough potassium-rich foods such as fresh fruits, vegetables, whole grains and legumes. When our genes were evolving, human diets contained little sodium and a lot of potassium. For example, eating an apple provides only 1 mg of sodium, but 310 mg of potassium. Eating a piece of modern apple pie provides 110 mg of sodium and only 80 mg of potassium, a drastic change.

Salt-rich diets force excess sodium into cells, disturbing the normal and healthy sodium/potassium balance. Among other problems, excess sodium interferes with cellular energy production, causing fatigue.

Salt/sodium is in your blood naturally. When additional salt is consumed, it absorbs into your blood stream. When the salt gets absorbed into your blood it makes your blood saltier than it should be. When the salt runs through your body and comes into contact with your cells, the salt in your blood makes the fluid on the outer part of your body's cells saltier then the cells that are meant to be. The cells notice this change immediately. As a reaction, the cells pull water out of the cells for protection. The cells in turn try to hold on to the water and then tell the brain of the change in quality of the water around them due to the additional salt that is added. When the brain notices that there is too much salt, the brain needs to sponge out the extra salt to prevent any harm. The way your brain does this is by obtaining water by having you feel thirsty. Another way your body gets rid of the extra salt is by slowing down the production of urine and retaining more water.

The constant balance of salt and water in the blood manages our blood pressure. Consuming salt isn't necessarily a bad thing; it just needs to be correctly proportioned throughout your diet.

Cells can be thought of as sacks of water containing dissolved salt and sugar. They are separated from the bloodstream by a plasma membrane, which surrounds cells and prevents salt and sugar from moving freely between cells and the bloodstream. Water, on the other hand, easily passes through the plasma membrane and naturally moves from where the concentration of salt and sugar is low to where their concentration is high. So, if salt and sugar are added to the bloodstream, for example, by eating salty or sugary foods, water will move out of cells and into the bloodstream. The result is that cells are left dehydrated.

The main reason why we are told to severely lower our intake of salt, especially if we suffer from hypertension, is because common table salt truly poses a big threat to our system. What we are rarely told, however, is that unrefined sea salt and rock salt are actually fundamental and beneficial to our health.

Water is the most important substance the body needs to live—every cell and every function in the body depends on it. This is why you need to drink 8–10 glasses of water per day, so it can be available for these functions 24/7. The second most important substance needed in the body is salt because salt has many other vital functions besides just holding water in the body.

You lose about a quart of water per day through respiration and another quart of water through kidney function. Most people either don't replace this water or try to replace it with soft drinks and other beverages that act like diuretics to remove more water than they contain. Thus, 75% of the population is dehydrated and doesn't realize it.

The reason the kidneys hold on to extra salt is because it retains water, and this is what the body is trying to do when you get dehydrated. When you take diuretics to remove the excess salt and water, the kidneys go into a hyper mode to replace the lost water and salt, and this is why diuretics aren't prescribed for long—the cycle never ends. Eventually, other drugs are prescribed to manipulate the arteries by holding them open, relaxing the muscles, etc.

Blood is naturally made up of 94% water and salt, and the "too much salt/too much water" theory on high blood pressure is wrong. If the arteries are getting too much water, why are blood thinners often prescribed? Blood thinners would be used on thickened blood and not watery blood, as there would be if the arteries contained too much water.

The reason the blood pressure rises is because dehydration removes 8% of the water from the blood, which causes the heart to work harder to pump thickened blood through the narrowed cardiovascular system.

Drinking more water and increasing (not decreasing) the salt intake slightly will lower the blood pressure without the need for medications.

White flour

Being part Italian, I love bread, I love Pasta, but your cells can find them burdensome if you are abusive. It is a shame that mostly all bread, pasta, and baked goods are made of white flour—an easy-to-use, easy-to-store, highly processed derivative of what was once a wheat grain. Wheat is a good and nutritious food, but by the time wheat gets ground up and processed into white flour, it bears little resemblance (physically or nutritionally) to wheat. However, the refining of flour, like sugar is refined, destroys most nutritional content. White flour contains little nutrition, is toxic, and is an antinutrient (like sugar). Yet the average American consumes in excess of 200 pounds of white flour every year.

Almost all of the nutrients once contained in wheat are lost in the process of creating white flour (including 60% of the calcium, 77% of the magnesium, 78% of the zinc, 89% of the cobalt, 98% of the vitamin E, 80% of vitamins B1 and B3, and 75% of the folic acid). These are vitamins we need and are robbing ourselves, thus creating a cellular deficiency.

When we consume white bread, basically all the essential fatty acids and fiber are lost. What complicates this is that many of the nutrients needed in order for your body to metabolize the flour for energy are not present. Fact of the matter is that because the flour does not contain those nutrients, your body is robbed of them, similar to what happens when you eat sugar; we will discuss sugar next.

In 1941, severe nutritional problems prompted our government to pass legislation requiring that certain nutrients be added back to the flour. "Enriched flour" was born. White flour has lost more than 25 known nutrients, a handful are added back, yet we still call flour "enriched" (instead of, perhaps, "impoverished").

We did not have nutritional deficiency in mind when we started making white flour. We made it because it doesn't spoil; it keeps practically forever, which makes white flour an ideal food to feed people in big cities. However, the malnutrition problem with flour is serious—our bellies are filled in the form of "hearty" pastas and breads, but all those empty calories do not even come close to fulfilling our needs for nutrients, thus contributing to deficiency.

Worse, flour also contributes to the other cause of disease—toxicity. White flour contains almost no fiber, which is essential for proper bowel movements and toxin removal. Eating too much flour (and not enough fiber) is associated with constipation, hemorrhoids, colitis, and rectal cancer.

Avoiding white flour is not easy because it is in virtually all breads, pastas, cakes, cookies, crackers, breakfast cereals, pizzas, and pastries. But when you realize that flour causes disease, cutting down on the refined flour products you consume is worth the effort. A plate of pasta with vegetables can no longer be considered a good meal. The vegetables are good, but the pasta is not; choose whole grains or beans instead. I substitute spaghetti squash for pasta.

The real health threat from white flour comes not from any single meal but from consuming so much of it on a daily basis—one or more meals a day, every day.

Grains frequently are refined (such as those in "multi-grain" breads and cereals) and are reduced to little more than empty calories. Any grain that is finely ground and "stripped" of fiber and other nutrients is a poor nutritional choice because essential nutrients have been lost, which most people do not realize. Eating processed foods of any kind is fundamentally different from and nutritionally inferior to eating whole, unprocessed foods. Keep it natural as often as possible

Beware of puff grains. The high heat and pressure used in the puffing process alters the molecular structure of proteins in the grains, making them toxic enough to kill laboratory animals. Absolutely avoid puffed wheat, puffed millet, and puffed rice (including rice cakes), and any other puffed grains. This warning does not include popcorn, which is not subjected to such high temperatures and pressures. In his book *Fighting the Food Giants*, Paul Stitt reported an experiment in which rats were fed either whole wheat or puffed wheat. The rats eating the whole wheat lived over a year while the rats eating puffed wheat died within two weeks.

To avoid health problems created by processed grains, choose whole grains such as millet, oats, quinoa, spelt, barley, amaranth, teff, kamut, and brown rice. Many people do not realize that white rice is also a processed grain and, therefore, a poor food choice. Buckwheat, not strictly a grain, can be cooked like whole grains. Organic whole grains are readily available at health food stores. In the real world, often we are forced to make less than ideal choices. At the very least, choose minimally processed whole grains (such as whole-wheat flour or oatmeal) instead of highly refined and stripped grains, such as white flour, white rice, and pasta made from white flour.

Gluten

Earlier in this chapter we discussed gluten. When I was in chiropractic school, we knew and studied nothing about gluten; now, however, I'm sure you know of someone who is gluten intolerant. More people today are experimenting with gluten-free diets than ever before. More people announce they have a gluten intolerance, despite not being tested by physicians or having a "real" diagnosis. And when you read the words "gluten-free" in a recipe or on the packaging to baked goods, you think it's healthy. Well hold on to your hats.

Let me explain to you what gluten intolerance is. It isn't a food allergy. It's a physical condition in your gut. Basically, undigested gluten proteins (prevalent in wheat and other grains) hang out in your intestines and are treated by your body like a foreign invader, irritating your gut and flattening the microvilli along the small intestine wall. Without those microvilli, you have considerably less surface area with which to absorb the nutrients from your food. This leads sufferers to experience symptoms of malabsorption, including chronic fatigue, neurological disorders, nutrient deficiencies, anemia, nausea, skin rashes, depression, and more—thus toxic to your cells. If you have any type of stomach ailment, try removing white flour and gluten from your diet. I did, and it worked great.

If you remove gluten, the toxin, from the diet, it allows the gut to heal and the myriad of symptoms disappears. Depending on the level and degree of the intolerance, which can range anywhere from a gluten sensitivity to a full-blown celiac disease, it may be possible to eventually re-introduce properly prepared grains (sourdough that has fermented for up to a month, sprouted grains, etc.) into the diet.

Every patient is different and you should discuss this with your doctor. Research has shown me some patients' guts may heal, but their bodies will never be able to digest gluten—even if it's been "bent" by traditional preparation methods. They have a genetic predisposition that causes gluten sensitivity, thus gluten is toxic to the cell and causes cellular malfunction.

Some doctors and scientists hypothesize that the quickly skyrocketing increase of wheat's share in the human diet over the last 150 years is part of why celiac disease has become so common. There is further conjecture that the newer strains of wheat further contribute to this because they are bred to contain higher gluten content than the wheat of ancient times.

Research over the past few decades has revealed that gluten intolerance can affect almost every other tissue and system in the body, including the brain, endocrine system, stomach and liver, nucleus of cells, blood vessels, and smooth muscle—just to name a few!

This explains why celiac disease is caused by a toxin to the cells, which occurs as a gluten intolerance. Gluten intolerance is now associated with several different diseases, including type 1 diabetes, thyroid disorders, osteoporosis, neurodegenerative conditions like Alzheimer's, Parkinson's and dementia, psychiatric illness, ADHD, rheumatoid arthritis, migraine, obesity, and more.

We know that only 1 in 8 people with celiac disease are diagnosed. We also know that those with celiac disease represent only a small fraction of the population of people with gluten intolerance. With this in mind, it's not hard to imagine that the number of people with gluten intolerance that have "undefined neurological disorders" (and other associated conditions on the list above) could be significantly higher than current research suggests. We also now know if we removed these toxins from our body, our cells would not malfunction and disease would be averted.

Whether we like it or not, gluten continues to proliferate in the human diet, including in regions that previously based their diets around other staples. Over time, research may show that such high gluten intake is not healthy for anyone, but what we already know for sure is that gluten continues to be truly toxic for people with celiac disease and can irritate the digestive systems of people with non-celiac gluten intolerances, irritable bowel syndrome, and other conditions.

Fortunately, delicious gluten-free foods are increasingly available across the developed world. We are seeing the history of gluten changed right before our eyes, and it's only continuing to get better.

I have concluded that the phenomenon of celiac disease and gluten intolerance has, in a way, come about rather suddenly. Why? Because gluten is far more prevalent in our society today than just 100 years ago.

I wanted to know how gluten came into existence; my parents' and grandparents' generations were never diagnosed with gluten problems. So it was back to the library.

What I learned was amazing: As the consumption of gluten has increased, the problems associated with gluten have, too. Wheat today is different than it was 100 years ago. It's got more gluten in it! Until the 1870s, almost all U.S. wheat production consisted of "soft wheat" varieties. A "hard spring wheat" variety (originally from Central Europe) with a higher protein content (aka gluten) was introduced in the U.S. in the mid-1800s. The flour made from the higher-gluten wheat resulted in fluffier bread and flakier baked goods, and of course the consumers liked that.

Thus, the demand for the new flour grew, but it wasn't so easy to get at first. Although some early types of wheat may have been grown as far back as 9000 B.C., people didn't eat much of it because it was difficult to eat in its raw form, and even when they figured out how to crack it open, to grind it, to sift it, and to cook with it, these processes were laborious because they had only primitive tools. Whole grains also went rancid rather quickly because of the high oil content in the bran.

It was eventually discovered that milling the grains (stripping away the germ and the bran) made it so the grains could be kept for longer and it also produced a soft, unadulterated white flour. By the early 1800s, many mills had equipment so that they could produce this refined flour. Demand for white flour grew as it became the desirable baking ingredient. Because it was more expensive than brown flour, it also became a status symbol.

It wasn't until the late 19th century that wheat production and consumption grew dramatically. One reason, as mentioned before, was the use of the new, hardier strains of wheat. Today food is shipped to us from all over the world; wheat can be grown every month of the year somewhere in the world. On top of this, great advancements have been made in the technology used to grow, harvest, mill, and transport wheat. Inventions such as the reaper, the steel plow, and high-speed steel roller mills helped produce huge quantities of finer, whiter flour. Historically, railroads provided better transport of the flour, making it available to more people, and better ovens allowed them to bake with it even more. With all of these advances, the masses had access to the refined wheat flour that was once a luxury of the wealthy.

Soy what?

Like cereal grains, soy is another toxin often promoted as a health food. It's now ubiquitous in the modern diet, present in just about every packaged and processed food in the form of soy protein isolate, soy flour, soy lecithin, and soybean oil.

For this reason, most people are unaware of how much soy they consume. You don't have to be a tofu-loving hippie to eat a lot of soy. In fact, the average American—who is most definitely not a tofu-loving hippie—gets up to 9% of total calories from soybean oil alone.

Whenever I mention the dangers of soy in my public talks, someone always protests that soy can't be unhealthy because it's been consumed safely in Asia for thousands of years. There are several reasons why this isn't a valid argument.

First, the soy products consumed traditionally in Asia were typically fermented and unprocessed—including tempeh, miso, natto, and tamari. This is important because the fermentation process partially neutralizes the toxins in soybeans.

Second, Asians consumed soy foods as a condiment, not as a replacement for animal foods. The average consumption of soy foods in China is 10 grams (about 2 teaspoons) per day and is 30 to 60 grams in Japan. These are not large amounts of soy.

Contrast this with the U.S. and other Western countries, where almost all of the soy consumed is highly processed and unfermented, and eaten in much larger amounts than in Asia.

How does soy impact our health? The following is just a partial list:

- Soy contains trypsin inhibitors that inhibit protein digestion and affect pancreatic function.
- Soy contains phytic acid, which reduces absorption of minerals like calcium, magnesium, copper, iron, and zinc.
- Soy increases our requirement for vitamin D, which 50% of Americans are already deficient in.
- Soy phytoestrogens disrupt endocrine function and have the potential to cause infertility and to promote breast cancer in adult women.

- Vitamin B12 analogs in soy are not absorbed and actually increase the body's requirement for B12.
- Processing of soy protein results in the formation of toxic lysinoalanine and highly carcinogenic nitrosamines.
- Free glutamic acid or MSG, a potent neurotoxin, is formed during soy food processing and additional amounts are added to many soy foods to mask soy's unpleasant taste.
- Soy can stimulate the growth of estrogen-dependent tumors and cause thyroid problems, especially in women.

Perhaps most alarmingly, a study at the Harvard Public School of Health in 2008 found that men who consumed the equivalent of one cup of soy milk per day had a 50% lower sperm count than men who didn't eat soy.

In 1992, the Swiss Health Service estimated that women consuming the equivalent of two cups of soy milk per day provides the estrogenic equivalent of one birth control pill. That means women eating cereal with soy milk and drinking a soy latte each day are effectively getting the same estrogen effect as if they were taking a birth control pill.

This effect is even more dramatic in infants fed soy formula. Babies fed soy-based formula have 13,000 to 22,000 times more estrogen compounds in their blood than babies fed milk-based formula. Infants exclusively fed soy formula receive the estrogenic equivalent (based on body weight) of at least five birth control pills per day.

The facts are that 99%, a very large percentage, of soy is genetically modified and it also has one of the highest percentages of contamination by pesticides of any of our foods.

Soybeans are high in phytic acid, present in the bran or hulls of all seeds. It's a substance that can block the uptake of essential minerals—calcium, magnesium, copper, iron, and especially zinc—in the intestinal tract, thus creating a cellular deficiency.

Only a long period of fermentation will significantly reduce the phytate content of soybeans.

Top 10 Reasons to Avoid Soy

WooMagazine | The Delicious Revolution

1. Soybeans contain large quantities of natural toxins or "antinutrients." First among them are potent enzyme inhibitors that block the action of trypsin and other enzymes needed for protein digestion.
2. These inhibitors are not deactivated during cooking & processing. Test animals fed these inhibitors developed enlargement and pathological conditions of the pancreas, including cancer.
3. Soybeans also contain haemagglutinin, a clot-promoting substance that causes red blood cells to clump together.
4. 99% of soy is genetically modified and is among the highest contamination by pesticides of any of our foods.
5. Soybeans are high in phytic acid, a substance that blocks the uptake of the essential minerals calcium, magnesium, copper, iron and especially zinc, in the intestinal tract.
6. Soy products contain high levels of aluminum, leached from the aluminum tanks in which they are acid washed and processed at high temperatures.
7. Nitrites, which are potent carcinogens, are formed during the spray-drying of soy.
8. Soy Protein Isolates are shown to enlarge the pancreas and thyroid and increase fatty acid deposits in the liver.
9. Soy contains toxic isoflavones.
10. Soy foods have a high concentration of goitrogens, which block production of thyroid hormones.

"The body is not built wrongly, but is being used wrongly," proposed T.L. Cleave, author of a 1974 book called *The Saccharine Disease*, which addressed health conditions that he believed to be caused by sugar and white flour. Rather than viewing people who are unable to tolerate gluten as defective, we need to recognize that it is the change in our environment—the increase in wheat consumption—that has led to our ill health.

Today, wheat is the single most cultivated crop worldwide. Most people in the United States eat wheat at almost every single meal, every single day, and for snacks and dessert, too. Bakers are adding in "vital wheat gluten" or high gluten flour to make fluffier loaves of bread. Vegetarian and vegan meat substitutes are made from extracted gluten. Wheat is everywhere and then some! It's no wonder we are not tolerating this food that has "suddenly" become our dominant food source.

In the 19th century, less than 1% of all deaths in the United States were caused by cancer, and even at the turn of the 20th century, only 3% of the population was affected. Today, it is estimated that more than 4 in 10 people will develop cancer in their lifetime, and 1 in 4 will die from cancer.

So what do we do? We provide the cell with toxic prevention and periodically cleanse our cells. Cleansing of the cells is important in removing as many toxins as possible. We will discuss this in detail in the next chapter so get ready to cleanse your cell.

"Men worry over the great number of diseases, while doctors worry over the scarcity of effective remedies."

—PIEN CH'IAO

Chapter 16

DEFICIENCY AND DISEASE

We have put much emphasis during this book, especially in prior chapters, on toxicity. Now we must begin to understand the second cause of disease, deficiencies, and how deficiencies affect our cells.

By eliminating toxins in our diet, this puts us halfway there to eliminating disease from our bodies. In the last chapter we studied toxins, their origin, and how to protect the cell from them. Let's study deficiency and how it affects our body and how we can eliminate any deficiency to our cells.

You will learn there are three major types of deficiency:

1. Nutritional
2. Nerve
3. Circulatory

Example: If your brain controls your body and your brain communicates throughout the body through the nervous system, what if that system gets blocked? In chiropractic we call this a subluxation, more commonly known as a pinched nerve. A pinched nerve can create a deficiency to the area it was in communication with. This is why both nutrition and chiropractic play an important part in this book.

Earlier in my education I had to take a course in cell biology, I thought it was boring. It wasn't until I became an intern and my professor and mentor, Dr. Donald Gutstein, taught me the importance of the cell and its importance to both health and disease. Earlier in this book I made you study the cell and hopefully by now you are beginning to understand its role in our everyday health. As a doctor, I have known many patients who were overweight yet suffered from cellular deficiency.

According to Wikipedia, "Nutritional diseases are diseases in humans that are directly or indirectly caused by a lack of essential nutrients in the diet. Nutritional diseases are commonly associated with chronic malnutrition." Malnutrition is a deficiency of the cell. If the cell does not get what it needs, it will weaken and disease will result.

A disease such as rickets or scurvy is caused by a dietary deficiency of specific nutrients, especially a vitamin or mineral. The disease may stem from insufficient intake, digestion, absorption, or utilization of nutrients. For instance, vitamin C deficiency leads to scurvy. Vitamin D deficiency can cause rickets and osteoporosis. Vitamin B deficiency causes a host of problems including pellagra and beriberi.

Some symptoms of short-term vitamin or mineral deficiencies include:

- Blurry vision
- Diarrhea
- Dizziness
- Fatigue
- Headaches
- Nausea
- Vomiting

To be healthy we need to include in our diets what our cells need and avoid what they don't need. A deficiency disease is caused by lack of some nutrient, or essential component, for proper bodily functioning. It means that an individual is not getting some really important vitamin or mineral. This can lead to severe consequences for growth, health, or proper bodily activities.

When does our journey to build healthy cells begin? It begins at conception and continues in the womb. If the embryo does get the proper nourishment to protect the cell and is also bombarded by toxins, the child may be born with a defect. Deficiency of the cells can begin as early as the early development of the fetus.

We learned earlier in this book how life begins with one cell, then these cells specialize. The human nervous system develops from a small, specialized plate of cells (the neural plate) along the back of an embryo. Early in fetal development, the edges of this plate begin to curl up toward each other and creates the neural tube—a narrow sheath that closes to form the brain and spinal cord of the embryo. As development progresses, the top of the tube becomes the brain and the remainder becomes the spinal cord. This process is usually complete by the 28th day of pregnancy. But if problems occur during this process, the result can be brain disorders called neural tube defects, including spina bifida.

Spina bifida, which literally means "cleft spine," is character-ized by the incomplete development of the brain, spinal cord, and/ or meninges (the protective covering around the brain and spinal cord). It is the most common neural tube defect in the United States, affecting 1,500 to 2,000 of the more than 4 million babies born in the country each year. There are an estimated 166,000 individuals with spina bifida living in the United States.

In many cases the disease can be prevented. Spina bifida is often a result of a deficiency. It is important to supplement during preg-nancy. Still to this day, not all pregnant mothers take folic acid. Folic acid, also called folate, is an important vitamin in the development of a healthy fetus. Although taking this vitamin cannot guarantee having a healthy baby, it can help. Recent studies have shown that by adding folic acid to their diets, women of childbearing age significantly reduce their risk of having a child with a neural tube defect like spina bifida.

Give the cells what they need and we increase our chances of being healthy. Cells will be healthy if we nourish them, protect them, and feed them.

Trouble in our bodies begins when our cellular factories have nutritional deficiency or toxic exposure, as you have learned we are exposed to thousands of toxins on a daily basis. If the cellular factories get overloaded or malnourished, they shut down. If our cells are unable to make sufficient amount of antibodies, we become susceptible to infections. When the cells cannot make sufficient neurotransmitters, our brain communication system suffers, and it shuts down. The brain as we know is the most important organ in our body because the brain controls every organ system in the body.

Although each cell is a living organism unto itself, its power is how it works and communicates with its neighboring cells. Cellular communication regulates everything from body temperature, digestion, immunity, memory, brain function and waste removal.

Toxins damage cells. Like sugar in a gas tank, or sand in a machine, toxins breakdown the ability for the machine to work. If the machine does not work at 100%, it will not produce healthy cells. If our cells are deficient, they are weakened. Studies have clearly shown that vitamins and other supplements that help us build healthy cells also help our telomeres. Telomeres, remember, are the structures at the ends of chromosomes that protect DNA. Telomeres shorten with age and disease and are especially susceptible to damage from oxidation and inflammation. We can reduce this shortening of our telomeres by providing our cells with the nourishment they need and protecting them from toxins.

Researchers evaluated the diets of over 500 women, aged 35 to 74, and measured the length of a particular white blood cell telomere that is a good indicator of age. Scientists found that telomeres in women who took a daily multi-vitamin were over 5% longer than telomeres of women who did not take multi-vitamins. Doctors also noted that those who got more vitamin C or vitamin E had longer telomeres than those who got less of these nutrients.

In a heart attack prevention study, doctors followed over 24,000 women who began the study without cancer, cardiovascular disease, or diabetes. Over a six-year period, researchers identified five major lifestyle and diet patterns that when combined, reduced the chances of having a heart attack by 92%. The three lifestyle patterns were: 1) non-smoking, 2) physically active, and 3) smaller waist size—indicating healthy weight. The two diet patterns were: 1) a very small amount of alcohol, less than 2/10ths of an ounce per day, and 2) high amounts of fresh vegetables, fruits, whole grains, legumes, and fish. Antioxidants were one of the key supplements used in reducing the risks for heart disease.

The best form of health insurance is cell insurance, insurance that the cells have what they need. If you can prevent toxicity or deficiency, you can even reduce your risk of heart disease. It remains important to decrease your risk factors using other proven methods along with vitamin supplementation. Some of the best methods include:

- Quitting smoking and using tobacco products
- Having your doctor check your lipid profile
- Getting treatment, if necessary, to reach a lipid goal of LDL less than 100 (those at high risk should reach a goal of less than 70) and HDL greater than 45
- Eat foods low in saturated fat and cholesterol and rich in fiber and nutrients (including antioxidants)
- Be active and exercise regularly
- Drink plenty of water
- Control high blood pressure and diabetes
- Achieve and maintain an appropriate weight

- Ask your doctor to do a blood test to detect high-sensitivity c-reactive protein, a general marker of arterial inflammation and indicator of heart disease
- Have regular check-ups with your doctor

Unbalanced body chemistry (called sulfhydrl chemistry) is a reflection of the response of thiols to your metabolism, food, stress, and health interventions. The value is changeable. As you raise your thiols, if necessary, then you express better health capabilities. If you have good values, then you may not need as much intervention as healthier individuals tend to respond poorly to taking antioxidants.

Tattered DNA gives rise to less healthy generations of cells, which translates to poorer health and faster aging. The healthier you are, the better your body is repairing your DNA holes, and the healthier generations of cells your body is birthing.

Your body makes DNA repair enzymes to unlock the DNA chain for repair.

When you have good thiol values, you can know two things:

1. This test has been correlated with research based DNA repair tests for accuracy.
2. When you are in a good health category, you are able to express more life and better health.

Measuring your thiol status makes you a player in your own health care for a very good reason. Each one of us is unique, having an individual variation to how we respond to food, the environment, and healthcare interventions. Personalized health care is more than a slogan when you know your own thiol score.

Also, if you consume nutritional supplements, you should know if they are beneficial or not. Generally, the healthier you are, the poorer your response will be to these products, so you may find that you are wasting your money.

Ten percent

Along my journey of cellular health, I have had the honor to work with many great doctors. One is Dr. Eric Nepute, a leader amongst healers. At my office in Florida one day he came to visit when he was lecturing in West Palm Beach. Here we sat, two professionals sharing information on the cells, and soon telomeres came into our subject. No wonder I thought he is the main doctor in St. Louis; his intelligence was beyond his years. We sat and talked this new paradigm of health with my partner Dr. Perry Bard. The three of us got excited and knew there was a new way to educate the masses toward health, toward living a better life.

Research has determined that an estimated 10% of you reading this will have very poor oxidative stress function and probably do need interventions, including nutritionals. This is the best way to see if you are part of that group.

Originally developed by a Cancer Pharmaceutical Company, you (and even your doctor) may never have heard of a thiol test—but it is the easiest way to assess your overall health and rate of aging. It is based on research dating back more than 30 years. The test was developed in the 1980s by a pharmaceutical company to measure DNA repair for cancer assessment and as a prognostic indicator for AIDS. Thiol testing has evolved since the 1990s to be seen as a reliable and trusted method for measuring overall human health status with 95% certainty.

Thiol measurement incorporates the PARP enzyme, a catalyst for DNA repair, and has been implicated not only in health disorders such as breast cancer, but also reflects reactions to air particles, food, and even stress. This activity occurs at the deepest level of your cell's life or death functional level. It is also involved in the maintenance of telomere length, a measure of longevity. PARP is best known for its role in cancer prevention as well as aging.

The MOST important thing to know is that there is a strong variation of PARP in people. This is why knowing your own thiol score is vital since your healthcare decisions may be affected by it. To learn more go to www.serumthiol.com, and tell them Dr. Kaplan and Dr. Nepute sent you.

Technology now allows us to live free of fear and confusion about our health and our level of independence as we age. Your individual thiol score and the ability to watch that score go up is the most empowering tool we can access. And if your doctor is a wellness practitioner, then your thiol score is the lens through which the two of you can structure and confirm a wellness strategy to achieve all of your healthcare goals.

How can we take rational control of our health if we lack a means for "real-time" comprehensive evaluation? Access to your thiol levels gives you comprehensive real-time tracking to know if your DNA repair measures at the levels of lowest risk. High thiol levels indicate a health risk of only 5% for all 9 major categories of disease.

Most the doctors I know take vitamins, yet not all of them recommend them to their patients. I find that strange. If they are good enough for the doctor, shouldn't they be good enough for the patient? The American Heart Association (AHA) continues to study the effects of vitamins and are learning that vitamins help prevent heart disease. The bad news is that it has taken them nearly 20 years to admit what I knew when I graduated professional school in 1978. AHA president, Dr. W. Virgil Brown of Emory University, told reporters, "Most of us in medicine have poo-pooed mega-doses of vitamins, but this research has a good ring to it."

The latest news is that Dr. Ishwarlal Jialal of the University of Texas Southwestern Medical Center in Dallas showed that vitamin E could block the adverse changes to low-density lipoprotein (LDL) that leads to plaque formation and blockages in arteries. The oxidation of LDL and/or high-density lipoprotein (HDL) causes most of the cases of heart disease.

Medical researchers can't help but see the many articles showing that the real heart disease culprit is oxidized lipoprotein, and now they will be seeing several articles on how antioxidant nutrients prevent these harmful reactions from occurring. Also, many researchers have read the recent article in the *American Journal of Clinical Nutrition* showing the single most reliable risk factor for heart disease is a deficiency of a key antioxidant: vitamin E.

If our bodies have deficiencies our cells will malfunction. One key vitamin of which many Americans are deficient is vitamin D. Over the past several years, the surprising prevalence of vitamin D deficiency has become broadly recognized.

Vitamin D deficiency is linked to:

- Osteoporosis
- Cardiovascular disease
- Cancer
- Autoimmune diseases
- Multiple sclerosis
- Pain
- Loss of Cognitive function
- Decreased strength
- Increased rate of all-cause mortality

Vitamin D determines how much inflammatory heat your immune system generates. When you are low in D then it is easy to overheat, generate a ton of free radicals, and damage your telomeres. Your ability to tolerate stress successfully is based in no small part on your vitamin D status, including your ability to fight infection. Researchers have now demonstrated in 2,100 female twin pairs, ages 19–79, that the highest levels of vitamin D were associated with the longest telomeres and the lowest vitamin D levels were associated with the shortest telomeres, a difference equating to five years of lifespan potential.

Approximately 50% of the healthy North American population and more than 80% of those with chronic diseases are vitamin D deficient. 80% of healthy infants are vitamin D deficient. Those with vitamin D deficiency experience 39% higher annual healthcare costs than those with normal levels of vitamin D.

Magnesium is present in all cells of the body and is involved in over 300 enzymatic processes, including energy production. Magnesium is essential for maintaining normal bone density, normal cardiac rhythmicity, normal pulmonary function, and normal blood glucose regulation. Magnesium is one of the most common worldwide deficiencies and it plays a role in most of the common health struggles people face every day.

Most doctors are not trained to detect magnesium deficiencies. Magnesium deficiency is often misdiagnosed because it does not show up in blood tests as only 1% of the body's magnesium is stored in the blood.

Dr. Norman Shealy, MD, PhD, an American neurosurgeon and a pioneer in pain medicine, says, "Every known illness is associated with a magnesium deficiency," and that, "magnesium is the most critical mineral required for electrical stability of every cell in the body. A magnesium deficiency may be responsible for more diseases than any other nutrient."

Research has shown that 68% of individuals in the U.S. do not consume the daily recommended amount of dietary magnesium and 19% do not even consume half of the RDA levels (310–420 mg daily). Most researchers believe this RDA level is far too low, and if it was raised to where it should be, we would see that roughly 80% of Americans are consuming insufficient quantities.

Magnesium is a basic element of life much like water and air. We need a lot of magnesium, roughly 1,000 mgs/day for a healthy active individual to keep up with the demands of the body. Magnesium is to the body like oil is to a car's engine, and if we are deficient, problems will arise.

Our current diet is rich in calcium but insufficient in magnesium. Our ancient ancestors had a a diet that was close to 1:1 whereas our present-day diets are more like 5:1 and up to 15:1. Having roughly ten times more calcium than magnesium is a serious problem.

This elevated calcium to magnesium ratio is a major player in conditions such as mitral valve prolapse, migraines, attention deficit disorder, autism, fibromyalgia, anxiety, asthma, and allergies. Wherever there is elevated calcium and insufficient magnesium inside of cells, the effects are muscle contractions, spasms, twitches, and even convulsions.

Without sufficient magnesium the body struggles to make and utilize protein and enzymes. It is also unable to properly methylate and detoxify and/or process and utilize antioxidants like vitamin C and E.

Magnesium is extremely critical for proper detoxification processes. As our world has gotten increasingly more toxic, our need for magnesium has increased. Meanwhile, the nutrition of our modern food has increasingly been diminished. This is due to overcropping, poor composting, and pesticide/herbicide chemical residue that reduces nutritional quality of the soil and produce.

If you fall prey to habitual symptoms of brain fog, you may be deficient in magnesium. Over 300 enzymes require magnesium to perform biological reactions essential to tissue and organ function. Magnesium supports optimal cognitive health by maximizing the various intricate functions of the brain.

Magnesium strengthens memory

Critical for age-related memory loss, magnesium is associated with memory potential. Studies show that low levels of brain magnesium directly correlate to poor memory function.

With the deteriorating health habits of our modern culture, it is not a surprise that Alzheimer's disease is associated with decreased levels of magnesium. Toxic plaque buildup is evident in patients with declining cognitive abilities symptomatic of the pathogenesis of Alzheimer's disease.

Restoring adequate levels of brain magnesium has been found to prevent the further decline of cognitive function. One study found that the supplemental treatment of magnesium over a 17-month period reduced amyloid plaque accumulation in the hippocampus region of the brain by 35.8% and by 36% in the prefrontal cortex. Some researchers even propose that the development of the disease may even be reversed following magnesium therapy.

Magnesium regulates mood and stress by nourishing the nervous system. Damage to the nervous system has been implicated as the cause of numerous health concerns, including dementia and depression.

Case studies show that treating magnesium deficiency has helped patients struggling with anxiety, irritability, confusion, hyperexcitability, postpartum depression, drug and alcohol abuse, as well as traumatic brain injuries. Magnesium has also been reported by the American Academy of Neurology and the American Headache Society as a "probably effective" treatment for preventing migraines and headaches that can be associated with stress.

Magnesium therapy can treat symptoms of anxiety by relaxing nerves, assisting in digestion, relieving muscle tension, and conducting healthy nerve responses. Unhealthy nerve impulses in the hippocampus can cause factors conducive to stimulating fear and anxiety. Magnesium therapy is not only found to strengthen the ability of nerves in the brain to function properly, but magnesium treatment also increases the selectivity of nerves to fire, which reduces one's risk of excitability and agitation.

Magnesium assists in detoxifying the body's tissue of acids, toxins, gasses, poisons, and other impurities. Environmental contaminants in our food expose our bodies to a higher amount of toxins and impurities than in the past. These impurities deplete our body of essential minerals.

Magnesium improves the motility of the gastrointestinal tract and colon and thereby stimulating the removal of contaminants by promoting a laxative effect. For this reason, magnesium is a primary ingredient in most laxatives used to relieve constipation.

Risks of magnesium deficiency

Magnesium deficiency is running rampant among Americans. One study sponsored by the National Institutes of Health shows that 68% of Americans are magnesium deficient. Other experts put the number closer 80%. Data from the 1999–2000 National Health and Nutrition Examination Survey suggests that substantial numbers of adults in the U.S. don't get even the minimal amounts of magnesium recommended.

In addition to magnesium, proper amounts of calcium are vital to your bodily functions and health. However, without magnesium, calcium cannot be properly used or absorbed by the body. This will often lead to arthritis.

Individuals at greatest risk of magnesium deficiency should pay special attention to health problems they are experiencing. Only 32% of Americans are believed to meet the recommended daily requirements for magnesium. Those at a higher risk of developing a magnesium deficiency include:

- Patients with gastrointestinal diseases such as Crohn's disease and celiac disease. These individuals are less able to absorb nutrients from dietary intake.
- Type-2 diabetics—A high concentration of blood glucose leads to increased urination and a higher risk of kidney damage.
- Alcoholics—Chronic alcohol abuse is likely to cause gastrointestinal problems, which further promotes the removal of magnesium in urine.

- Elderly—As the body ages, the gastrointestinal tract becomes less efficient at absorbing minerals. Older adults are more likely to be taking medications that can interfere with the absorption of magnesium.

There are two causes of disease: deficiency and toxicity. Many deficiency conditions to the body are caused by stress and how stress reacts upon the cell. Remember, when the body is not at ease, the body is at dis-ease and this leads to disease. Stress is associated with diseases such as cardiovascular disease, insulin resistance, diabetes, hypertension, atherosclerosis, and even dementia. All of these affect telomere length. Correcting subclinical nutritional deficiencies that may contribute to such diseases is crucial for telomere maintenance and this is why proper supplementation is so important. Do supplements heal you? No. The body is a self-healing organism. *The power that creates the body has the power to heal the body.* But supplements do help the body cope with deficiency in our diets and the toxins that trigger stress inside our bodies.

Summary deficiency

Consult the table below for the role of each vitamin and mineral, along with the associated health problems that can result from a deficiency of that particular nutrient.

Type of Nutrient	Role of Nutrient	Associated Deficiency Diseases
Vitamin A	Vitamin A is essential to bone, eye and liver health.	Reproductive problems, infertility, certain types of cancer, weakened immune system
Vitamin B12	B12 promotes metabolism, as well as blood and overall nerve system health.	Nerve damage, anemia, blood clotting disorders

Vitamin C	Vitamin C is important to the immune system and general skin health.	Anemia, depression, arthritis, scurvy, ulcers, weakened immune system
Calcium	Calcium is one of the main nutrients essential to bone health.	Osteoporosis, loss of teeth
Vitamin D	Vitamin D not only promotes skin and liver health, but it is also essential to ensuring that the body properly absorbs and uses calcium.	Rickets, general fatigue, muscle weakness
Vitamin E	Vitamin E is crucial to healthy cell reproduction.	Certain types of cancers, skin problems, wrinkles
Iron	Iron is key to maintaining overall blood health.	Anemia, muscle weakness, general fatigue
Vitamin K	Vitamin K ensures that the blood clots after injury.	Excessive bleeding, blood clotting disorders
Magnesium	Magnesium is key to promoting bone health, as well as to producing healthy cholesterol and proteins.	Asthma, general fatigue, diabetes, attention deficit disorder (ADD)
Zinc	Zinc ensures blood health, proper calcium absorption by the body and the production of reproductive hormones.	Bone weakness, infertility, hair loss, slowed growth and development

The above chart should act like a guide, if you are experiencing any of the symptoms associated with any of the vitamins mentioned, talk to your health professional.

Please keep in mind that the above table lists the long-term, chronic effects of various types of vitamin deficiencies. Short-term symptoms of vitamin deficiencies tend to be general, making them easy to confuse with a variety of other health problems.

If you think you're starting to experience any symptoms related to vitamin deficiencies, see your doctor immediately for a thorough exam and a proper diagnosis. Early diagnosis is key to getting immediate treatment and warding off the potentially irreversible effects of vitamin deficiencies.

It's important that we emphasize that this book is a guide, not a replacement for medical advice. Nor will we claim that we are offering all the answers—nobody can. Anyone who claims to have the definitive word on healthcare is sure to eventually wind up in deep water, as the following story by Charles Tremendous Jones illustrates.

"Once there was a boy rowing an old-timer across a wide river. The old-timer picked a floating leaf from the water, studied it for a moment, and then asked the boy if he knew anything about biology. 'No, I don't,' the boy replied. The old-timer said, 'Son, you've missed twenty-five percent of your life.'

"As they rowed on, the old-timer took a rock from the bottom of the boat. He turned it in his hand, studying its coloration, and asked the boy, 'Son, do you know anything about geology?' The boy sheepishly replied, 'No, I don't, sir.' The old-timer said, 'Son, you've missed fifty percent of your life.'

"Twilight was approaching and the old-timer gazed at the North Star that had begun to twinkle. After a while he asked the boy, 'Son, do you know anything about astronomy?' The boy, head bowed and brow furrowed, admitted, "No, I don't sir' The old-timer scolded, 'Son, you've missed seventy-five percent of your life!'

"Just then the boy noticed a huge dam upstream beginning to crumble and torrents of water pouring through the break. Quickly he turned to the old-timer and shouted, 'Sir, do you know how to swim?' the old-timer replied, 'No,' to which the boy shouted back, 'Old-timer, you just lost your life!'"

You do not have to know everything about nutrition to enjoy good health. You simply need to be willing to learn before it's too late. We never stop growing until we stop learning, and people who are learning this simple truth will grow old but never get old.

Here is a list by Mary West on various actions you can take to increase your telomere lengths and therefore life expectancy:

1. Lead a healthful lifestyle.

In 2008, scientists evaluated the effect of a healthful lifestyle on telomerase levels. Telomerase is an enzyme that plays a vital role in the maintenance of telomeres. Without adequate levels of this enzyme, telomeres become progressively shorter. The participants in the study were requested to make several lifestyle changes, including eating a diet plentiful in whole foods, fruits, and vegetables but low in refined sugar and fat. Additionally, they were to regularly engage in moderate workouts, breathing exercises and relaxation techniques. The healthful lifestyle caused the blood levels of telomerase to increase by 29%.

2. Consider calorie restriction.

This practice may lessen the natural telomere shortening process that occurs over the years, says Dr. Theodore S. Piliszek of King's College School of Medicine of the University of London.

3. Enjoy a glass of non-alcoholic red wine daily.

A 2011 study showed resveratrol, a component of red wine, increased telomerase, which delayed the deterioration of cells. In addition, a 2012 study showed the compound increased the lifespan of mice. A daily glass on non-alcoholic red wine could be helpful.

4. Incorporate plenty of fish into your diet.

In 2010, a study published in JAMA found that individuals with the highest level of dietary omega-3s had the lowest rate of telomere shortening, while those with the least levels had the fastest rate of telomere shortening.

5. Eat dark chocolate.

Some studies suggest that the polyphenols contained in dark chocolate may slow telomere shortening.

6. Drink three cups of tea a day.

A Chinese study in 2009 found that those who drank three cups of tea per day had significantly longer telomeres than those who drank only a small amount. Green tea has a much higher percentage of valuable nutrients called polyphenols than black tea.

7. Abstain from smoking and excessive alcohol consumption.

Shorter telomeres correlate with both of these practices.

8. Deal with stress.

Some research suggests stress accelerates the telomere shortening process. Practices such as massage, exercise, and relaxation techniques can help siphon off anxiety.

Circulatory deficiency

Blood circulates through a network of vessels throughout the body to provide individual cells with oxygen and nutrients and helps dispose of metabolic wastes. The heart pumps the blood around the blood vessels.

Functions of blood and circulation:

- Circulates OXYGEN and removes Carbon Dioxide
- Provides cells with NUTRIENTS
- Removes the waste products of metabolism to the excretory organs for disposal

- Protects the body against disease and infection
- Clotting stops bleeding after injury
- Transports HORMONES to target cells and organs
- Helps regulate body temperature

Blood

Blood is made up of about 45% solids (cells) and 55% fluids (plasma). The plasma is largely water, containing proteins, nutrients, hormones, antibodies, and dissolved waste products.

General types of blood cells: (each has many different sub-types)

Erythrocytes (red cells) are small red disk-shaped cells. They contain hemoglobin, which combines with oxygen in the lungs and is then transported to the body's cells. The hemoglobin then returns carbon dioxide waste to the lungs. Erythrocytes are formed in the bone marrow in the knobby ends of bones.

Leukocytes (white cells) help the body fight bacteria and infection. When a tissue is damaged or has an infection, the number of leukocytes increases. Leukocytes are formed in the small ends of bones. Leukocytes can be classed as granular or nongranular. There are three types of granular leukocytes (eosinophils, neutrophils, and basophils), and three types of nongranular (monocytes, T-cell lymphocytes, and B-cell lymphocytes).

Thrombocytes (platelets) aid the formation of blood clots by releasing various protein substances. When the body is injured, thrombocytes disintegrate and cause a chemical reaction with the proteins found in plasma, which eventually create a thread-like substance called fibrin. The fibrin then "catches" other blood cells which form the clot, preventing further loss of blood and forms the basis of healing.

Arteries carry oxygenated blood away from the heart. They are thick hollow tubes that are highly elastic, which allows them to dilate (widen) and constrict (narrow) as blood is forced down them by the heart. Arteries branch and re-branch, becoming smaller until they become small arterioles, which are even more elastic. Arterioles feed oxygenated blood to the capillaries. The aorta is the largest artery in the body, taking blood from the heart, branching into other arteries that send oxygenated blood to the rest of the body.

Capillaries distribute the nutrients and oxygen to the body's tissues and remove deoxygenated blood and waste. They are extremely thin, the walls are only one cell thick and connect the arterioles with the venules (very small veins).

Venules (very small veins) merge into veins, which carry blood back to the heart. The vein walls are similar to arteries but thinner and less elastic. Veins carry deoxygenated blood towards the lungs where oxygen is received via the pulmonary capillaries. The pulmonary veins then carries this oxygenated blood back to the heart.

The heart

The heart is a hollow muscular organ that beats over 100,000 times a day to pump blood around the body's 60,000 miles of blood vessels. The right side of the heart receives blood and sends it to the lungs to be oxygenated, while the left side receives oxygenated blood from the lungs and sends it out to the tissues of the body. The heart has three layers: the endocardium (inner layer), the epicardium (middle layer), and the myocardium (outer layer). The heart is protected by the pericardium, which is the protective membrane surrounding it.

The heart has four chambers, in the lower heart the right and left Ventricles, and in the upper heart the right and left Atria. In a normal heart beat, the atria contract while the ventricles relax, then the ventricles contract while the atria relax. There are valves through which blood passes between ventricle and atrium, these close in such a way that blood does not backwash during the pauses between ventricular contractions. The right and left ventricles are divided by a thick wall (the ventricular septum). Babies born with a "hole in the heart" have a small gap here, which is a problem since oxygenated and deoxygenated can blood mix. The walls of the left ventricle are thicker as it has to pump blood to all the tissues, compared to the right ventricle which only pumps blood as far as the lungs.

Exercise—The key to circulation

The beauty of any deficiency is provide what the cells need and you are back on the road to health and recovery. A sedentary lifestyle is one of the 5 major risk factors (along with high blood pressure, abnormal values for blood lipids, smoking, and obesity) for cardiovascular disease, as outlined by the AHA. Evidence from many scientific studies shows that reducing these risk factors decreases the chance of having a heart attack or experiencing another cardiac event, such as a stroke, and reduces the possibility of needing a coronary revascularization procedure (bypass surgery or coronary angioplasty). Regular exercise has a favorable effect on many of the established risk factors for cardiovascular disease. For example, exercise promotes weight reduction and can help reduce blood pressure. Exercise can reduce "bad" cholesterol levels in the blood (the low-density lipoprotein [LDL] level), as well as total cholesterol, and can raise the "good" cholesterol (the high-density lipoprotein level [HDL]). In diabetic patients, regular activity favorably affects the body's ability to use insulin to control glucose levels in the blood. Although the effect of an exercise program on any single risk factor may generally be small, the effect of continued, moderate exercise on overall cardiovascular risk, when combined with other lifestyle modifications (such as proper nutrition, smoking cessation, and medication use), can be dramatic.

Benefits of Regular Exercise on Cardiovascular Risk Factors

- Increase in exercise tolerance
- Reduction in body weight
- Reduction in blood pressure
- Reduction in bad (LDL and total) cholesterol
- Increase in good (HDL) cholesterol
- Increase in insulin sensitivity

There are a number of physiological benefits of exercise; Two examples are improvements in muscular function and strength and improvement in the body's ability to take in and use oxygen (maximal oxygen consumption or aerobic capacity). As one's ability to transport and use oxygen improves, regular daily activities can be performed with less fatigue. This is particularly important for patients with cardiovascular disease, whose exercise capacity is typically lower than that of healthy individuals. There is also evidence that exercise training improves the capacity of the blood vessels to dilate in response to exercise or hormones, consistent with better vascular wall function and an improved ability to provide oxygen to the muscles during exercise. Studies measuring muscular strength and flexibility before and after exercise programs suggest that there are improvements in bone health and ability to perform daily activities, as well as a lower likelihood of developing back pain and of disability, particularly in older age groups.

Patients with newly diagnosed heart disease who participate in an exercise program report an earlier return to work and improvements in other measures of quality of life, such as more self-confidence, lower stress, and less anxiety. Importantly, by combining controlled studies, researchers have found that for heart attack patients who participated in a formal exercise program, the death rate is reduced by 20% to 25%. This is strong evidence in support of physical activity for patients with heart disease. Although the benefits of exercise are unquestionable, it should be noted that exercise programs alone for patients with heart disease have not convincingly shown improvement in the heart's pumping ability or the diameter of the coronary vessels that supply oxygen to the heart muscle.

How much exercise is enough exercise?

Being appointed as an advisor to the President's Council on Sports and Physical fitness was one of the highlights of my career. I had the opportunity to work with Dr. Jocelyn Eldrer and was featured in the USA Today newspaper. While working with Nutrisystem I got to meet former surgeon general, C. Everet Koop. Both were so educated, so aware, and so in the belief of prevention of disease. This made me continue to do my homework and follow these dedicated leaders.

In 1996, the release of the Surgeon General's Report on Physical Activity and Health provided a springboard for the largest government effort to date to promote physical activity among Americans. This historic turning point redefined exercise as a key component to health promotion and disease prevention, and on the basis of this report, the federal government mounted a multi-year educational campaign. The Surgeon General's Report, a joint CDC/ACSM consensus statement, and a National Institutes of Health report agreed that the benefits mentioned above will generally occur by engaging in at least 30 minutes of modest activity on most, preferably all, days of the week. Modest activity is defined as any activity that is similar in intensity to brisk walking at a rate of about 3 to 4 miles per hour. These activities can include any other form of occupational or recreational activity that is dynamic in nature and of similar intensity, such as cycling, yard work, and swimming. This amount of exercise equates to approximately five to seven 30-minute sessions per week at an intensity equivalent to 3 to 6 METs (multiples of the resting metabolic rate*), or approximately 600 to 1200 calories expended per week.

Note that the specific phrase "...30 minutes of accumulated activity..." is used in the above-mentioned reports. It has been shown that repeated intermittent or shorter bouts of activity (such as 10 minutes) that include occupational and recreational activity or the tasks of daily living have similar cardiovascular and other health benefits if performed at the moderate intensity level with an accumulated duration of at least 30 minutes per day. People who already meet these standards will receive additional benefits from more vigorous activity.

Many of the studies documenting the benefits of exercise typically use programs consisting of 30 to 60 minutes of continuous exercise 3 days per week at an intensity corresponding to 60% to 75% of the individual's heart rate reserve. It is not usually necessary, however, for healthy adults to measure heart rate diligently because substantial health benefits can occur through modest levels of daily activity, irrespective of the specific exercise intensity. In fact, researchers estimate that as much as a 30% to 40% reduction in cardiovascular events is possible if most Americans were simply to meet the government recommendations for activity.

One need not be a marathon runner or an elite athlete to derive significant benefits from physical activity. In fact, the Surgeon General's physical activity recommendations seem surprisingly modest. One reason for this is that the greatest gains in terms of mortality are achieved when an individual goes from being sedentary to becoming moderately active. Studies show that less is gained when an individual goes from being moderately active to very active.

First, if you currently have heart disease or are over 45 years of age and have 2 or more risk factors (immediate family member with heart disease before age 55, cigarette smoking, high blood pressure, abnormal cholesterol levels, diabetes, sedentary lifestyle, or obesity), you should consult your physician before starting any type of exercise. Clearly, most people can derive significant benefits from integrating a half hour of moderate activity into their day. If you know you simply cannot or will not set aside a half hour of activity on a given day, then try to work more activities into the day by taking the stairs rather than the elevator, or try walking rather than driving a short distance to the store. Try to work several shorter periods of activity, such as 10 minutes, into your schedule. The most important thing is to get started. There is mounting evidence in the scientific literature that physical activity and physical fitness have a powerful influence on a host of chronic diseases, a fact underscored by the recent Surgeon General's report on Physical Activity and Health. Reducing the risk of heart disease through greater physical activity could have an enormous impact on health in the United States.

Nerve deficiency

Like any deficiency, remove the cause and you are again on your way to health. I am excited my son, Dr. Jason Kaplan, and his future wife, Dr. Stephanie Lyons, will continue to treat patients in Wellington, Florida. Daily, they deal with nerve deficiencies. Although I have an entire chapter dedicated to this subject (Chapter 38) let's just get a simple basic understanding for now.

The master control system for your body is your nerve system, consisting of the brain, spinal cord, and peripheral nerves. While the practice of medicine is defined as the diagnosis and treatment of disease, chiropractic is dedicated to restoring the body's ability to regulate and heal itself through normalized nervous system function. Rather than treating sickness with drugs or surgery, chiropractors examine and correct interference to the nervous system (called *vertebral subluxation*), ensuring that their patients have a healthy and functioning nerve supply to the body. **If your nerve system is not**

functioning fully free of interference, it is impossible to be truly healthy.

You might think of your spine as simply a series of bones, but the spinal column is actually a complex organ system. At its core, literally inside your spine, your spinal cord and nerve tissuetransmitsinformation, allowing your brain to monitor and coordinate the function of every cell, tissue, organ, and organ system in your body. A chiropractor's purpose is ensuring that the flow of vital information from your brain to your body occurs without interference.

The role of a healthy spine is to protect the nerve system from stress, allowing it to transmit information. Freely flowing information across your nerve system is an essential element for health. If not properly cared for, trauma or repetative stress to the spine will interfere with this flow of information. An unhealthy spine will create stress on the nerve system. This is why chiropractors have had such success with conditions as diverse as constipation, headaches, asthma, fertitily issues, ear infections, and many other diseases that can be caused by nerve or structural deficiencies.

'*Chiro*' is greek for 'by hand,' so chiropractic literally translates into 'practice by hand.' It is important to understand why everyone who wishes to be truly healthy needs to be checked by a chiropractor regularly. Chiropractic focuses on the relationship between the spine, the nervous system, and healthy body functions. Chiropractors correct subluxation, allowing for proper nerve supply. Through chiropractic adjustments, chiropractors are able to correct subluxations, restoring functionand increasing positive body signals, therefore decreasing stress. See Chapter 38 for more details.

Although adequate exercise, perfect nutrition, perfect genes, a pure environment, and ideal behavior probably do not readily exist, these factors write the story of your life, including not only how many chapters you will finish, but the sheer quality of your story. My book, my life, has had a few scary moments, some chapters I wish I could rewrite. However, life is about change. My book, my life, seems to get better each day, and I am now excited for the upcoming chapter on my book of life.

The key to health is often the interaction between inherited genes, nutritional intake, the environment, and our beliefs. These determine our current state of health or disease, including how long we live.

Once I started to do my homework, my research, it amazed me how rapidly the human understanding of our own aging process is expanding. It is only a matter of time before we're able to take control over that process and literally *Awaken the Wellness Within*.

"*A wise man should consider that health is the greatest of human blessings, and learn how by his own thought to derive benefit from his illnesses.*"

—Hippocrates

Chapter 17

YOUR CELLS NEED
ANTIOXIDANTS

To live a long healthy life, your telomeres must remain long. We now know that long telomeres are associated with optimal biological age—it should be everyone's goal to look and feel much younger than your chronological age. Without certain supplements, especially antioxidants to help your telomeres remain long, your cells will experience deficiency. By removing the deficiencies, we are on the path of prevention.

The good news is that supplements can assist our bodies in avoiding these deficiencies. Antioxidant supplements have tremendous influence on oxidative damage. However, targeted supplementation is the key, as antioxidants work synergistically and must be balanced to work most effectively.

Antioxidants are a cornerstone to any wellness and prevention program. Antioxidants are natural substances that exist in the foods we eat. They are recognized for their benefits and ability to help prevent disease by fighting free radicals, substances that harm the body when left unchecked. Free radicals are formed by normal bodily processes such as breathing, and by environmental contaminants like cigarette smoke. Without adequate amounts of antioxidants, these free radicals travel throughout the body, damaging cells.

Earlier in the book we spoke of oxidative damage to the cells and their telomeres. This oxidative damage is offset with antioxidants. Take an apple and slice it open. Leave one half out to the air, and squeeze lemon juice from a freshly cut lemon on the other half. Notice which portion of the apple browns first? The lemon half that was preserved from oxidative damage from the antioxidant value of the lemon will brown at a much slower pace. You may have heard of antioxidants and free radicals, but you may not know exactly what they are and how they relate to your overall health.

In simple terms, free radicals are highly reactive, unstable molecules that roam around your body. These molecules are unstable because they are missing an electron and they want to "steal" electrons from other healthy cells in your body. When a free radical steals an electron from a healthy cell, that healthy cell then becomes a free radical, and a chain reaction occurs. This chain reaction, called oxidation, can cause damage to the cells of the body.

So where do these free radicals in our bodies come from? Just the simple act of breathing results in the production of free radicals. During respiration, some electrons leak away from the normal respiratory pathway during electron transport. These electrons latch on to free oxygen molecules, resulting in the production of free radicals. Under normal conditions, approximately 1% to 3% of oxygen molecules are converted into free radicals.

The air that we breathe is polluted with toxins, which can increase free radical production during respiration. Other environmental toxins, such as alcohol, cigarette smoking, and radiation can also lead to an increase in free radical formation. Free radicals damage our cells and over time will shorten our telomeres. Antioxidants are germane to anti-aging.

Many people don't not know that our bodies actually produce a certain amount of free radicals on purpose. For example, the body's immune system purposely creates free radicals to destroy unwelcome organisms, such as infections. This is the yin and yang of the body, the universe.

Fortunately for us, our bodies have a defense system to protect our cells from oxidative damage. Antioxidants, which are manufactured within our body or extracted from the food we eat, help neutralize the free radicals in our bodies. But in the chemical age we live in, our bodies just don't produce enough of them.

The term antioxidant means "against oxidation." Antioxidants work by giving up one of their electrons to free radicals, but unlike free radicals, antioxidants don't become harmful and reactive when they lose an electron.

Free radicals are toxic to our cells, and antioxidants prevent them from harming us. To *Awaken the Wellness Within*, you must protect and repair the cells in your body; it is important to get enough antioxidants through our diet and nutritional supplements.

Some common antioxidants

In order to protect and repair the cells in your body, it is important to make sure you are getting enough antioxidants through the food you eat and/or nutritional supplements. The most studied antioxidants are vitamin C, vitamin E, beta-carotene, and selenium. Vitamin C, which is a water-soluble vitamin, cannot be stored in the body, so it is important to get some regularly in your diet. Sources of vitamin C include citrus fruits, green peppers, broccoli, green leafy vegetables, and strawberries.

Vitamin E is a fat-soluble vitamin, which means that it can be stored in the liver and other tissues of the body. Sources of vitamin E include wheat germ, nuts, seeds, whole grains, and green leafy vegetables.

Beta-carotene, which is converted to vitamin A in the body, is a scavenger of a particular type of free radical and has been found to decrease free-radical damage associated with HIV. Food sources of beta-carotene include green leafy vegetables, carrots, and other yellow and orange fruits and vegetables.

Selenium is a trace element with antioxidant properties. A selenium deficiency is associated with immune dysfunction and decreased CD4+ counts. Food sources of selenium include seafood, brazil nuts, eggs, meats, and whole grains. In our toxic world we must supplement our cells.

My four ACES, are vitamins A, C, E, and Selenium.

It is important to get as many antioxidants as you can from the foods you eat by choosing a well-balanced diet including whole grains, lean meats, and 5 to 10 servings of fruits and vegetables every day.

There are many authorities—including the American Heart Association, the American Cancer Society, the World Cancer Research Institute in association with the American Institute for Cancer Research, and the World Health Organization's International Agency for Research on Cancer—that recommend getting beta-carotene and other antioxidants from food instead of supplements, at least until research finds out whether supplements offer the same benefits. Eating 5 servings of fruits and vegetables daily provides 6-8 mg of beta-carotene.

Most vitamin labels provide minimum daily requirements. Not all vitamins are the same. This is where a doctor or anti-aging specialist can help you design your own regimen. The key word is minimum. When we are deficient we need more than the minimum.

When conditions of higher inflammatory stress exist, cells will then increase their rate of replicating and dividing in order to restore themselves. Remember, the body works to heal itself. The body will fight to heal itself and this need to recover from cellular damage will eventually speed up the loss of telomeres. This is a result of increased cell turnover. This is compounded by the free radicals that are generated during the inflammatory situation, which results in further damage to existing telomeres. To protect our cells, we must do everything we can to reduce cellular inflammation.

Increasing antioxidant capacity at the cellular level is critical to maintaining telomere length. Recent evidence suggests that even a high-quality balanced multivitamin helps maintain telomere length. Specifically, studies have linked longer telomeres with levels of vitamin E, vitamin C, vitamin D, omega-3 fatty acids, and the antioxidant resveratrol.

People with lowered immune systems have a higher need for vitamins, minerals, and antioxidants. A supplement regimen may be beneficial, including a multivitamin/mineral supplement (without extra iron) with antioxidants and trace elements.

Inflammation sets off a chain reaction of free radical damage, a problem that can magnify if inflammation remains high. Quenching inflammation naturally is a key role that nutrition plays in preserving telomeres. Nutrients such as quercetin, green tea, grape seed extract, curcumin, and resveratrol Natural phenol or type of antioxidant found in red grapes, red wine. Research has shown beneficial effects as anti-cancer and anti-inflammatory agents along with supporting healthy blood sugar and cardiovasculature function. all show specific ability to help preserve telomeres, with grape seed extract and curcumin showing the ability to generate longer telomeres.

Scientists today recognize that contrary to the wear and tear of inanimate objects, people age differently if we protect our cells. Certainly, cells can suffer from damage akin to wear and tear, but remember our skin is constantly replacing itself. *The power that creates the body has the power to heal the body.* Our bodies are always undergoing change and our bodies can repair damaged tissue and cells. When not compromised, our body has the ability to repair and regenerate any damaged cells. This is what makes us so unique. The key is not being deficient in the nutrients the cells need or they will not have the tools to repair themselves. From this day forward, look at your vitamin cabinet as a tool chest for you cells, and you'll build something special and something to pass the test of time.

This book will help you develop a lifestyle that avoids toxicity from free radical damage.

Kaplan's Key Cellular Supporters

1. Astragalus Root

A chemical in astragalus root, TAT2, stimulates the production of telomerase, an enzyme that aids telomere repair. Short telomeres indicate damaged DNA and are the key contributors to increased cellular aging. Astragalus root also supports the liver's toxin-removing actions by acting as a diuretic. The increased urine flow flushes the kidneys and prevents toxin buildup.

2. Resveratrol

The French Paradox made resveratrol famous for its role in promoting longevity. Present in red wine, chocolate, and peanuts, resveratrol is unique among antioxidants for its ability to cross the blood-brain barrier and deliver potent soothing properties and free radical scavenging actions directly to brain cells. Its effect mimics caloric restriction, a proven anti-aging dietary strategy.

3. Pterostilbene

Similar to resveratrol in function, pterostilbene may actually be a more powerful antioxidant. Like resveratrol, it mimics caloric restriction, which slows aging and promotes healing. Researchers have found it very effective for protecting and rejuvenating brain cells, balancing blood sugar, and maintaining healthy cholesterol levels.

4. Pyrroloquinoline Quinone (PQQ) Disodium Salt

Often called PQQ Na, this non-protein co-enzyme facilitates cellular metabolic processes and stimulates mitochondrial regeneration, an essential factor in slowing the aging process. It also neutralizes free radicals and reactive oxygen species (ROS), compounds that expedite physical aging.

5. Digestive and Systemic Enzymes

Digestive enzymes work only in the digestive tract, while systemic enzymes support digestion and also enter the bloodstream to clear toxins, fibrins, and allergens. Systemic enzymes, also called proteolytic enzymes, support immune function, target and reduce inflammation, and improve circulation.

6. R-lipoic Acid

Alpha-lipoic acid comes in two forms, r-lipoic acid (the most bioavailable and bioactive form) and s-lipoic acid. Lipoic acid plays a crucial role in mitochondrial energy creation, which makes it an important part of the cellular life cycle. Inadequate levels lead to faster aging, and like other factors in mitochondrial processes, lipoic acid possesses a strong antioxidant effect.

7. Pomegranate Extract

Anthocyanins give pomegranates their red color and offer a powerful dose of antioxidants. Punicalagins specifically support cardiovascular well-being, neural synaptic health, and possibly reduce AGEs (advanced glycation end products). AGEs are associated with type II diabetes and Alzheimer's disease and are just one of the accelerators to the aging process.

8. Tibetan Rhodiola

Tibetan monks consider Rhodiola the supreme herb. Two potent compounds in the herb—salidroside and rosavin—act as antioxidants, protect nerves and brain cells, extend physical performance, and increase feelings of well-being.

9. CoQ10

Every cell in the body requires coenzyme Q10 to produce ATP. As a factor in the metabolic process, it acts as an antioxidant to neutralize free radicals protecting the cell, DNA, and mitochondria from oxidative damage. Although the body naturally produces CoQ10, supplementation alleviates the symptoms of chronic disease and fatigue and supports general cardiovascular health.

10. Folate

This B vitamin is important for DNA and RNA structure and function, and it plays a major role in DNA maintenance. But it's also important to DNA methylation, a process that regulates cell development and suppresses viral genes. These are all crucial to telomere length. If you are getting enough folate, your DNA should be running smoothly. But a deficiency can cause direct damage to telomeres. Skip the supplements for this one. The telomere benefits only come from naturally occurring folate. Some great sources are beef liver, spinach, asparagus, and avocado.

11. Vitamin B12

In conjunction with folate, this B vitamin is important for the methylation, or detoxification, of homocysteine. Higher levels of homocysteine are associated with increased oxidative stress.

12. Niacin (nicotinamide)

Can influence telomere length through its multiple regulatory and coenzymatic activities.

13. Vitamin A and Beta-Carotene

These antioxidants reduce concentrations of harmful signaling molecules and increase beneficial ones to help reduce oxidative stress.

14. Vitamin D

There doesn't seem to be any limit on the benefits of vitamin D. Lengthening telomeres is no exception. One study finds that women with higher concentrations of D3 in their blood have longer telomeres. In fact, women with the highest levels of this vitamin showed up to five less years of telomere aging. Of course, you can get vitamin D3 from being out in the sun, but getting it from supplements or foods like eggs, mushrooms, and cold-water fish is more practical.

15. Vitamins A, C, E and Selenium

These antioxidant vitamins are widely acknowledged for limiting oxidative stress and its damage on DNA and telomeres. *My four ACES, for the winning hand of health.*

16. Magnesium

Telomerase is an enzyme that keeps telomeres long and stable, and it's completely dependent on magnesium, which promotes DNA replication and stability. If you don't get enough, cells age faster and telomeres shorten. And the longer you go on with a magnesium deficiency, the more damage you can do to your telomeres. So seek out foods that are high in magnesium. Leafy green vegetables like spinach are good sources, but you can also get magnesium from nuts like almonds and cashews, too. Just don't go overboard with magnesium. **Too much of it can be dangerous, especially if you have kidney problems, so before adding any supplement regime speak to your physician.**

17. Zinc

This mineral is necessary for a variety of enzymes including DNA polymerases, which are important for DNA and telomere maintenance.

18. Iron

In contrast to the other nutrients, iron supplementation is associated with shorter telomeres. This is likely because of iron's pro-oxidant ability to stimulate free radical generation. While iron supplements may increase oxidative stress, iron from diet or multivitamins (containing less iron) is not negatively associated with telomere length.

19. Omega-3s

Omega-3 oils, especially DHA, are routinely in the headlines for their extensive science, demonstrating the ability to reduce heart disease, lower triglycerides, improve brain function, help weight management, and reduce the chronic low-grade inflammation associated with virtually any disease of aging. The omega-3 oils protect our cells and that is germane to cellular health.

A new study published in the *Journal of the American Medical Association* shows for the first time that omega-3 oils also possess a powerful anti-aging characteristic—the preservation of telomeres.

In one study, researchers were trying to find reasons why heart patients live longer when they take fish oil. They measured telomere length and the concentration of omega-3 fatty acids (DHA and EPA) in blood cells (leukocytes). Five years later they repeated the measurements. Individuals with the lowest amount of omega-3 oils had the shortest telomeres, whereas the group with the highest concentration of DHA and EPA had the longest telomeres. Each 1-standard deviation increase in DHA+EPA levels was associated with a 32% reduction in the odds of telomere shortening. While this study was conducted in a population of cardiovascular patients, there is no reason to assume the finding would not also apply to the general population. This is a major anti-aging benefit of fish oil consumption.

It should be pointed out that in the case of omega-3 fatty acids, you are what you eat. Omega-3 oils accumulate in the membranes of your cells in direct response to how much of them you consistently consume.

20. Curcumin and turmeric

Turmeric, and its primary component curcumin, are common dietary spices that stimulate synthesis of antioxidants, thereby protecting against oxidative stress. Mice fed diets containing curcumin had a trend for longer telomeres compared with controls. I also reccoemnd this as an anti-inflamatory, which Peter Kash outlines in his book *Take Two Tablets: Medicine From The Bible*. Disease puts the body in an inflammatory state. Curcumin, turmeric, makes for a great prophylactic to disease.

21. Polyphenols

Polyphenols from grape seed and green tea provide additional protection for DNA and telomeres from oxidative stress. Those who drink tea regularly have longer telomeres while mice fed grape seed polyphenols had longer telomeres compared to controls

22. Astaxanthin

Telomeres are extremely vulnerable to oxidative stress. Studies show that women who take multivitamins with antioxidants have 5% longer telomeres. But if you want super-charged antioxidant power (and you do), forget the multi. There's nothing stronger than astaxanthin. It's over 50 times more potent than vitamins C and E at fighting oxidative stress. You can find it as a supplement. But we recommend that you get it from wild-caught salmon. A six-ounce serving contains about four milligrams of astaxanthin.

I am often asked, "How can I get more antioxidants in my diet?"

- **Vitamin C** is found in citrus, kiwi, strawberries, bell peppers, and broccoli.
- **Vitamin E** is contained in almonds, avocados, and olive oil.
- **Beta-carotene** creates vitamin A, important for vision and bone health. Good sources are carrots, sweet potatoes, kale, chard, and papayas.

- **Lycopene** is found in red fruits and vegetables like tomatoes, papaya, and watermelon.
- **Lutein and zeaxanthin** are found in dark green leafy veggies like spinach, kale, collard greens, and broccoli and may help slow the progress of age-related macular degeneration in the eyes.
- **Anthocyanins** are found in blue and purple foods like blueberries, raspberries, plums, pomegranates, eggplant, and red cabbage.

Posted on WebMD, Charlotte E. Grayson Mathis, MD: "USDA scientists analyzed antioxidant levels in more than 100 different foods, including fruits and vegetables. Each food was measured for antioxidant concentration as well as antioxidant capacity per serving size. Cranberries, blueberries, and blackberries ranked highest among the fruits studied. Beans, artichokes, and Russet potatoes were tops among the vegetables. Pecans, walnuts, and hazelnuts ranked highest in the nut category.

"USDA chemist Ronald L. Prior says the total antioxidant capacity of the foods does not necessarily reflect their health benefit. Benefits depend on how the food's antioxidants are absorbed and utilized in the body. Still, this chart should help consumers trying to add more antioxidants to their daily diet."

Rank	Food Item	Serving Size	Total anti-oxidant capacity per serving size
1	Small Red Bean (dried)	half cup	13,727
2	Wild Blueberry	1 cup	13,427
3	Red Kidney Bean (dried)	half cup	13,259
4	Pinto Bean	half cup	11,864
5	Blueberry (cultivated)	1 cup	9,019

6	Cranberry	1 cup	8,983
7	Artichoke (cooked)	1 cup (hearts)	7,904
8	Blackberry	1 cup	7,701
9	Prune	half cup	7,291
10	Raspberry	1 cup	6,058
11	Strawberry	1 cup	5,938
12	Red Delicious Apple	1 whole	5,900
13	Granny Smith Apple	1 whole	5,381
14	Pecan	1 ounce	5,095
15	Sweet Cherry	1 cup	4,873
16	Black Plum	1 whole	4,844
17	Russet Potato (cooked)	1 whole	4,649
18	Black Bean (dried)	half cup	4,181
19	Plum	1 whole	4,118
20	Gala Apple	1 whole	3,903

WebMD Public Information from the United States Department of Agriculture

People who eat diets rich in fruits, vegetables, legumes, nuts, and fish generally have a strong and healthy immune system that is fueled by the nutrients, minerals, and antioxidants found in the foods they eat. Nutritious foods have the ability to boost your health and preserve your DNA, and in some cases, can even help repair your damaged DNA.

As you begin to age, your body may start to accumulate a higher number of damaged cells and molecules that can interfere with the DNA repair process—and the function of telomeres. To *Awaken the Wellness Within* we must feed our cells with foods they need and avoid toxins at all costs.

Before changing your diets or adding any supplement regime, speak to your physician.

"Health is merely the slowest possible rate at which one can die."

—Anonymous

Chapter 18

AWAKENING OUR WELLNESS

As Americans, we have been taught through experience and media that disease is a normal part of the aging process. When I watch television, I'm amazed by the amount of drug advertisements. The scary part is listening to the sweet voice mentioning a long list of side effects that should cause anyone with common sense to avoid ever taking that drug. But our culture has learned to treat the symptoms, not the cause of disease.

Drugs are now big business. As the former president and chief operating officer of Nutrisystem, I learned all about big business, and I know how it works. I enjoyed working on Wall Street, and I learned almost everything there is to learn about weight loss and how health fits into corporate America. For your stock to go up, your revenues and profits must go up. For drug companies to make more money, more people have to use their drugs. The more drugs they sell, the higher their stock price.

These commercials urge you to take Lunesta to get to sleep, Lyrica to battle aches and pains, Cymbalta when "depression hurts." And if the commercials seem more pervasive than ever, that's because they are. Drugmakers spend nearly $5 billion a year to make sure you're hearing about their products—a sound investment considering that every $1,000 they spend translates to 24 new prescriptions, according to the House Commerce Committee. But, as industry spending has soared, so has public scrutiny. At a day-long House subcommittee hearing, lawmakers pushed for tougher regulations, taking aim at seemingly deceptive ads by drug companies such as Pfizer and Merck. The U.S. Food and Drug Administration (FDA), which mandates and monitors the content of drug ads, has also convened to discuss the issue.

Prescription drug spending is the third most expensive cost in our healthcare system, and spending seems to grow larger every year. Just last year, the average American got 12 prescriptions a year, as compared with 1992 when Americans got an average of seven prescriptions. In a decade and a half, the use of prescription medication went up 71%. This has added about $180 billion to our medical spending.

While there are more medicines on the market today than in 1992, researchers estimate that around 20% of the $180 billion increase has absolutely nothing to do with the number of medications available or increases in the cost of that medication.

How do our children learn the difference between good drugs and bad drugs? Drugs are big business. We are raised thinking that with aging, disease is accepted. Older people are typically seen as the helpless victims of the inevitable and natural process we call aging. Especially when we were raised thinking that aging and disease are acceptable and unavoidable. We are seen as the helpless victims to the inevitable and natural process we call aging. When the symptoms of aging and disease develop, I'm amazed by how people feel surprised and victimized.

We live in a world where poor diets and the toxic environments are part of our society. Living this way not only affects how we view our world but also creates a toxic environment within our bodies. This affects the cells, making them deficient and toxic—the two causes of disease.

Although painful to acknowledge, those who suffer from disease invariably (if unknowingly) have made poor choices leading to illness. In the case of sick children, it's often the parents who have made the poor choices. We learned earlier that breakfast cereals full of sugar do not build healthy cells. Children often are not taught that we have the ability to and, in fact, the need to consistently make meaningful choices about our health. Health is not a part of our education system. We teach our children how to memorize the parts of the body, but we don't teach them how they can heal their own bodies.

We live in a drug culture; we look for a magic pill or potion for health. When we get ill, we look to the outside for solutions when the problems and solutions lie within us.

We must take responsibility for our health. However, accepting this responsibility for our health and aging can be enormously empowering. The overall healing powers and the cells' competence and effectiveness are determined by relative levels of deficiency and toxicity within our cells. Toxicity and deficiency are the sole determinants of health. The goal of this book is to teach you, the reader, how to embrace health and avoid illness by educating yourself in how to make healthful choices that lower your levels of deficiency and toxicity and promote your cellular health and well-being. To Awaken the Healer within we must understand the importance of cellular health.

In review:

1. There is only one disease—cytopathology.
2. There are only two causes of cytopathology—toxicity and deficiency.
3. There is only one cure—treat the cause by healing the weakened cells.

We begin by protecting the cells, which in return lengthens our telomeres, which in return protects our health.

There is only one way to stop aging—protect and nourish your cells, thereby protecting your telomeres. Clearly, if you could stop your telomeres from shrinking after cell division, you could slow down the aging process and protect yourself from disease. The key to *Awakening the Wellness Within* is to awaken and preserve our telomeres. Scientists have reported, in numerous publications and in study after study, that if you promote the production of telomerase, the enzyme that makes telomeres in the body, you can slow the rate of telomere degradation and even reverse it. In other words, if short telomeres are the problem, then telomerase may be the best solution.

We discussed earlier how scientists have introduced telomerase into cells in tissue culture and extended the length of their telomeres, and I found this simply amazing. They reported that the cells then divided for 250 generations—that's correct, 250 generations past the time they normally would stop dividing, and they are continuing to divide normally, giving rise to normal cells with the normal number of chromosomes. By extending the telomeres with telomerase, scientists will literally be able to turn back the clock of aging.

Now imagine if you could promote the production of telomerase in your healthy cells. You could theoretically slow down the aging process. This is something scientists are actively working on. It appears every year the product formulation improves and provides better results. We're not there yet, but we're getting close.

We are aware how toxins and deficiencies affect the cell. Stress speeds up the rate that telomeres shorten, in turn speeding up the rate of biological aging. Many conditions and diseases associated with aging are associated with short telomeres. Modern research done continues to demonstrate that telomereA telomere is a repeating sequence of DNA at the end of a chromosome. Each time a cell replicates and divides the telomere loses some of its length. Eventually the telomere runs out and the cell can no longer divide and rejuvenate, triggering a poor state of cell health that contributes to disease risk and eventual cell death. length is very important, but equally important is telomereA telomere is a repeating sequence of DNA at the end of a chromosome. Each time a cell replicates and divides the telomere loses some of its length. Eventually the telomere runs out and the cell can no longer divide and rejuvenate, triggering a poor state of cell health that contributes to disease risk and eventual cell death. quality.

Look at telomeres like a chain. If you have a weak link, then you have a weak link in your DNA, thus a weaker cell. Cells damaged must be repaired; yet they lack the repair efficiency of other DNA. This results in an accumulation of partially damaged and poorly functioning telomeres of lower quality, regardless of length.

One way to influence the aging process of any person is simply to slow down the rate of reproduction. In the context of telomeres, this means you would have strategies to slow down the rate they are shortening, while helping to protect and repair them so that their quality is better maintained. Many experts agree that it is possible to do this today.

Although influential in our destiny, our genetics don't determine the totality of our future. Genes are pliable to some degree and nutrition can excel at offsetting gene weaknesses. We studied how protecting the cell membrane can protect the cell and how antioxidants help our immunity. We can protect the cell and we can protect our telomeres from shortening. This is not genetic altering, it is protecting. Yes, modern medicine gets some credit for people living longer, but so does exercise, diet, and smart nutrition.

How simple our healthcare system would be if they embraced the truth of One Disease, Two Causes, One Cure. If we find the cause and we treat it, we could literally *Awaken the Wellness Within*. By treating and protecting the cells, we preserve our health and our telomeres. The cure to aging and disease is in many ways essentially the same. The cure deals directly with the cell's health by protecting and nourishing the cell and lengthening our telomeres. A secret to ageless aging is to protect the telomere, slow down the process of telomere shortening, and thereby lengthen your life.

The *American Journal of Clinical* Nutrition (*AJCN*) study was among the first to document the relationship between diet and telomere length. The authors of the study concluded that the results provided more support that an improved diet and lifestyle would indeed help to slow the aging process. "Telomere shortening is accelerated by oxidative stress and inflammation, and diet affects both of these processes," the authors report.

As previously discussed, the most important basic supplement to help your telomeres is a good quality multi-vitamin that is properly formulated with the right amount of antioxidants. Now combine these vitamins along with adequate dietary protein (I prefer whey), especially sulfur-containing proteins.

Your brain also has a high need for methyl donors, especially for your mood to feel good. If you are stressed out or depressed, you are typically lacking methyl donors. This means that your telomeres are also running low of nourishment and prone to accelerated aging. This is a major reason why stress ages a person.

The more demands you are under and/or the worse you feel, emotionally or mentally, then the more you need to pay attention to adequate support of basic nutrients that will not only help your nerves and brain but also help your telomeres. Conversely, if you feel pretty good most of the time with a good energy level and mostly positive mood, and you have basic B vitamins and adequate dietary protein, then you are doing a good job of covering the nutrient needs of your telomeres.

Many nutrients can help protect and enhance the repair capacity of your cells, including your telomeres. A lack of antioxidants, as we discussed earlier, leads to increased free radical damage and more risk for damage to telomeres. Remember, one of the causes for disease is deficiency. You must supply the cells with what they need or they will become deficient.

Your cells are daily under constant free radical attack. In a healthy person there is an adequate antioxidant defense system that is fueled by nutrition. These antioxidants help reduce damage from toxins as well as preserve function of healthy cells.

The body knows how to heal itself

The brain and the spinal cord are very delicate tissues, more delicate than the tissue in your eye. Nature had to develop a way to protect this system. Now, in the case of the brain, the solid piece of bone called the skull protects the brain. In the case of the spinal cord, a solid piece of bone would not do because if it were solid, it would afford no movement except for your arms and your legs. So, instead of having a solid bone, bones were stacked one on top of the other, each with a joint and a disc in between to provide a little bit of movement. Discs are like shock absorbers. They are able to alter their shape in response to movement.

Everything you need, your body already has. For example, there is the stomach. There are nerves that go to the stomach. When you eat something, there are signals sent from the stomach up to the brain, which tells the brain what the food is. Then, there is a signal sent back to the stomach telling it to secrete the correct enzymes to digest the food. Now, suppose there is an interruption or interference with that system and the brain thinks there is food and there isn't because of some nerve malfunctioning. The stomach starts to digest itself, thus forming an ulcer. It only takes one cell out of line to put the whole body out of tune. The key is to heal the cell, to "Awaken" our "Inner Healer." To do this we must begin to treat the cause of of the disease and not just the symptoms.

To give you an idea of how complex the nervous system is, in the brain and the spinal cord there are at least 12–18 billion nerve cells, all of which are present at birth. There are 100,000 miles of nerves in your body and each of these nerves can carry 1,000 separate messages in a second, some of them up to speeds of 200 miles per hour. The brain can record a trillion bits of information. We marvel at the computer and how complex it can be, yet it is nothing in comparison to the complexity of our own nervous system.

So now you can see why the brain and the nervous system are so important. The nervous system is the system that maintains health, and any interference with this nervous system will produce a signal that we all learn to respect because that means that the body is no longer in control. That signal is pain and that pain signal is a symptom. Yet, we are taught to treat pain as the symptom, and not the cause of the pain. This could be dangerous if you only treat the symptom. Nerves are part of our alarm system signaling that something has been damaged. Remove the cause of the pain and the cell will heal. This is the essence, the foundation of chiropractic.

Think of this in terms of a fire in a building. The symptom or signal is the fire alarm. You don't simply stop the alarm and expect the cause, the fire, to magically disappear. Instead, you put out the fire and remove the cause of the alarm.

Remember, the amount of pain does not relate to the type of problem or to the severity of the problem. Keep this in mind. A little splinter in your finger can be very painful and yet it's a very minor problem. On the other hand, you could have serious health problems developing in your body and have very, very little pain. Suffice it to say that pain or symptoms alone, or the lack thereof, do not really show one's state of health or sickness. Just because you aren't sick doesn't mean you're healthy.

To treat aging, we don't just treat the symptoms of aging—we treat the cause of aging. Yes, toxins and deficiency affect aging, but now we can turn back the clock of aging by protecting the cells and preserving our telomeres. This is a monumental discovery.

Most scientists now agree that aging is, at least in part, the result of accumulating damage to the molecules—such as proteins, lipids, and nucleic acids (DNA and RNA)—that make up our cells. If enough molecules are damaged, our cells will function less well, our tissues and organs will begin to deteriorate, and our health will decline. We age like our car does: Our parts start to wear out, and we gradually lose the ability to function.

It's important to realize that growing old is a relatively new phenomenon in humans. If you go back only 100 years, or for that matter, 99.9% of the time humans have roamed the Earth, average life expectancies have topped out at 30 or 40 years. The most dramatic leap in life expectancy occurred in the past century with the advent of improved sanitation, nutrition, medical, and alternative care in developed countries. For example, in 1900, the average lifespan in the United States was 47 years, while just a century later it had skyrocketed to 77 years.

In contrast to the average life expectancy, the maximum human life expectancy has always hovered around 115 to 120 years. This apparent inborn maximum intrigues scientists who study aging. Does there have to be a maximum? What determines it?

Our increased lifespan is because our cells are living longer. Cells don't retire as quickly, and we are protecting our cells through antioxidants and other nutrients essential to the cell and the telomere. Some researchers speculate that after cells divide about 50 times, they quit the hard work of dividing and enter a phase in which they no longer behave as they did in their youth.

How do our cells know when to retire? Do we have a clock inside our cells? How does this clock work? We learned through Hayflick, Blackburn, Andrews, and other top scientists that each cell has approximately 92 internal clocks—one at each end of its 46 chromosomes. These ends we know know are the telomeres. Before a cell divides, it copies its chromosomes so that each daughter cell will get a complete set. But because of how the copying is done, the very ends of our long, slender chromosomes don't get copied. It's as if a photocopier cut off the first and last lines of each page. As a result, our chromosomes shorten with each cell division. Once a cell's telomeres shrink to a critical minimum size, the cell takes notice and stops dividing. Telomere health and cell preservation is a key to *Awakening the Wellness Within.*

As we learned throughout this book, life is not just about living longer but about living a healthier and more active life. It's about ageless aging. It's about staying active as the years go by so you can continue to do the things you love. After all, would you really want to reach 100 if you were going to feel 100? At that age, I want you to feel like you're 50 or 60.

In our chapter discussing the history of telomeres, we discussed that in 2009 the Nobel Prize in Physiology for Medicine was awarded for the discovery of how chromosomes are protected by telomeres and the enzyme telomerase. Why a Nobel Prize? Because modern science now knows that the enzyme telomerase extends telomeres, rebuilding them to their former lengths. In most of our cells, the enzyme is turned off before we're born and stays inactive throughout our lives. But theoretically, if turned back on, telomerase could pull cellular retirees back into the workforce. Isn't this what we all want? To live better, longer, healthier, and happier? We can and let me explain how.

According to Wikipedia, "A telomere is a region of repetitive DNA at the end of chromosomes, which protects the end of the chromosome from destruction." Now this may sound complex, but it really isn't. The key to protecting our telomeres is cell division, which is happening as you read this very sentence. It's during our cell division that the enzymes that duplicate the chromosome and its DNA can't continue their duplication all the way to the end of the chromosome. When duplication is not complete, our telomeres will become shorter and we begin to show the characteristics of aging. If cells divided without telomeres, they would lose the end of their chromosomes, and the necessary information it contains. In 1972, James Watson named this phenomenon the "end replication problem."

The telomere, as we learned, is a disposable buffer, which is consumed during cell division and is replenished by the enzyme telomerase. Hopefully by now we understand that the significance of telomeres is that they protect a cell's chromosomes from fusing with each other or rearranging. This is important to our total health as well as our aging. If our cells are not protected, they can become abnormal. These chromosome abnormalities can lead to cancer, so cells are normally destroyed when telomeres are consumed. Most cancer is the result of cells bypassing this destruction. Biologists speculate that this mechanism is a tradeoff between aging and cancer.

Telomeres have been the life's work of many scientists. They brought to the mainstream the importance of telomeres and cellular duplication. Telomeres, which some considered nothing more than a relatively long strand of excess DNA at both ends of every chromosome in the human body, we now know are vital to the health and aging of the cell. Telomeres have an effect on not just aging, but also disease.

Even as we age, our bodies are growing, changing, and replicating. Our cells and our bodies are replicating at an amazing pace—a few billion cells per day. When chromosomes divide and multiply, instead of losing DNA that matters, chromosomes only lose some of the telomere's DNA. The telomeres protect the rest of the DNA and allow it to replicate error free. But what if you could also protect the telomeres and not allow them to shorten?

With each and every replication of our DNA, part of the telomere sequence is chopped off and eliminated. Nature does this to protect the DNA in a chromosome. When telomeres become too short (less than 5,000 base pairs) cells can no longer divide. Then, the cell either enters a state of paralysis called senescence or it simple commits suicide (apoptosis) and dies.

Scientists pursuing genetic engineering reactivated the enzyme in human cells grown in the laboratory. As hoped, the cells multiplied with abandon, continuing well beyond the time when their telomerase-lacking counterparts had stopped.

A telomere as we learned prior, is the part of your DNA chromosome that controls aging. Whenever your DNA multiplies to form a new cell, the telomeres get a little bit shorter. When they get too short, your DNA knows it can't make accurate copies anymore, so the cell stops dividing and dies. The more cells that stop dividing, the older your body acts.

But here's the good news. Your body uses an enzyme called telomerase to rebuild the telomeres at the end of your DNA. Every one of your cells has this enzyme—but it's turned off. If you activate telomerase, you can help slow the aging process in these cells.

Dr. Bill Andrews states, "Obviously, there must be a way for our bodies to re-lengthen telomeres. Otherwise, our sperm and egg cells would contain telomeres the same length as the rest of our cells, which would yield embryos as old as we are. Because so much cell division takes place in the womb, our children would then be born much older than us. Humanity could not exist more than a generation or two if this were the case.

"However, our reproductive cells do not exhibit telomere shortening and show no signs of aging. They are essentially immortal. They are our germ line—the same one that has been dividing since the beginning of life on this planet.

"The reason these cells are immortal is that our reproductive cells produce an enzyme called telomerase. Telomerase acts like an assembly line inside our cells that adds nucleotides to the ends of our chromosomes, thus lengthening our telomeres.

"In a cell that expresses telomerase, telomeres are lengthened as soon as they shorten; it's as though every time the "telomere clock" inside our cells ticks once, telomerase pushes the hands of the clock back one tick.

"Telomerase works by filling the gap left by DNA replication."

Living younger than your years

So how did we learn how to activate telomerase?

According to Dr. Andrews, "Inserting the gene directly into our DNA, through the use of viral vectors, is not a viable option. The main problem with this approach is that inserting genes into cells often causes cancer. That's because the gene gets inserted into our chromosomes at random sites, and if the wrong site is chosen, the gene can interrupt and disable cancer suppressor genes or turn on cancer-inducing genes. And you only need one out of the hundred trillion cells in your body to become cancerous in order to kill you.

Fortunately, the telomerase gene already exists in all our cells. That's because the DNA in every one of our cells is identical: A skin cell, muscle cell, and liver cell all contain exactly the same genetic information. Thus, if the cells that create our sperm and egg cells contain the code for telomerase, every other cell must contain that code as well. The reason that most of our cells don't express telomerase is that the gene is repressed in them. There are one or more regions of DNA neighboring the telomerase gene that serve as binding sites for a protein, and if that protein is bound to them, telomerase will not be created by the cell. However, it is possible to coax that repressor protein off its binding site with the use of a small-molecule, drug-like compound that binds to the repressor and prevents it from attaching to the DNA. If we find the appropriate compound, we can turn telomerase on in every cell in the human body."

TA-65 was developed by the Geron Corporation, utilizing a single unique molecule that's extracted from astragalus, an ancient Chinese herb. According to Wikipedia, "Astragalus propinquus (also known as Astragalus membranaceus) has a history of use as an herbal medicine and is used in traditional Chinese medicine."

The biotechnology firms Geron Corporation and TA Therapeutics of Hong Kong have been working on deriving a telomerase activator from astragalus. The chemical constituent cycloastragenol (also called TAT2) is also being studied to help combat HIV.

In a study published in the November 2008 *Journal of Immunology*, researchers shed light on the antiviral and anti-aging benefits of Astragalus, which we mentioned in our last chapter. In their paper, a team of researchers from the UCLA AIDS Institute described how their work with a new drug derived from astragalus root reduces the aging process of immune cells and enhances how these cells respond to viral infections. The compound works by boosting production of telomerase that allows for the replacement of the short ends of DNA (the telomeres) that play a key role in cell replication, cancer, and human aging.

The astragalus root has been used for centuries to stimulate the creation of new cells to activate and support your immune system. This is important to the aging process as the UCLA study showed astragalus may help prevent your telomeres from shortening. In some cases, preliminary lab studies suggest it may help lengthen telomeres, extending the useful life of those cells.

Researchers tested a group of people and measured the number of white blood cells that looked old and the number that looked young. They then gave them a supplement containing the extract from astragalus. After three months, the participants were found to have a ratio of young-looking cells to old-looking cells that a younger person would have.

In an interview, Dr. Andrews said, "Short telomeres are bad. Short telomeres will cause cancer, so keeping the telomeres long will prevent that cell from becoming a cancer. It is well known that a cell requires eight to ten mutations before it can become a cancer. I believe that most of those mutations are induced by short telomeres. Keeping telomeres long is a way to prevent cancer, and it can also help fight the cancer.

"I believe a telomerase inducer will help you fight cancer. If you already have a cancer, taking a telomerase inducer is not going to help your cancer cells stay immortal, but it will boost your immune system. When the telomeres in immune cells get really short, they lose the ability to fight. But if you take a telomerase inducer, you can keep the telomeres in your immune cells long and maintain the ability of your immune cells to fight the cancer.

"The immune system is actually pretty effective at fighting cancers. This is one of the reasons cancers are a lot more prevalent in the elderly, it's because older people have shorter telomeres in their immune cells.

"The reason reproductive cells are immortal is because they produce the telomerase enzyme which in turns lengthens telomeres as soon as they are shortened. It's as though every time the "telomere clock" inside reproductive cells ticks once, telomerase pushed the hands of the clock back one tick."

The science of telomeres is specific and the facts are in that all of our cells have the potential to produce telomerase, it's just that the genetic code for doing so is repressed.

How to lengthen your telomeres

Research is just starting on this topic. However, scientists have found the following so far:

1. Vigorous exercise. In young people, exercise is not helpful. But in those over about age 40 to 50, short periods of vigorous exercise called the "Peak 8" or other types of vigorous exercise is helpful to slow the process of telomere shortening. Exercise probably helps because it can increase oxygenation, circulation, and hydration in an aging body.

Unfortunately, vigorous exercise has many problems, such as possibly stressing the joints and tendons, and it is somewhat more difficult for older people to do, especially if they are disabled. However, some exercise is helpful for the telomeres.

2. Antioxidant supplements. Scientists have found that antioxidants are extremely important to maintain and grow your telomeres. Go back to our last chapter for a comprehensive review.

3. Reduce oxidant damage. Oxidant damage is one reason for the shortening of the telomeres. This means that anything that can help prevent oxidant damage is helpful to preserve your telomeres.

Anything that increases glutathione is helpful. Selenium, one of my four ACES, is required to make glutathione, along with several amino acids. An excellent idea is to eat plenty of sulfur-containing amino acids. These are found in meats, eggs, cooked green vegetables, and few other foods.

Besides adding antioxidants to your diet, it is equally important to get rid of the oxidants in the body, which are often mineral oxides. This can be done with a nutritional balancing program, but not with most other nutrition, chelation, herbal, homeopathic or other healing programs.

4. Increase yang energy in the body. Another aspect of healing that apparently helps lengthen the telomeres is to make the body more yang. The opposite—making the body more yin—seems to damage the telomeres even more.

This concept is not yet accepted medically. However, personally as chiropractor and acupuncturist, I can tell you the Chinese have understood this for over 5000 years and counting Alternative health care is the primary care of the future and will be appreciated and accepted more in the future.

5. Resolve mental and psychological traumas. This way of lengthening the telomeres, or slowing their shortening, is mentioned in the book *The Immortality Edge*. This book is a research report on telomeres and is a very good read.

Many methods can be used to undo traumas and psychological stress that simply wears out the body faster. Nutritional balancing is a powerful bio-energetic method for releasing all types of traumas; it uses a diet, certain supplements, mild exercise, more rest and sleep, and meditation.

The problem with many stress-release techniques such as vigorous exercise and homeopathy, herbs, vitamins and others, is they have other undesirable effects. This must be recalled at all times when considering these approaches.

6. More rest and sleep. This is also helpful to slow the shortening of the telomeres. The bottom line is you need a lifestyle and nutrition intake that can offset wear and tear and prevent free radical damage.

Nutritional strategies are an important part of your telomere preservation toolbox. The healthier you are, the less you need to do. The worse off your health, the more you need to make changes. Even if you are healthy, general aging takes its toll on your telomeres, and you want to do everything you can to maintain your fitness and health while preserving them. This means that more nutritional support is needed as you grow older, simply as an attempt to minimize the common wear and tear of aging.

7. Avoid processed meats. One study follows the eating habits of 840 people. The ones who ate one or more serving of processed meat per week had 7% shorter telomeres than the rest of the group. Surprisingly, other junk foods in the study, like soda, did not affect telomere length. (But please don't think that makes them okay!) You'll want to avoid anything that comes in a can, lunch meat, and hot dogs. Instead, look for grass-fed meat. It's free of grain, preservatives, and other nasty surprises.

Your lifestyle should be fairly balanced, avoiding known behaviors and substances that cause wear and tear on your cells and speed telomere loss. Our telomeres reflect the vitality of our bodies, which works diligently to keep up with demands and challenges of our everyday life. As cells are bombarded with toxins and remain deficient of nutrients, our telomeres shorten and/or become functionally impaired, thus our body struggles to keep up. When toxins are rampant, damaged cells accumulate in your body, hampering repair processes and accelerating disease and aging. This sets the stage for the early onset of any number of health issues, based on whatever your weak spots may be.

Nutrient or lifestyle intervention that takes stress off of telomeres improves lifespan potential. This is one main reason why antioxidants, which deactivate free radicals, are considered anti-aging nutrients.

The choice is yours. Feed your cells with what they want, what they need, and you have the ability to "Awaken" your "Inner Healer" and *Awaken the Wellness Within*. You better start making lifestyle changes now because your clock is ticking and if you are reading this, time is still on your side.

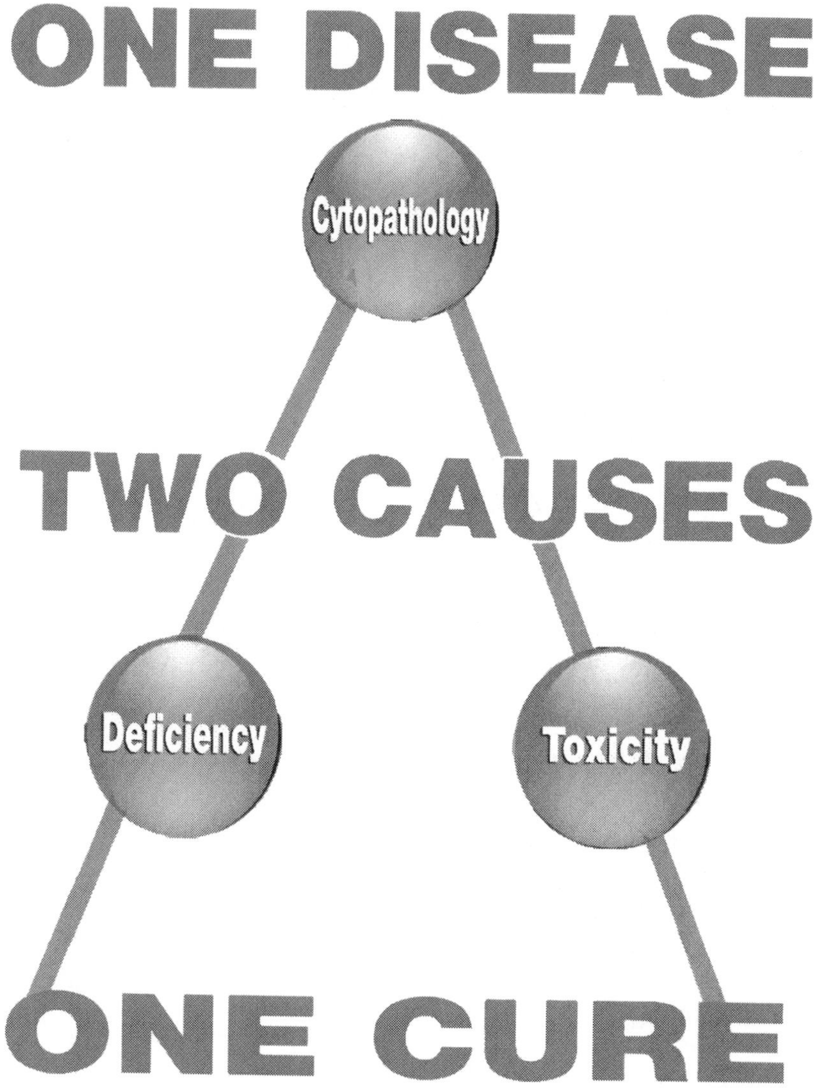
ONE DISEASE
Cytopathology
TWO CAUSES
Deficiency
Toxicity
ONE CURE

"Today, more than 95% of all chronic disease is caused by food choice, toxic food ingredients, nutritional deficiencies, and lack of physical exercise."

—MIKE ADAMS

Chapter 19

<hr/>

THE DISEASE KNOWN AS AGING

Aging is a term we use to define our body's normal aging processes, which contribute to health deterioration and ultimately to death with the passage of time. To *Awaken the Wellness Within*, to age gracefully and healthfully, we must understand the aging process of the cell. To fully understand aging, we must review any and every process that contributes to age-related decline in our body's performance, productivity, or health. Any change in our body's health is often a component of the aging process that deserves our attention and intervention.

You can think of aging as a group of processes responsible for such manifestations as increasing risk of frailty, disability, morbidity (for age-related degenerative diseases in particular), and ultimately increasing mortality rates.

In Greek mythology, the prince Tithonus's wife prayed to Zeus to grant him eternal life, but forgot to specify that she would also like him to receive eternal youth. So she was cursed to watch him grow impossibly old, withering away further every day, until finally his frail and desiccated body was transformed into a cicada.

This is a potent illustration of a misconception some people have about aging. When some people hear about research to cure aging, they look horrified and ask "You plan to keep people immortal, just getting older and sicker forever?" Some people see old age as something that will kill you if you avoid all the other diseases, that if you can make it through your 70s and 80s without succumbing to heart disease or cancer or any other number of ailments, then and only then will you have old age to contend with. This book proves that is not the case any longer.

Aging does not have to be a merciful release from the natural decline of our bodies during the aging process. Nothing could be further from the truth. Aging is a disease that has been slowly eating away at all of us since we were a tiny embryo, since the embryonic stem cells that once comprised our body first began to differentiate. Now we can make a choice how we age. We have learned throughout the last few chapters that Drs. Andrews and Blackburn, along with some of the world's scientific leaders work on telomerase, has shown that you can extend both the quality and quantity of your life. We have learned our cells are the key to our future.

Most doctor's view that disease later in life is simply the natural result of a lifetime of wear and tear on the body and this is partially true. It is clear to me and hopefully you that now telomere evidence shows us that often our choices of food, diet, and exercise also affect the rate at which we age. We now know that if we protect the cell and protect and lengthen our telomeres, we can live a healthier and longer life.

My opinion is that the biggest causes of aging are:

- Excessive consumption of all sugars and artificial sweeteners
- Environmental toxins
- Smoking
- Lack of exercise
- Vitamin deficiency
- Refined and processed foods (contain harmful chemicals that can cause premature aging through disease and illness)
- Chronic stress and inflammation
- Free radical damage
- Poor nerve supply

- Bad spinal health
- Elevated homocystine levels (caused by a lack of B6, B12, and folate)
- Telomere shortening (caused by free radicals and toxins)

We only have One Disease and Two Causes. It doesn't take an organism 60, 70, or 80 years to develop a cancer or heart disease. Mice tend to get cancer after just two or three years and our household pets tend to develop these kinds of maladies near the end of their species and their breed's lifespan. Disease develops over time due to weakening and malfunctioning cells—a malfunction caused by either too many toxins or too great a deficiency for the cells to overcome. Disease does not simply happen, it manifests.

Several studies have shown that mean leukocyte telomere length is a more accurate risk factor for disease than chronological age. It's clear that the way our bodies break down with age is not a passive process, like a car that's been driven too many miles. It is an active process.

We've learned that if we take better care of our cars, change the oil, etc., we can extend its life significantly. Let's do the same for our bodies. Why do we so often take better care of our cars then we do our bodies?

If we care for our cell, protect our telomeres, and turn on our telomerase, good things will happen. Turning telomerase on in the human body affects far more than just our lifespan. It has a beneficial effect on practically every disease you can think of, from heart disease to Alzheimer's.

Why do human beings have an aging process?

After years of research, science is beginning to uncover just what the aging process is, what it does, why we have it. And the more that is learned, the more all the evidence points to the conclusion that yes, aging is something we can eliminate.

Aging is something we all do but understand very little. We could list things that change as we age (memory loss, wrinkles, muscles loss, balance trouble, etc.) but no one really understands what aging is, why it happens, or how to stop it. Aging, then, is the impact of time on our bodies.

Let's review:

Cellular Aging: Cells' age based on the number of times they have replicated. A cell can replicate around 50 times before the genetic material is no longer able to be copied accurately because of the shortening of telomeres. The more damage to your cells (through toxin, deficiency, free radicals, and other factors), the more your cells need to replicate.

Hormonal Aging: Without a doubt, hormones play a big factor in aging, especially in childhood growth and adolescent maturity. Hormone levels change through life, leading to menopause and other age-related changes.

Accumulated Damage: Toxins, deficiencies, the UV radiation from sunlight, harmful foods, pollution, and other toxins all take their toll on our bodies. Over time, these toxins can lead to tissue damage and the body falls behind in maintaining and repairing your cells, tissues, and organs.

Metabolic Aging: As you go through your day, your cells are turning food into energy, which produces byproducts that can be harmful. This process of metabolizing and creating energy results in damage to your body over time. Some believe that slowing the metabolic process (through practices such as calorie restriction) may slow aging in humans.

Our body is a complex of specialized cells that cooperates to accomplish basic tasks of life: move, eat, digest, make energy to run on, reproduce, and die. This tremendous array of cells has an equally vast spread of life spans. One cell may last a day, another a lifetime.

"The fully differentiated neutrophil dies within a day," says Gail Sullivan, assistant research professor of medicine at the University of Virginia Health Science Center. Neutrophils are white blood cells that find, engulf, and destroy foreign microbes.

Red blood cells, on the other hand, last longer—120 days for humans. They cannot, however, reproduce themselves. That's the price these cells pay for specialization. They must rely on another kind of cell (undifferentiated stem cells) to replace dead red blood cells.

And that brings us to an example of a long-living cell: Stem cells last a lifetime, maintaining a lifelong supply of both red and white blood cells for an individual. When cells die, they replace themselves, but will an unhealthy cell replace itself with a totally healthy cell? No, we must preserve and maintain our cells as we do our cars.

What's the "natural" life span of a car? Most cars last about 100,000 to 150,000 miles before they become more trouble than they're worth and their owners throw them away. I drove my last car 125,000 miles and it still had life left in it because I took very good care of it. You can replace every part of your car as it goes bad, and cars can continue to function after 50 years and a million miles. There's no theoretical limit—if you're willing to maintain a car forever, it will last forever.

You don't have the luxury of saying your body has become more trouble than it's worth and you want to trade it in for a new model. We have one body, and we're stuck with it. The good news is that there's no reason it can't last longer and be more productive with monitored maintenance. If you accept that there is one disease and one cure, you can maintain your body and revitalize your cells, which will repair your telomeres. No one wants to age prematurely, but it's okay to age if we age with grace, dignity, and health.

We are all born undamaged, and every day we're alive on earth, we're vulnerable to accumulate damage. We eat, drink, and breathe toxins, we abuse the sun, we take too many drugs—life puts pressure on our bodies. Every step we take puts strain on our bones and muscles and eventually we break down if we do not take care of ourselves.

This is exactly how a car ages. Drive it for 10 years with no maintenance, and it will accumulate damage until it breaks down. If you keep a car in a cool garage, however, it won't age as fast. You can wheel it out thirty years later, and although you might have to change the battery, it will run fine. But does this analogy extend to humans, too? I want to be a classic. I want to play with my grand-children, not just watch them play. I want to continue to hit greens in regulation; I don't want to play the senior tees.

Aging and disease

Obviously, non-age-related diseases do exist in childhood and early adulthood, but the majority of the time we don't get cancer or heart disease simply because something in the human machine broke. We get cancer because our bodies received a signal to stop fixing things as they break. That signal is telomere shortening and bad things happen when telomeres get short. The litany of diseases that are more common at age 80 than at age of 20 are all very good examples of those "bad things."

Keeping telomeres long could be a treatment or a cure for most of the worst ravages of age we humans face. It is not an exaggeration to say that it could be the beginning of medical science providing humans with a disease-free existence on earth.

You can observe that elderly individuals are at a higher risk for a vast range of degenerative and infectious diseases than younger indi-viduals. The hypothesis that controlling telomere length could treat most, if not all, of this wide variety of diseases has not been proven false and is supported by the scientific literature. Essentially, it may be possible for an 80-year-old to be no more susceptible to disease in general than a 20-year-old.

The bottom line here is that environmental damage along with nutritional deficiencies can accelerate aging, but telomere shortening and damage are not independent actors. Free radical damage causes telomere shortening; telomere shortening causes free radical damage. They work like two gears pushing against each other—turn one gear and the other turns as well. In other words, solve the cell problem, the telomere problem, and you may literally be returning to the same low risk of disease that you enjoyed in your 30s. You can do this by making lifestyle changes, exercising; meditating by adding antioxidants to your diet to offset the free radical damage. You will commence to *Awaken the Wellness Within*.

Cardiovascular disease

The relationship between heart disease and telomere length has been studied extensively. Heart disease is the most common cause of death in the Western world. To offset heart disease, our omega-3 fatty acids are vital to protecting our cell, and thus our telomeres. Scientists have been highly interested in studying its association with telomere length and unfortunately, there is no short supply of patients to study:

- A pilot study in 2001 found evidence that patients with severe chronic artery disease had shorter telomeres in their blood cells—about 300 base pairs shorter than patients without the disease. Their telomeres were equivalent in size to individuals 8.6 years older.
- In a broader study in 2003, the telomeres in patients who had suffered a heart attack were measured. On average, they were as short as individuals 11.3 years older. The study additionally concluded that individuals with the shortest telomeres for their age had about a three times higher risk of heart attack than individuals with the longest telomeres.

- A 2007 study on about 500 individuals with heart disease showed that average telomere length in blood cells is a reliable predictor of coronary heart disease. The risk for heart disease in individuals with the shortest telomeres was nearly double the risk of individuals with longer telomeres, regardless of their biological age.

It has been established beyond any doubt that short telomeres are a risk factor for cardiovascular disease. It stands to reason that inducing telomerase could prevent, and possibly treat, cardiovascular disease. Cardiovascular disease is just another symptom of aging. Cure the disease; cure the symptom.

Chronic obstructive pulmonary disease (COPD)

Just as with cardiovascular disease, a French study in 2009 reported that patients with COPD had significantly shorter average telomere lengths than either non-smokers or smokers without COPD. This study reconfirms the correlation between short telomeres and a disease. But correlation is not causation; just because two things occur together doesn't mean that one caused the other. So, the question arises: Do short telomeres cause COPD or does COPD cause short telomeres? Or does some third factor cause them both?

Short telomeres are a risk factor for COPD, and it's probably not much of a stretch to say that short telomeres are a likely cause of COPD. If that's true, control of telomere lengths could prevent or reverse this condition, even for smokers.

Degenerative disc disease and other degenerative diseases

I am honored to be the co-chairman of the International Medical Advisory Board on Spinal Decompression. The honorary chairman, Dr. Norman Shealy MD, a neurosurgeon who taught at Harvard

Medical School and the developer of the Tens unit is probably the most published in the world on this modality. Studying under him and his works has been life changing and am honored to teach at Parker University in Dallas Texas, as an adjunct professor. What is more exciting is that my son, Dr. Jason Kaplan, teaches along with myself and Dr. Perry Bard.

Daily, we are learning that cell health has an affect on our bones and our pain. Discs consist of 87% water. Doesn't it make sense to keep those with back cases hydrated?

Avoiding toxins and abnormal stress will help keep our telomeres long as well as keep our bones healthy, which should allow us to be more athletic at any age. In 2007, a University of Manchester study established that the telomere length of disc cells decreased with every progressive stage of disc degeneration, and hypothesized that degenerative disc disease is caused by cellular senescence as a result of telomere shortening. This is exciting news and along with chiropractic care shows that back pain can now be treated and controlled. I am so excited about this subject I have written an entire chapter on it.

I have had back issues, it really does seem like one of those "wear and tear" diseases; but thanks to spinal decompression and chiropractic I am jogging and golfing again.

But all you have to do is look to other animals to realize that it doesn't take decades for a spine to wear out. Dogs that are genetically susceptible to degenerative disc disease tend to show symptoms, on average, by the time they're seven years old. Have you ever seen a seven-year-old human child with a bad back? Since I started taking Product B from Isagenix, my back has improved. Now some would say it is in my head, but it's definitely in my back.

The American Association of Neurological Surgeons in an article titled, "High-Dose Omega-3 Oils used to Treat Non-Surgical Neck and Back Pain Doctors Guide," by Cameron Johnston reported, "Investigators at the University of Pittsburgh have treated chronic pain patients with high doses of omega-3 fatty acids—the ingredient found in many cold-water fish species such as salmon. The researchers say their findings suggest that this could be the answer to the adverse effects seen with non-steroidal anti-inflammatory drugs (NSAIDs), including cyclooxygenase (COX)-2 inhibitors, which have been associated with potentially catastrophic adverse effects."

One study I touched on earlier was by Dr. Joseph Maroon, neurosurgeon and specialist in degenerative spine disease at the University of Pittsburgh, who reported the findings April 19th at the 73rd meeting of the American Association of Neurological Surgeons. Patients who took high doses of omega-3 oils were impressed enough with the outcomes that they chose to continue using the oils and forego the use of NSAIDs. The 250 study patients suffered from chronic neck or back pain but were not surgical candidates, and they had been using daily doses of NSAIDs. After 75 days of taking high doses of omega-3s, 59% had stopped taking prescription drugs from their pain, and 88% said they were pleased enough with the outcomes that they planned to continue using the fish oils. No significant adverse effects were reported.

In addition to the degenerative diseases discussed previously, short telomeres have been identified as a risk factor for osteoarthritis, rheumatoid arthritis, osteoporosis, macular degeneration, liver cirrhosis, and idiopathic pulmonary fibrosis. These days, it seems like not a week goes by when some lab isn't confirming the theory that diseases of aging are actually symptoms of the disease of aging. They're saying, "Hey, you know this disease that's often associated with the elderly? Well, we're seeing shortened telomeres." The good news is we can reverse disease by increasing the length of our telomeres.

Alzheimer's disease

Alzheimer's disease is arguably one of the diseases most closely associated with the physical and mental deterioration that occurs toward the end of life. Scientists have naturally been interested to see what role, if any, telomere shortening plays.

Researchers at the University of Adelaide in 2007 compared the telomere lengths in several different kinds of cells in Alzheimer's patients to those of age-matched controls without Alzheimer's. They observed significantly lower telomere lengths in several cell types, including white blood cells, but higher telomere lengths in hippocampus cells. The researchers concluded that Alzheimer's was related to important differences in the mechanisms of telomere maintenance. A 2009 study similarly showed an association between Alzheimer 's disease and shorter mean leukocyte telomere length.

There does appear to be a relationship between Alzheimer's disease and telomere length, but this one hasn't seemed like as much of a slam-dunk as other disease targets. I'm not as confident saying, "If you lengthen telomeres, you'll probably cure it." However, one very promising study suggesting that lengthening telomeres could treat brain disease comes in the form of Dr. DePinho's study at Harvard Medical School. In that study it was determined that when mice were forced to age due to artificial telomere shortening, their brain weight shrunk. When telomeres were lengthened by turning on telomerase, their brains grew back to a normal size.

If the same thing happens in humans, would it cure Alzheimer 's disease? It's too soon to say, but it seems possible that telomerase could be part, if not all, of the solution.

Infectious diseases

Infectious diseases are not typically thought of as diseases of aging. When we're talking about AIDS, we're talking about a disease that a 20-year-old can get just as easily as an 80-year-old. So how can it be possible that this is a disease of aging?

There is evidence that AIDS is a disease of aging in that it ages the body incredibly quickly. When we get an infection, the cells of the immune system spring into action, dividing rapidly. They divide at a rate rarely seen in any other system of the body. For this reason, chronic or latent infections, or any virus that hangs around in the bloodstream for a long time can cause premature aging of the immune system, reducing its capacity to fight disease, much like psychological stress can.

This phenomenon has been observed in studies of HIV-positive patients who displayed significantly shorter telomeres in their CD8+ T cells than healthy individuals. In studies of identical twins, this held true compared to the patients' HIV-negative twins. HIV shortens the telomeres of the immune system

HIV is a virus; AIDS is a disease. So when does HIV become AIDS? That transformation occurs when immune cells lose their ability to fight the HIV infection, allowing symptoms to start manifesting for the first time. The studies on HIV and telomere length suggest that the reason our immune cells lose the ability to fight back is the result of replicative senescence in the immune system. In other words, our white blood cells fight back so hard and divide so frequently that they age themselves to death. They go through generation after generation after generation of cell division, until they've divided more times than a white blood cell typically divides in the lifespan of a centenarian.

So, inducing telomerase in the immune system holds the promise of preventing HIV from ever developing into AIDS. If white blood cells can divide forever, they can be essentially locked in an eternal struggle with HIV, which is not exactly an ideal situation. But it is certainly better than having the struggle end with HIV crowned the victor.

The idea of an immune system aging itself to death isn't limited to HIV. Lengthening telomeres won't cure the common cold, but it is well known that catching a cold as a teenager is very different than catching a cold when you're very old. In an elderly individual, a simple head cold can drag on for weeks or months, and can even be life-threatening. Restoring telomeres to their youthful state could make a cold at age 90 no more of an inconvenience than a cold at age 20.

Diminished wound healing

It is common knowledge that our capacity for wound healing decreases as we age. A cut that would have disappeared in days when we were young gradually takes longer and longer to close and heal. Wound healing requires a lot of cell division; the longer telomeres are, the more efficiently the body can perform that cell division. Experiments on telomerase-deficient mice confirm that shortened telomeres reduce the capacity for wound healing. So, control of telomere length would almost certainly increase the healing capacity of the aged, presumably restoring it to what it was when the individual was young.

For the same reason, therapies that prevent telomere shortening could prove vital to the success of tissue transplants in the elderly. In a proof of concept experiment in 2000, scientists at the Baylor College of Medicine artificially "telomerized" cow tissue, splicing the telomerase gene into the DNA of the tissue. They then transplanted the cow tissue into the kidney capsules of immunodeficient mice. The mice survived, the transplant was successful, and there were no indications of malignant transformation of the tissue.

Along similar lines, skin aging is thought to be controlled primarily by progressive telomere shortening. It is likely that control of telomere length could stop skin aging dead in its tracks. Whether such a therapy could reverse the appearance of aging in a living human being is unknown, but there is hope. Experiments by Geron Corporation made skin cells more youthful by the introduction of the telomerase gene, providing evidence that such a therapy may be possible.

Of course, this would be the biggest revolution in the history of cosmetics—the ability for anyone, of any age, to revert to the exact appearance they had when they were young. This is just another indicator of the massive size of the market for telomerase-inducing drugs. A product like this could put every anti-aging skin cream out of business overnight.

Congenital disorders

A congenital disorder is, by definition, a disease that you're born with, meaning that congenital disorders really cannot be diseases of aging. But several congenital genetic disorders are characterized by prematurely short telomeres, including muscular dystrophy, progeria, dyskeratosis congenita, Fanconi's anemia, tuberous sclerosis, and Werner syndrome. Maternal telomere length has also been associated with the prevalence of Down syndrome. It is still unknown whether inducing telomerase could treat and/or cure any or all of these conditions, but it is not unreasonable to hypothesize that such a therapy could be beneficial. These are all tragic diseases that affect the very young, and we would all like to see them cured.

Some of us seem to attempt to preserve themselves better than others. I live in Florida and people stay active here. They walk, go to the gym, the beach, or the golf course. They stay active, and they age better as a result. Yet we all know people who spend the majority of their lives lying on a couch in an air-conditioned room, watching television and eating potato chips. The body is different than a car. It likes activity. Running a car for too many miles shortens its lifespan, but keeping a human in motion lengthens our lifespan.

If the "everyone ages the same" theory were correct, then people from different parts of the world would all look and act the same the same age. Generally, most of us are able to look at someone and place their age within ten years. Humans age at a consistent, steady rate, not one determined by our environment. The key is to age healthily and happily.

Dr. Kaplan's Top Ten Tips for Healthy Aging

1. No Smoking
2. Maintain a positive attitude
3. Cleanse daily
4. Exercise daily
5. Practice healthy sleep habits
6. Reduce stress. This is not always easy, but finding ways to solve the cause of stress in your life is absolutely necessary.
7. Take antioxidants, omega-3s, vitamins, minerals, and other quality nutrients that fight aging and support your body.
8. Get enough protein. Shakes are allowed daily to replace meals low in nutrition and protein. It's proven that nutrient density and low caloric intake is helpful in slowing aging and ensuring proper weight control. Adkins is one company whom I utilize.
9. Drink eight, 8-ounce glasses of water minimum per day.
10. Get regular chiropractic adjustments to remove nerve deficiency.

"Now there are more overweight people in America than average-weight people. So overweight people are now average. Which means you've met your New Year's resolution."

—Jay Leno

Chapter 20

CELLULAR CLEANSING

If your cells are toxic, you need to cleanse them. I shower my cells daily. When you hear the word cleanse, the most popular forms of cleansing are what probably come to mind: a liver flush or a colon cleanse. If you're doing either of these, you better hope you work from home because the toilet will become your best friend—and I don't mean that in a good way. I'm happy to tell you that cellular cleansing is neither of those. A healthy cleanse cleanses the whole body, instead of just one organ, and its benefits far exceed those of a colon or liver cleanse

Cellular cleansing accelerates the removal of toxins and impurities from the body's cells. Remember, there are 50 to 100 trillion cells in the human body. If you were to count one number per second, it would take you over 31,000 years to count to 1 trillion, so 50 to 100 trillion is almost unimaginable. When you cleanse your colon or your liver, you're merely cleansing one area of the body. A whole body cellular cleanse, however, does just what the name implies—it removes toxins from the whole body instead of just one organ. Most people can attest to feeling better after just one organ is cleansed. Imagine what a whole body cleanse can do. Not only does a good cleanse rid the body of impurities; it also replenishes each one of those 50 to 100 trillion cells with vital nutrients to rapidly revive your body's health

When toxins enter the body, it wraps fat around them to protect itself from long-term cellular damage. It's no wonder people have so much trouble losing weight and keeping it off. These toxins not only contribute to fat buildup and obesity, they also contribute to decreased levels of energy and mental clarity, as well as to the many health problems that we as a nation face more and more each day.

The ultimate long-term benefits of cellular cleansing:

- The liberation of the body's own natural healing mechanisms
- Body systems are restored to their perfect state and are free from disorders
- Internal acidic and alkaline environment of the body is balanced
- Natural vibrant energy returns
- Weight is balanced
- Radiate skin tone and strong healthy hair is visible
- Excess fat cells begin to deflate as the acidic waste is released

Kaplan's Daily Cell Detox

- **Drink water.** Pure, clean water with lemon helps flush out unwanted toxins. It is important to drink the proper amount of water per your body weight. Remember, 8 glasses of water for a man who weigh 300lbs is extremely low. On the same token 8 glasses of water a day for a man who weighs 125lbs is too much. To determine the amount of water you need to drink a day, simply divide your body weight in half. The answer is the amount you need to drink in ounces every day.
- **Eat a healthy cleansing detox diet.** A natural body detox cleansing diet provides cellular nutrition to your trillions of cells. All cells require quality protein, essential fatty acids found in whole grains, nuts, seeds, extra virgin olive oil, and omega-3 fish oil from cold-water fish like salmon, tuna, mackerel, and snapper. To ensure that toxins don't build up

in your system, include plenty of fresh vegetables, raw fruit, beans, whole grains, and other nutritious high-fiber foods for better elimination.

- **Exercise and stretch your body daily.** Regular physical activity helps you to detox naturally. At least a half-hour of daily exercise and stretching will improve blood circulation, burn calories to break down toxins stored in fat cells, and help you to excrete toxic residue through sweat.

- **Stimulate your skin to detox naturally.** Massage can boost your lymphatic system to naturally detoxify your body. I love my massages and get at least one per week. Drink water afterwards to increase toxin elimination. Dry brushing skin before bathing can also improve circulation and stimulate natural body detox cleansing.

- **Sweat for perspiration waste elimination.** Besides daily physical activity, saunas and warm baths with Epsom salts or sea salt can be used to induce sweating and eliminate toxins and heavy metals.

- **Reduce stress.** Since hanging on to negative thoughts and feelings can be toxic too, it's important to focus on positive thinking and behavior. Even crying is a way to naturally detoxify. I suggest meditation, visualization, self-hypnosis, and yoga to release stress.

With these tips you can give yourself the gift of health by helping your body detox naturally.

Green tea and Telomere length

Dr. Andrew Weil, when asked about green tea and telomeres, reported: "A recent a study in Hong Kong suggested that people who drink green tea regularly may be younger, biologically, than those who don't drink green tea or consume only small amounts. The science here is somewhat complex, so bear with me while I summarize this fascinating new study. The researchers looked at the length of telomeres, repeating DNA sequences at the ends of chromosomes. (One expert suggests thinking about telomeres as the caps on the ends of shoelaces that prevent the laces from unraveling.) In cells, telomeres prevent chromosomes from fusing with one another or rearranging—undesirable changes that could lead to cancer and other life-threatening diseases.

"Research has shown that as cells replicate and age, telomeres get shorter and shorter and that when telomeres finally disappear, the cells can no longer replicate. Some experts have suggested that the length of telomeres may be a marker for biological aging. The shorter your telomeres, the "older" you are. Earlier studies have suggested that telomeres are highly susceptible tooxidative stress.

"Now, for the Hong Kong study findings: researchers looked at telomere lengths of 976 Chinese men and 1,030 Chinese women, all over the age of 65. All the study participants completed a food frequency questionnaire.

"The researchers reported that telomere length was associated only with tea drinking – participants with the highest intake, three cups per day of tea, had longer telomeres than participants who drank an average of only one quarter of a cup of tea daily. Most participants drank green tea while a few drank black tea. The investigators reported that the average difference in telomere length corresponded to "approximately a difference of five years of life" and that the "antioxidative properties of tea and its constituent nutrients may protect telomeres from oxidative damage in the normal aging process." The study was published online on August 12, 2009.

A group of scientists, led by Ruth Chan, noted an association between green tea drinkers and longer telomeres. This was reported by scientists from the Chinese University of Hong Kong last year. In a study published in the *British Journal of Nutrition*, the researchers said that telomeres of people who drank an average of three cups of tea per day were about 0.46 kilobases longer than people who drank an average of a quarter of a cup a day.

Dr. Chan and her scientists stated, "This average difference in the telomere length corresponds to "approximately a difference of five years of life."

There are so many supplements that aid our cells. A nutrient like curcumin, mentioned above, is being extensively studied for its ability to help repair DNA, especially epigenetic malfunction, and prevent and help treat cancer, making it one of the best documented nutrients you could take.

If our body is deficient, our cells malfunction, where do we begin? We begin with a good multi-vitamin formulation. Each of the mechanisms by which these nutrients and bioactives work in harmony may help explain why taking multivitamins is associated with longer telomere length.

With the large number of recent studies attributing the shortening of telomeres to aging, Ligi Paul, PhD, of the USDA Human Nutrition Research Center on Aging at Tufts University, has reviewed the types of nutrients that may influence telomere length. "Of interest to nutritionists, telomere length has been shown to be associated with nutritional status in human and animal studies. Healthy lifestyles and diets are positively correlated with telomere length," Dr. Paul wrote.

"Twelve different vitamins, minerals and bioactives have been identified to enhance telomere protection and keep aging at bay. They include the B vitamins folate and B12, niacin, vitamin A, vitamin D (which lowers levels of CRP, a harmful protein), vitamins C and E (which limit oxidative stress to telomeres), magnesium (which is a required mineral for DNA replication and repair), zinc, iron (which is only good in small doses), the spice turmeric and omega-3 fatty acids (which both stimulate antioxidants), and polyphenols (from grape seeds and green tea, which also protect DNA from oxidative stress)."

"Those who take multivitamins," Dr. Paul notes, "are also more likely to follow a healthy lifestyle. For example, they are more likely to combine a diet high in fruits and vegetables with exercise, to not smoke, and to maintain a healthy weight—factors all associated with longer telomeres. Since diet and lifestyle can influence inflammation, oxidative stress and psychological stress, all of which cause telomere attrition [shortening], they could also influence telomere length."

We now know that short telomeres are reflective of a "worn out" DNA repair and rejuvenation capacity that increases risk for cancer and heart disease. The key is not to let the cells become worn out. This is why it is so important to understand how and why antioxidants will help the cell. We will focus on the value of antioxidants throughout the remainder of this book.

One study I found very interesting tracked 662 people from childhood until age 38, measuring their HDL levels (the protective form of cholesterol). Those with the highest HDL levels had the longest telomeres. The researchers believed this was due to less cumulative inflammatory and free radical damage in their life up to this mid-life point. This study shows that a low HDL level is not only predictive of a longer-term lifestyle of not being healthy, but also of the toll those health issues have taken on telomeres. Of course, any chronic health problem has increased inflammation and free radical damage as features and is likely to be associated with shorter telomeres, as has been demonstrated for COPD (chronic obstructive pulmonary disease).

The bottom line is that you need a lifestyle and nutrition intake that can offset wear and tear and prevent free radical damage. Nutritional anti-inflammation strategies are an important part of your telomereA telomere is a repeating sequence of DNA at the end of a chromosome. Each time a cell replicates and divides the telomere loses some of its length. Eventually the telomere runs out and the cell can no longer divide and rejuvenate, triggering a poor state of cell health that contributes to disease risk and eventual cell death. preservation toolbox. The healthier you are, the less you need to do. The worse your health, the more you need to make changes. Even if you are healthy, aging is taking its toll on your telomeres and you want to do everything you can to maintain your fitness and health while preserving them. This means that more nutritional supported is suggested as you grow older simply as an attempt to minimize the common wear and tear of aging.

Every cell in our body generates waste that must be removed to preserve normal function. This process is called autophagy and is known to decline in efficiency as we age.

When excess cellular debris is allowed to accumulate in our cells, normal function is altered and the cell begins to deteriorate. This paves the way for accelerated aging and chronic illnesses including many cancer lines and neurological disorders such as Alzheimer's disease.

Cutting edge research underscores the importance of natural nutrients such as resveratrol and curcumin, and a diet rich in berries and leafy greens to induce autophagy and lower the risks associated with premature aging. Here's a summary of what some of the recent research has shown.

3 simple ways to cleanse your cells

1. Resveratrol triggers natural cellular housekeeping.

Resveratrol is a powerful nutrient that has been shown to directly influence genes that regulate metabolic mechanisms and promote longevity. In addition to mimicking the effect of calorie restriction, resveratrol is emerging as a compound that can be used to assist the removal of cellular debris and improve efficiency.

The result of a study published in the *Impact Journal on Aging* demonstrates how resveratrol triggers autophagy in otherwise dormant cells. Resveratrol is shown to activate a series of proteins known as SIRT 1 that protect the delicate functional structures within the cell body and stimulate waste removal. This action effectively sets off a chain of events that leads to improved cellular efficiency and anti-aging characteristics. This is my wifes and my personal favorite. Who knew a cellular cleanse could be so much fun?

2. Curcumin is a powerful anti-cancer agent.

We talked about tumeric and curcumin earlier. Curcumin has a long history as an effective weapon in the fight against cancer and as an anti-aging nutrient. Derived from curry powder, curcumin has been shown to initiate normal cell death in abnormal cancer cells in a process called apoptosis. The nutrient works on cellular DNA to stimulate the removal of waste debris and can target precancerous tumor cells to undergo programmed destruction.

Information published in the *British Journal of Cancer* explains that curcumin targets several death pathways in cancer cells that can become disabled, allowing uncontrolled growth and proliferation. Researchers found the turmeric extract to be particularly effective in cancers of the digestive tract and esophagus and concluded, "it is likely that curcumin and indeed some of its bioavailability-enhanced analogues are realistic options to be considered in the future for targeted molecular cancer prevention and treatment."

3. Berries and leafy greens found to be neuroprotective.

Blueberries, strawberries, and spinach are natural foods that exhibit a strong protective shield to the aging brain. An analysis published in *The Journal of Neuroscience* demonstrates the capacity of these super foods to induce autophagy. Berries and leafy greens are packed with polyphenols and anthocyanins that convey powerful antioxidant and anti-inflammatory properties to these foods.

The study authors found that compounds in berries and spinach were able to cross the blood-brain barrier and directly influence the functional capacity of neurons. The lead study author noted that the findings from this research suggest that nutritional intervention with fruits and vegetables may play an important role in reversing the deleterious effects of aging on neuronal function and behavior.

Cellular housekeeping is an essential task that determines our rate of aging and risk of developing chronic disease. In addition to proper diet and regular exercise, health-minded individuals can take advantage of natural nutrients such as resveratrol and curcumin and foods like berries and spinach to maximize cellular autophagy and extend our natural lifespan.

Telomeres reflect the vitality your body displays to keep up with demands and challenges. As telomeres shorten and/or or become functionally impaired, your cells struggle to do their jobs. In this situation, damaged molecules accumulate in your body and repair processes are hampered—aging is accelerated. This sets the stage for cellular malfunction and the early onset of poor health, making disease is more likely as the quality of health and energy declines. Good health and anti-aging is for everyone, not just for the old people. The earlier we begin, the better our cells grow and the longer our telomeres stay. Keeping your body healthy is easy when you know how and why. Remember, there is only One Disease, Two Causes, and One Cure. Now we know the formula that can help our innate healing powers combat disease and assist our bodies in building healthy, happy cells, while maintaining and supporting our telomeres.

"Our bodies are our gardens—
our wills are our gardeners."

—WILLIAM SHAKESPEARE

Chapter 21

HEALING AND HELPING
OUR CELLS

I n life, we never want to "cell" ourselves short. You may look at that as a pun, but there is truth in those words. If we could stop our telomeres from shrinking after cell division, we could slow down the aging process and protect ourselves from disease. There are a number of ways to do that, yet so many people aren't doing it. What would you pay for even one more year of life? You must pay the price by protecting your cells, and we do this by promoting the production of telomerase, the enzyme that makes telomeres in the body. With telomerase you can naturally—without drugs, surgery, or chemicals—slow the rate of telomere degradation, and we even know how to reverse it. In other words, if short telomeres are the problem, then telomerase is the answer. In the laboratory, scientists daily continue to "awaken cells" by introducing telomerase into cells in tissue culture with the objective of extending the length of telomeres. Some results have had cells dividing for 250 generations past the time they normally would stop dividing. They are continuing to divide normally, giving rise to normal cells with the normal number of chromosomes. Once we have the ability to extend our telomeres with telomerase, the mortal cell begins to become immortal. By awakening our cells we *Awaken the Wellness Within.*

Dr. Blackburn, recently published, along with her colleagues at the University of California, San Francisco, a study that showed intakes of the omega-3 fatty acids DHA (docosahexaenoic acid) and EPA (eicosapentaenoic acid) protect telomere length in people with cardiovascular disease.

The study, which was published in the January 2010 edition of *the Journal of American Medical Association*, looked at telomere length in blood cells of 608 outpatients with stable coronary artery disease. The length of telomeres was measured at the start of the study and again after 5 years. The researchers compared levels of DHA and EPA with subsequent change in telomere length. The researchers found that individuals with the lowest average levels of DHA and EPA experienced the most rapid rate of telomere shortening, while people with the highest average blood levels experienced the slowest rate of telomere shortening.

During their research, they primarily looked at the immune system, and more specifically at leukocytes (white blood cells). These cells play a critical role in protecting the human body against microbes, bacteria, and viruses.

Cellular health is the place to begin, as health and aging relate to the health of the cell. If we can heal the cell, we can age better and more naturally. I recommend the following:

Lifestyle Change—Positive lifestyle changes may also prevent telomere shortening. These include proper nutrition, weight control, stress reduction, exercise, the withdrawal of substances of abuse (simple sugar, tobacco, alcohol, illicit drugs), elimination of unnecessary prescriptions and over the counter medications, and the restoration of normal sleep patterns.

Dietary Supplements—There are a number of nutraceuticals associated with supporting telomere structure and function, including: extracts of ginkgo biloba, astragalus, ginger root, vitamins B, C, D,

E, folate, folic acid, and B12, CoQ10, selenium, chromium, nicotinamide, and omega-3 fatty acids. Current studies clearly prove that taking a basic multivitamin or antioxidant may be associated with enhanced telomere length or prevention of telomere shortening. This alone is a good place to begin.

Life is about choices. By making better choices and developing healthier habits, you can avoid largely preventable chronic diseases such as diabetes and heart disease. You can avoid smoking and obesity, which are risk factors for cardiovascular disease and other diseases that are the leading causes of death in the U.S.

You can avoid not only catastrophic diseases and premature death, but also financial devastation. Americans making healthy lifestyle changes can soften the blow of high healthcare costs in the U.S. This can save millions of lives and billions of dollars in healthcare costs.

When toxic foods and stimulants are suddenly stopped, headaches are common and a letdown occurs. These sources in excess put stress on the body and are viewed as toxins to the body or stressors. This is due to the body discarding toxins like caffeine and theobromine that are removed from the tissues and transported through the blood stream. Toxins will cause disease and will cause symptoms. As these noxious agents reach their final destination for elimination, these irritants may give us a signal to our consciousness as pain—a headache. The let-down is due to the slower action of the heart. The resting phase follows the more rapid heart and may be experienced as depression and last for 3 to 10 days. After that the symptoms vanish and we feel stronger. Symptoms are the body's way of communicating, and we should not always mask the symptoms with other drugs. We need to trust our bodies.

Change is good but often it has side effects. Don't be worried, but don't hesitate to discuss these with your health expert. Often after continuing with an improved dietary regimen for any length of time, one may expect to experience "retracing."

Retracing is a good thing, and remember—the body knows what it is doing. The cellular intelligence says something like, "Look at all those fine building materials coming in to our factory. Once we have a chance to get rid of old garbage, we can build a beautiful new cell. Let's get this excess bile out of the liver and gallbladder and send it to the intestines for elimination. Let's get this sludge moving out of the arteries, veins, and capillaries. These smelly, gassy, brain-stupefying masses have been here too long. These arthritic deposits in the joints need to be cleaned up. Let's get these irritating food preservatives, aspirins, and drugs out of the way, along with these other masses of fat that have made life so burdensome for us for so long. Let's get going and keep going until the job is done, until we have a healthy body comprised of healthy cells." This is why when ill, the need to detoxify is so important. During the beginning of any detoxification phase the key concentration of the cell is on elimination, or breaking down of tissue. The body begins to remove the garbage deposited in all the cells and tissues. As wastes are rapidly discarded, you'll experience frequent bowel movements that are often foul smelling or toxic. This is the body's way of letting you know you are on the right track, the body's way of healing itself.

Any phase of detoxification begins when the amount of waste material being discarded is equal to the amount of new cells and tissues being formed. The old you is replaced by the newer, more vital nutrients you are taking in.

Once you give the cell what it needs or remove what it doesn't need, then you begin to build healthier cells. I call this phase the "restoration phase." It's during the restoration phase that much of the toxic waste has already been discarded, and the cell and tissues that were formed since the diet was raised in quality are more durable. Also, new cells and tissues are now being formed faster due to the improved assimilation of nutrients. These new cells are maintaining their telomere length. Once this happens, the body's need for the usual amounts of food decreases and we are able to maintain our weight with less food.

The telomere restoration phase is a rebuilding phase. During rebuilding, you may experience an inner feeling of calm and peace. This is a healing feeling that you should see as an encouraging sign. This is important for health and should not be interfered with.

As the body gains strength, it will occasionally clean house with a vengeance. If this happens, don't be alarmed. If your body is toxic, let your body remove the toxic waste. When this happens we may experience other symptoms that will vary according to the materials being eliminated, the health of the organs involved in the elimination, and the amount of energy you have available. Headaches, fever, colds, and your skin breaking out are all normal.

Never hesitate to speak with your health professional during any health change. It's not uncommon for there to be a short interval of bowel sluggishness or diarrhea. Feelings of tiredness and weakness, disinclination to exercise, nervousness, irritability, and depression are all common. Be happy you are having these symptoms; the body is eliminating toxins and is beginning to heal itself. The more rest you give yourself, the more quickly the symptoms will be alleviated and the more beneficial the healing path will be.

This is nature's way of cleaning house. Understand that these actions are constructive even though the symptoms may be unpleasant. Don't try to stop the symptoms by the use of drugs. These symptoms are part of the healing process and not allergic manifestations or symptoms that should be suppressed. Don't try to cure a cure.

Once you realize that your body is becoming younger and healthier because you are throwing off more and more wastes that eventually would have brought pain, disease, and suffering you will realize that you can turn back the clock without drugs or surgery.

We age when we don't take care of our cells. We age because our cells are deficient or toxic. Once we restore deficiencies the cell gains strength to remove toxins. These toxins that the body eliminates help save you from more serious diseases that might have resulted if you had kept them in your body, including high cholesterol, lung disorders, kidney disorders, hepatitis, blood disease, heart disease, or tumors. Be happy you are paying your bill now in a less costly method. The key to less expensive health care is preventive health care.

You possess a precious gift. The human body is a magnificent, self-healing machine that is capable of enabling you to maintain optimal health, rejuvenation, and overcome any disease. You have a built-in healing ability, and you can learn to activate it through natural means.

Your body is designed so that when you cooperate with nature and put in place the conditions for healing and rejuvenation, your body will spontaneously begin healing and eventually complete the job.

As you begin the journey toward ageless aging, health, and wellness, marvel at the wondrous way in which the human body works. Marvel at its ability to regenerate and heal when given the proper fuel. Welcome to the beginning of ageless aging. When you begin to turn back the clock, you begin to accept and appreciate healing. Once you experience what is meant by total health and vitality, your strength will make it easier to eliminate harmful foods and toxins from the diet while welcoming the many benefits of nature's housecleaning efforts.

Celling resveratrol

In the last chapter, one of my "big three" was resveratrol. I briefly mentioned resveratrol and told you it was my favorite, but I didn't tell you why. My wife and I like our occasional glass of red wine and this is good news in the world of cellular health. There is much research that says moderate drinkers tend to have better health and live longer than those who are either abstainers or heavy drinkers. In addition to having fewer heart attacks and strokes, moderate consumers of alcoholic beverages (beer, wine, and distilled spirits or liquor) are generally less likely to suffer strokes, diabetes, arthritis, enlarged prostate, dementia (including Alzheimer's disease), and several major cancers. Alcohol has been used medicinally throughout recorded history; its medicinal properties are mentioned over 100 times in the Old and New Testaments. As early as the turn of the century there was evidence that moderate consumption of alcohol was associated with a decrease in the risk of heart attack. And the evidence of health benefits of moderate consumption has continued to grow over time.

Resveratrol is an active ingredient in red wine. Now if you avoid alcohol, and many of you do, you can supplement your body with resveratrol. The key to longevity is to help fortify the cells. Whether it is dark chocolate or wine, moderation is the key.

Resveratrol can protect you from the damages of aging while helping to switch on your anti-aging genes. That's because resveratrol is a type of phytoalexin containing a key enzyme called stilbene synthase. Not all plants can make resveratrol. Plants produce phytoalexins for one reason—self-defense. Whether it's bad weather, or an attack by insects or microbes, plants use phytoalexins to protect themselves when they're under stress from their environment.

Resveratrol works the same way in humans. It does this by activating certain proteins called sirtuins that your body produces naturally to extend life under conditions of stress (like starvation). Sirtuins transmit signals to every cell in your body, including telomeres, that cancel out the effects of aging. They bring the processes that lead to cell death and telomere shortening to a crawl, buying your body more time to repair DNA damage. This is great news for cellular health; resveratrol can induce cell repair all by itself.

One study found that resveratrol actually causes cells to make new mitochondria (remember, these are the power plants in your cells that give your cells their energy). Resveratrol can help keep you young by improving your body's response to exercise. Researchers gave mice resveratrol and turned them into extraordinary athletes. Resveratrol was shown to improve the oxygen use in their muscles.

Resveratrol also improved their aerobic capacity and gave them significantly increased endurance. It's for this reason we are recommending adding foods rich in resveratrol to your diet.

Cell me more

I was personally happy to read that one recent study showed that men who drink one glass a wine a day are likely to reduce their risk of the most aggressive forms of prostate cancer by 50% according to a cancer research study. The cancer-fighting compound, resveratrol, is found in the red grapes that are used to make red wine. Resveratrol is also found in peanuts and raspberries. Upon testing other liquors such as beer and hard liquor, researchers found they produced no significant effects.

Because it is an antioxidant, resveratrol has the ability to clear dangerous cancer-inducing radicals from the body. Its anti-inflammatory properties prevent certain enzymes from forming that trigger tumor development. It cuts down cell reproduction, which helps reduce the number of cell divisions that could contribute to the progression of cancer cell growth. It may play a similar role to estrogen by its ability to reduce testosterone levels, which promote the cancer growth. The study involved interviewing two groups of men: 753 recently diagnosed prostate cancer patients and 703 healthy patients, who acted as the control group.

The goal of the study was to evaluate the possible benefits of drinking red wine. The participant's ages ranged from 40 to 64, with the majority under the age of 60. This youthful range was considered one of the strong aspects of the study due to the fact that the risks of prostate cancer are lower in younger age groups. This factor also allowed researchers to hone in on specific environmental factors of cancer risk, such as wine consumption.

Future studies are being planned to further research the relationship between resveratrol and prostate cancer.

So enjoy your glass of wine with some peanuts tonight with your favorite loved one. Wine and related beverages are good sources of concentrated resveratrol, which protect our cells and assist in maintaining the length of our telomeres.

Snacking can be beneficial for your health and for weight control. According to the Mayo Clinic, eating healthy snacks between meals can keep you from binge eating and satisfy cravings. Just remember to snack in moderation and add regular exercise to your day. So go ahead, allow yourself a little time to be a couch potato and snack without the guilt.

These are many simple ways to live younger and live longer, and each one begins with healthy cells. Bottoms up!

"If you can't pronounce it, don't eat it."

—COMMON SENSE

Chapter 22

LET'S BEGIN TO HEAL

Our society's basic understanding of sickness and disease is based on the symptom treatment model. We wait until we get symptoms before we focus on health. We treat the symptoms, not the cause. With a host of symptoms, the doctor will name a disease. This is called symptomology. We all know, however, that there is only one disease (cytopathology) with many names.

The symptom model is the current utilized model, as it allows the doctor to supposedly differentiate one disease from another. But it's like a dog chasing its tail. Drugs often don't cure, they just mask the symptoms. Only the body can heal; the body is a self-healing organism. In this chapter we focus on prevention. If toxins are one of the two causes of disease and if deficiency is the other, then we must learn how to prevent and cope with both.

In today's world, almost the entirety of modern medicine and everything we have ever learned about disease is based on symptomology. The concept of only one disease may seem unacceptably simplistic. The symptomology concept is flawed and far too complex. If the symptomology approach was valid, we could simply enter the symptoms into a computer and the computer would then spit out the diagnosis. Medicine is not that simple. When we focus on health, we can treat disease. Since we now know that shorter telomeres make us more prone to disease, wouldn't it make sense to focus on the telomeres?

Symptomatology is based on a fundamental misconception, one held by health practitioners in Western society. The misconception is that thousands of different diseases exist, each with different symptoms, causes, and treatments. This misconception stems from the many different ways that cells can malfunction, and therefore the thousands of different symptoms that can be produced. The modern medical treatment of almost all disease focuses on the management of these symptoms (the effects of disease), rather than eliminating the causes of deficiency and toxicity.

Diagnosis by symptoms is the process by which modern medicine gives each collection of symptoms a particular name. Medicine views symptoms as enemies; I see them as little helpers. They allow us to know that our cells are weak and need special care.

In truth, each collection of symptoms—each specific "disease"—is just a different expression of malfunctioning cells. However, with all of our different types of cells, and all of the different ways in which each cell can malfunction, the number of possible combinations of symptoms becomes vast. In other words, when cells malfunction, we may feel sick in many different ways. Toxicity and deficiency of the cell will both yield symptoms. If our cells start to malfunction because of a vitamin C deficiency, they will exhibit different symptoms than those malfunctioning because of a zinc deficiency. The solution would be to remove the deficiency by treating the cause of the symptoms, not the symptoms alone.

In the case of toxicity, if the cells were malfunctioning because of lead toxicity, they would exhibit different symptoms from those malfunctioning because of mercury toxicity. Again remove the toxin and the cell will heal. There are various combinations of deficiencies and toxicities producing a host of separate diseases. However, treating the symptoms alone is not relevant. To solve any problem, you have to address the causes, not the symptoms. Modern medicine, by placing the focus on symptoms, has yet to develop any theory regarding the relationship between health and disease. Medicine looks at these as if they are two different states, while health and disease are really different sides of the same coin.

Drugs and surgery are not the answer to everything. Healthcare costs are spiraling out of control. Our model simply does not work. Dr. Julian Whitaker, a leader in alternative healthcare states, "If the only tool you have is a hammer, so the saying goes, then every problem looks like a nail." If you go to a conventionally trained physician, then medicine's hammers—surgery and drugs—are what you receive. Unfortunately, these tools are designed to manage and suppress symptoms, not to cure disease.

For a more meaningful understanding of disease (cellular malfunction), we must consider the health of our cells. Noticeable health problems begin when first one cell and then eventually a large number of cells malfunction. As this happens, important cellular chemicals are not produced, cell-to-cell communications break down, and eventually the body ceases to function properly. Our cells, and thus our tissues, organs, and muscles, suffer and noticeable symptoms appear such as allergies, headaches, sinus problems, obesity, weakness, fatigue, aches and pains, colds, flu, depression, anxiety, diabetes, cancer, or any of thousands of other complaints we call symptoms. All revert back to the one disease—cytopathology.

When you get sick, your immune system makes copies of its disease-fighting white blood cells called T-cells. These cells divide over and over again to fight off the bacteria or virus that's invading your body. The more often these cells reproduce, the shorter their telomeres become until they stop copying. This happens because the older you get, the fewer active T-cells you have because they've fought off as much sickness as they can. The bottom line is that when your telomeres are short, your immune system looks and acts old. Like our copy machine metaphor, your copier needs ink. We get new cells; we need new healthy cells. If we reproduce weak cells, like weak copies, your risk for infection and disease grows much higher.

Study after study shows that people who had shorter telomeres were three or more times likely to die from disease.

Shortened telomeres are associated with many chronic diseases like:

Diabetes. When you eat too many carbohydrates, your pancreas is asked to create more insulin than it's supposed to. And to get the job done, the pancreas has to create more of a factory to create the insulin it needs by making more cells. If the pancreas is continually challenged to produce more and more insulin, the cells have to continue to divide. When their telomeres are too short, they can't reproduce anymore. And your body can't make the insulin you need. This is what causes diabetes.

Atherosclerosis. One study I read looked at reviews men with high blood pressure. Those with shorter telomeres in their white blood cells were more likely to get heart disease.

Alzheimer's disease. Alzheimer's patients' glial cells, the maintenance cells of the brain, have short telomeres. It is believed by researchers that some kind of toxic environmental hazard caused those cells to replicate to defend themselves.

Pulmonary Fibrosis. According to the *American Journal of Respiratory and Critical Care Medicine*, significant fraction of individuals with pulmonary fibrosis have short telomere lengths that cannot be explained by coding mutations in telomerase. Telomere shortening of circulating leukocytes may be a marker for an increased predisposition toward the development of this age-associated disease.

Depression. A *ScienceDaily* article summarizes new research showing a link between depression and telomere length in white blood cells. Telomeres are the end-caps on chromosomes. If telomeres become too short, DNA becomes unstable, genetic integrity is lost during cell division, and cells become senescent (crippled beyond hope of recovery) or commit apoptosis (suicide). The study went on to say that. It turns out that in depressed people, white blood cell telomeres are *shorter* than in normal people, even though telomerase is *more active*. Moreover, for a given telomere length, the more telomerase activity, the more depressed the patient. It summarized that telomerase activity predicts which patients will recover: Patients who recovered from depression had the highest telomerase activity along with their short telomeres.

Viral Infections. *Oncogene* reported, "The Epstein-Barr virus (EBV) is carried by more than 90% of the adult world population and has been implicated in several human cancers. EBV disrupts the caps of telomeres, creating dysfunctional telomeres." BMC Neuroscience reported that, "HIV also showed a statistically significant telomere shortening. Interestingly, telomere shortening by HIV was reversed by providing N-acetylcysteine, suggesting that NAC should be beneficial for AIDS and possibly other chronic viral infections." Research shows that connections between viruses and telomere loss run deep. In fact, it has been proposed that cellular senescence, the usual outcome of telomere loss, evolved as an anti-viral defense mechanism.

Cardiovascular Disease. I was pleased to find the study by Nakashima H, Ozono R, Suyama C, Sueda T, Kambe M, Oshma T, that I mentioned prior, that showed that white blood cell telomeres were shorter in heart disease patients.

The list of diseases goes on, but we are blessed in that our immune system does a remarkable job of defending us against disease-causing microorganisms. But sometimes it fails: A germ invades successfully and makes you sick. The idea of boosting your immunity is enticing but it takes work and must have your cells working in harmony with each other. The immune system is a system, not a single entity. Why does it weaken? How can we protect it? If there are two causes of disease, deficiency and toxicity, our goal is to remove the area of concern.

Categorizing and suppressing the symptoms of malfunctioning cells does not fix the problem. The only cure is to restore our cells and tissues to health. If there is only one disease and one cure, it's best we focus on the cure.

I believe the science of cells offers the most exciting and viable possibility for extreme life extension—the kind of anti-aging strategy that can actually allow you to regenerate and in effect "grow younger." Naturally, researchers are hard at work devising pharmaceutical strategies to accomplish this, but there's solid evidence that simple lifestyle strategies and nutritional intervention can do this, too.

Throughout this book we discussed that there is only One Disease and Two Causes. I have taken you to toxic city along our road to wellness. Other health practitioners throughout the world are working on wellness through cellular health. Here is one whose work I enjoy. Let me share with you his top 12 supplements.

Best-Selling Author, Dr. Joeseph Mercola, authored three *New York Times* Best Sellers: *The Great Bird Flu Hoax*, *The No-Grain Diet*, and *Effortless Healing*.

Dr. Mercola's Top 12 Supplement Healers

1. Vitamin D

In one study of more than 2,000 women, those with higher vitamin D levels were found to have fewer aging-related changes in their DNA, as well as lowered inflammatory responses. Women with higher levels of vitamin D are more likely to have longer telomeres, and vice versa. This means that people with higher levels of vitamin D may actually age more slowly than people with lower levels of vitamin D.

Your leukocyte telomere length (LTL) is a predictor for aging related diseases. As you age, your LTL's become shorter, but, if you suffer from chronic inflammation, your telomeres decrease in length much faster because your body's inflammatory response accelerates leukocyte turnover. Your vitamin D concentrations also decrease with age, whereas your C-reactive protein (a mediator of inflammation) increases. This inverse double-whammy increases your overall risk of developing autoimmune diseases such as multiple sclerosis and rheumatoid arthritis.

The good news is that vitamin D is a potent inhibitor of your body's inflammatory response, and by reducing inflammation, you diminish your turnover of leukocytes, effectively creating a positive chain reaction that can help protect you against a variety of diseases. In essence, it protects your body from the deterioration of aging. Researchers have found that subsets of leukocytes have receptors for the active form of vitamin D (D3), which allows the vitamin to have a direct effect on these cells. This may also explain the specific connection between vitamin D and autoimmune disease.

The absolute best way to optimize your vitamin D levels would be through safe sun exposure. I am fully aware that many will not be able to implement this recommendation due to lifestyle constraints, but I feel I would be reprehensibly negligent if I did not emphasize how superior photo vitamin D is compared to oral.

The role of vitamin D in disease prevention

A growing body of evidence shows that vitamin D plays a crucial role in disease prevention and maintaining optimal health. There are about 30,000 genes in your body, and vitamin D affects nearly 3,000 of them, as well as vitamin D receptors located throughout your body.

According to one large-scale study, optimal vitamin D levels can slash your risk of cancer by as much as 60%. Keeping your levels optimized can help prevent at least 16 different types of cancer, including pancreatic, lung, ovarian, prostate, and skin cancers.

2. Astaxanthin (derived from the microalgae Haematococcus pluvialis)

In the 2009 study on multivitamin use and telomere length, longer telomeres were also associated with the use of antioxidant formulas. According to the authors, telomeres are particularly vulnerable to oxidative stress. Additionally, inflammation induces oxidative stress and lowers the activity of telomerase (again, that's the enzyme responsible for maintaining your telomeres).

Astaxanthin has emerged as one of the most potent and beneficial antioxidants currently known, with potent anti-inflammatory and DNA-protective capabilities. Research has even shown that it can protect against DNA damage induced by gamma radiation. It has a number of unique features that make it stand out from the crowd.

For example, it is by far the most powerful carotenoid antioxidant when it comes to free radical scavenging: astaxanthin is 65 times more powerful than vitamin C, 54 times more powerful than beta-carotene, and 14 times more powerful than vitamin E. It's also far more effective than other carotenoids at "singlet oxygen quenching," which is a particular type of oxidation. It is 550 times more powerful than vitamin E, and 11 times more powerful than beta-carotene at neutralizing singlet oxygen.

Astaxanthin crosses both your blood-brain barrier AND your blood-retinal barrier (beta carotene and lycopene do not), which brings antioxidant and anti-inflammatory protection to your eyes, brain and central nervous system.

Another feature that separates astaxanthin from other carotenoids is that it cannot function as a pro-oxidant. Many antioxidants will act as pro-oxidants (meaning they start to cause rather than combat oxidation) when present in your tissues in sufficient concentrations. This is why you don't want to go overboard taking too many antioxidant supplements like beta-carotene, for example. Astaxanthin, on the other hand, does not function as a pro-oxidant, even when present in high amounts, which makes it highly beneficial.

Lastly, one of its most profound features is its unique ability to protect the entire cell from damage—both the water-soluble part and the fat-soluble portion of the cell. Other antioxidants affect just one or the other. This is due to astaxanthin's unique physical characteristics that allow it to reside within the cell membrane while also protecting the inside of the cell.

3. Ubiquinol (CoQ10)

Coenzyme Q10 (CoQ10) is the fifth most popular supplement in the United States, taken by about 53% of Americans, according to a 2010 survey by ConsumerLab.com. This is a good thing as one in every four Americans over 45 is taking a statin and every single one of these individuals needs to be taking it.

CoQ10 is used by every cell in your body. In fact, it is so important for your body's daily functions that it is also known as "ubiquinone" because it's 'ubiquitous' in the human body.

What you may not know, however, is that to benefit from the form of the nutrient needed to produce cellular energy and help you reduce the typical signs of aging, your body must convert the ubiquinone to the reduced form, called ubiquinol—and research is showing that this reduced form may actually be superior for your health in a number of ways. If you're under 25 years old, your body is capable of converting CoQ10 from the oxidized to the reduced form. However, if you're older, your body becomes more and more challenged to convert the oxidized CoQ10 to ubiquinol.

Premature aging is one primary side effect of having too little CoQ10 because this essential vitamin recycles other antioxidants, such as vitamin C and E. CoQ10 deficiency also accelerates DNA damage, and because CoQ10 is beneficial to heart health and muscle function, this depletion leads to fatigue, muscle weakness, soreness, and eventually heart failure.

4. Fermented Foods / Probiotics

It's quite clear that eating a diet consisting of high amounts of processed foods will shorten your life. Part of the problem is that these processed, sugar- and chemical-laden foods effectively destroy your intestinal microflora. Your gut flora has incredible power over your immune system, which, of course, is your body's natural defense system. Antibiotics, stress, artificial sweeteners, chlorinated water, and many other factors can also reduce the amount of probiotics (beneficial bacteria) in your gut, which can predispose you to illness and premature aging. Ideally, you'll want to make traditionally cultured and fermented foods a staple in your daily diet.

You can use a probiotic supplement, but getting your probiotics from food is definitely better as you can consume far more beneficial bacteria, in many cases up to 100X more. Fermented vegetables are an excellent alternative as they are both delicious and simple to make.

5. Krill Oil

According to Dr. William Harris, an expert on omega-3 fats, those who have an omega-3 index of less than 4% age much faster than those with indexes above 8%. Therefore, your omega-3 index may also be an effective marker of your rate of aging. According to Dr. Harris' research, omega-3 fats appear to play a role in activating telomerase, which, again, has been shown to be able to actually reverse telomere shortening.

Although this research is preliminary, I would suggest that optimizing your omega-3 levels above 8% would be a good strategy if you're interested in delaying aging. (Your doctor can order the omega-3 index test from a lab called Health Diagnostic Laboratory in Richmond, Virginia.) After all, you have nothing to lose and a lot to gain by doing so, since omega-3 has proven to be extremely important for your health in so many respects.

My favorite animal-based omega-3 is krill oil, as it has a number of benefits not found in other omega-3 supplements such as fish oil. Aside from higher potential for contamination, fish oil supplements also have a higher risk of suffering oxidation damage and becoming rancid. Dr. Rudi Moerck has discussed these risks at great length in a previous interview. Krill oil also contains naturally occurring astaxanthin, which makes it nearly 200 times more resistant to oxidative damage compared to fish oil.

Additionally, according to Dr. Harris' research, krill oil is also more potent gram for gram, as its absorption rate is much higher than fish oil. You get somewhere between 25 to 50% more omega-3 per milligram when you take krill oil compared to fish oil, hence you don't need to take as much.

6. Vitamin K2

Vitamin K may very well be "the next vitamin D" as research continues to illuminate a growing number of benefits to your health. While most people get enough vitamin K from their diets to maintain adequate blood clotting, they're NOT enough to offer protection against more serious health problems. For example, research over the past few years suggests that vitamin K2 can provide substantial protection from prostate cancer, which is one of the leading causes of cancer among men in the United States. And research results are similarly encouraging for the benefits of vitamin K to your cardiac health: In 2004, the Rotterdam Study, which was the first study demonstrating the beneficial effect of vitamin K2, showed that people who consume 45 mcg of K2 daily live 7 years longer than people getting 12 mcg per day.

In a subsequent study called the Prospect Study, 16,000 people were followed for 10 years. Researchers found that each additional 10 mcg of K2 in the diet resulted in 9% fewer cardiac events.

K2 is present in fermented foods, particularly cheese and the Japanese food natto, which is by far the richest source of K2.

7. Magnesium

According to the featured research, magnesium also plays an important role in DNA replication, repair, and RNA synthesis, and dietary magnesium has been shown to positively correlate with increased telomere length in women. Other research has shown that long-term deficiency leads to telomere shortening in rats and cell cultures. It appears the lack of magnesium ions has a negative influence on genome integrity. Insufficient amounts of magnesium also reduce your body's ability to repair damaged DNA, and can induce chromosomal abnormalities. According to the authors, it's reasonable to hypothesize that "magnesium influences telomere length by affecting DNA integrity and repair, in addition to its potential role in oxidative stress and inflammation."

8. Polyphenols

Polyphenols are potent antioxidant compounds in plant foods, many of which have been linked to anti-aging benefits and disease reduction. Here are but a few examples of these potent antioxidant compounds:

Grapes (resveratrol)—Resveratrol deeply penetrates the center of your cell's nucleus, giving your DNA time to repair free radical damage. Research dating back to 2003 showed that resveratrol, a powerful polyphenol and anti-fungal chemical, was able to increase the lifespan of yeast cells.

The findings showed that resveratrol could activate a gene called sirtuin1, which is also activated during calorie restriction in various species. Since then studies in nematode worms, fruit flies, fish, mice, and human cells have linked resveratrol to longer lives.

Resveratrol is found in grapes, and there are numerous products on the market containing resveratrol. I recommend looking for one made from muscadine grapes and that uses whole grape skins and seeds, as this is where many of the benefits are concentrated.

Cocoa—Quite a few studies have confirmed the potent antioxidant properties, and subsequent health benefits, of raw cocoa powder. Dark, organic, unprocessed chocolate has been found to benefit your glucose metabolism (diabetic control), blood pressure, and cardiovascular health.

Green tea—Polyphenols in tea, which include EGCG (epigallo-catechin gallate) and many others, have been found to offer protection against many types of cancer. The polyphenols in green tea may constitute up to 30% of the dry leaf weight, so, when you drink a cup of green tea, you're drinking a fairly potent solution of healthy tea polyphenols.

Green tea is the least processed kind of tea, so it also contains the highest amounts of EGCG of all tea varieties. Keep in mind, however, that many green teas have been oxidized, and this process may take away many of its valuable properties. The easiest sign to look for when evaluating a green tea's quality is its color: If your green tea is brown rather than green, it's likely been oxidized.

My personal favorite is matcha green tea because it contains the entire ground tea leaf, and can contain over 100 times the EGCG provided from regular brewed green tea.

9. Folate (aka Vitamin B9 or Folic Acid)

According to the featured study in the *Journal of Nutritional Biochemistry*, plasma concentrations of the B vitamin folate correspond to telomere length in both men and women. Folate plays an important role in the maintenance of DNA integrity and DNA methylation, both of which influence the length of your telomeres.

It is useful for preventing depression, seizure disorders, and brain atrophy. In fact, folate deficiency can lead to elevated homocysteine levels, which can be a major contributor to heart disease and Alzheimer's disease. One unfortunate and preventable reason why some believe folate numbers are slipping is the increased prevalence of obesity, which negatively affects the way most people metabolize this important vitamin. The ideal way to raise your folate levels is to eat plenty of fresh, raw, organic leafy green vegetables, and beans.

Please note that it is the natural folate from food that has been found to be beneficial. This may not be true for the supplement folic acid.

10. Vitamin B12

Vitamin B12 is fittingly known as "the energy vitamin," and your body requires it for a number of vital functions, such as energy production, blood formation, DNA synthesis, and myelin formation. (Myelin is insulation that protects your nerve endings and allows them to communicate with one another.) Unfortunately, research suggests about 25% of American adults are deficient in this vitally important nutrient, and nearly half the population has suboptimal blood levels.

Vitamin B12 is found almost exclusively in animal tissues, including foods like beef and beef liver, lamb, snapper, venison, salmon, shrimp, scallops, poultry, and eggs. It's not readily available in plants, so if you do not eat meat or animal products you are at risk of deficiency. The few plant foods that are sources of B12 are actually B12 analogs. An analog is a substance that blocks the uptake of true B12, so your body's need for the nutrient actually increases.

If you aren't getting sufficient B12 in your diet, I recommend you begin supplementation immediately with this vital nutrient with either an under-the-tongue fine mist spray or vitamin B12 injections. Ensuring your body has adequate B12 can vastly improve the quality of your life and prevent debilitating, even life-threatening diseases that result from a deficiency of this all-important nutrient.

11. Curcumin (Turmeric)

Curcumin—the active ingredient in the spice turmeric—acts both as an immune booster and potent anti-inflammatory. But perhaps its greatest value lies in its anti-cancer potential, and it has the most evidence based literature backing up its anti-cancer claims of any other nutrient. It affects over 100 different pathways once it gets into a cell—among them, a key biological pathway needed for development of melanoma and other cancers.

The spice actually stops laboratory strains of melanoma from proliferating and pushes the cancer cells to commit suicide by shutting down nuclear factor-kappa B (NF-kB), a powerful protein known to induce abnormal inflammatory response that leads to an assortment of disorders such as arthritis and cancer.

To get the full benefits that curcumin has to offer, you will want to look for a turmeric extract with at least 95% curcuminoids that contains only 100% certified organic ingredients. The formula should be free of fillers, additives, and excipients (a substance added to the supplement as a processing or stability aid), and the manufacturer should use safe production practices at all stages: planting, cultivation, selective harvesting, and then producing and packaging the final product.

12. Vitamin A

According to the featured study in the *Journal of Nutritional Biochemistry*, telomere length is positively associated with dietary intake of vitamin A in women who do not take multivitamins. It plays an important role in your immune response, and if you're deficient, you become predisposed to infections that can promote telomere shortening. However, vitamin A does not appear to have a dose-dependent effect on telomere length, so you don't need high amounts.

Key lifestyle strategies that affect telomere length

While a nutritious diet accounts for about 80% of the benefits derived from a healthy lifestyle, exercise cannot be ignored, and there's evidence suggesting that exercise protects against telomere shortening as well. Another lifestyle strategy that can have a beneficial impact is intermittent fasting.

Exercise—Like my former friend and mentor, Jack LaLanne, I have no love for exercise, but I know I must do it; you can't hide from the research on its healing powers. One recent study on postmenopausal women suffering from chronic stress found that "vigorous physical activity appears to protect those experiencing high stress by buffering its relationship with telomere length (TL)." In fact, among the women who did not exercise, each unit increase in the Perceived Stress Scale was related to a 15-fold increase in the odds of having short telomeres. Those who did exercise regularly showed no correlation between telomere length and perceived stress!

High-intensity exercise appears to be the most effective all-natural approach to slow down the aging process by reducing telomere shortening. In fact, research has shown there's a direct association between reduced telomere shortening in your later years and high-intensity-type exercises: Greta Blackburn's book *The Immortality Edge: Realize the Secrets of Your Telomeres for a Longer, Healthier Life* further details the importance of high-intensity exercise to prevent telomere shortening.

Intermittent Fasting—Previous research has shown that you can extend your lifespan by reducing your caloric intake, and I've written about this technique in the past. The problem is that most people do not understand how to properly cut calories, because in order to remain healthy, you have to cut out the right kind of calories—namely carbohydrates. Research by Professor Cynthia Kenyon has shown that avoiding carbs will activate genes that govern youthfulness and longevity.

So what have we learned?

To *Awaken the Wellness Within* you must embrace several key concepts that are at the heart of our present understanding of cellular health and aging, which we discussed and have been around for many years.

One example was the "wear and tear" theory of cell degeneration (August Weismann, 1891) which showed that the higher the metabolic rate of a species, the shorter the lifespan (rate of living theory, Rubner, 1908; Raymond Pearl, 1928); that oxygen damage could be caused by free radicals (Rebecca Gerschnian, 1954); and that free radicals generated during oxidative metabolism cause cellular damage leading to aging and death (free radical theory).

Denham Harman, 1956). James Fleming, with the mitochondrial theory of cell aging in 1982, has integrated rate of living and free radical theories by focusing on the mitochondria, the energy factory of the cell where oxidative metabolism takes place.

In 1961 Leonard Hayflick overturned the notion that embryonic cells contain a substance that renders them immortal and demonstrated that cultured human cells go through a set number of divisions, usually about fifty, before they undergo a series of degenerative changes and die. In contrast to the "Hayflick limit," Roy Walford's pioneering work on caloric restriction has demonstrated that animals that eat fewer calories are healthier, suffer less cancer and live significantly longer. In one experiment published in 1986, the longest-lived 10% of mice on his regime far exceeded all records for mouse longevity. Walford is currently extending his research to humans in the Biosphere project in Texas. Ron Hart of the NIH, whose research has demonstrated that the lifespan of a species is directly related to its ability to repair damaged DNA, believes that caloric restriction lowers body temperature, reduces DNA damage, inhibits free radicals, and results in increased metabolic efficiency.

Our present-day understanding is that aging is a tiered process, caused by the accumulation of innumerable damaging and degenerative events at a cellular and whole body level. The single most responsible entity for inflicting such damage that leads to a multiplicity of degenerative conditions is the free radical, which appears to be the root trigger of so many conditions, including heart disease, cancer, diabetes, arthritis, skin wrinkling, memory loss, even perhaps Alzheimer's.

Free radicals = #1 cause of aging

Free Radicals we learned are extremely unstable molecules with an unpaired electron that can wreak havoc upon every level of the cell. Free radical molecules are generated in respiration and normal cellular chemistry as byproducts of energy production and by immune cells as powerful antimicrobial weapons to protect against infectious disease. Hence they are natural byproducts of life processes. Free radicals are also generated by many activities and facets of modern life, including UV radiation, smoke, stress, pollutants, iron, lead, mercury, rancid unsaturated fatty acids, intense exercise, alcohol, and nitrites used to prepare smoked meats.

The prominent position accorded to free radicals is illustrated by expert Professor Denham Harman, from the University of Nebraska Medical Center, who says that, "Chances are 99% that free radicals are the basis for aging." According to a growing consensus of research, our ability to resist disease, stay young, and live a long life is dependent upon our optimum capacity to repair free radical damage. Indeed, free radical damage can be prevented and even reversed if there are sufficient concentrations in the body of free radical scavengers called antioxidants. There are numerous such scavenger species, either working together or specialized within specific niches, to nullify or repair damage by toxic free radical species.

The discovery and confirmation of the central role played by free radicals in our cells is responsible for degenerative diseases, which themselves contribute to cellular malfunction and aging. Understanding this is a significant milestone in the search of healthy options to achieve optimum longevity. At long last we have obtained a unifying conceptual understanding of how so many diverse nutrients and therapeutic practices can enhance our health and life expectancy. Although the arguments concerning the ultimate human lifespan are still fiercely ongoing within the scientific community, most people would agree that what really matters to all of us is the quality, rather than the quantity of our lives. Sensible implementation of these nutritional and lifecycle guidelines may indeed enable us to live to an "ageless" and healthy age.

Diet

Throughout this book we talked about the importance of lifestyle, the importance of diet, of supplements to supplement your diet to avoid any deficiencies. The simple fact is, what we eat and drink provides the nutrients that strengthen the immune system, build protein, muscle, and connective tissue, and fuel every metabolic process from thinking, breathing, digestion, elimination of waste, to the prevention and repair of free radical damage. Unfortunately, in stark contrast to our farming ancestors, who had a rather spartan diet of homegrown food replete with an abundance of soil nutrients, we of the modern era live in highly polluted environments and tend to gorge on an abundance of junk and adulterated food. In order to live a long, healthy, and vigorous life, we must limit free radical damage to our bodies, which we can do by carefully choosing the foods we eat. Therefore, the over-riding emphasis must be to choose "pure" water and a wide variety of whole, fresh produce that is not refined, processed, or adulterated. Several highly important guidelines for a health-promoting diet include:

- Eat a diet that contains about 50–55% complex carbohydrates, obtained from fruits and vegetables and some whole grains. We want to eat foods that are rich in fiber, proteins, vitamins and minerals, and are low in fat. Eat a lot of raw food, green vegetables are best. Raw foods supply the body with vitamins and minerals and fiber. You must avoid raw sugar or any sugar products, especially anything with corn syrup. Lastly, try to avoid fruits after 6 PM. Fruits eaten during the day will supply natural energy.

- Obtain essential fatty acids through eating oily fish (tuna, mackerel, salmon, sardines) or omega-oils in nuts, seeds and oils.
- Consume low levels of saturated fat, hydrogenated margarine, processed polyunsaturated fats, and deep-fried foods. These fat products favor the synthesis of leukotrienes, which promote inflammatory conditions and are also the source of free-radical formation.
- Minimize salt, caffeine, alcohol, and refined sugar intake, and don't smoke.

Supplements

The supplements listed throughout this book and below are recommended for their anti-free radical or antioxidant activities.

- Vitamin A beta-carotene, vitamin B complex, vitamin C, vitamin D, vitamin E, zinc, chromium, magnesium, selenium, omega-3s, & conzyme Q-10 to start.

Lifestyle

Nutrition is not the full story of how to stay young. Stress, as researched by Hans Selye during the 1950s, has a profound influence on the entire metabolic system, and how we respond to stress has a major impact at the cellular level. Research has shown that people who have a say in decisions about their work and personal life suffer less stress than those who have no responsibility in making decisions about their lives. Extensive research has also demonstrated that enjoyable exercise is an effective stress-buster, combats free radicals, promotes lymphatic drainage, promotes circulation of endorphins and enhances our sense of well-being. However, intense and high impact forms of exercise actually generate free radicals. Excellent choices of exercise include what is most enjoyable for the person, whether that is walking, swimming, cycling, golf, yoga, Tai Chi, or dancing. Hence, the key to *Awakening the Wellness Within* is the achievement of optimum cell health and longevity, which requires health-promoting lifestyles including relaxation, optimum nutrition, avoidance of toxins and daily moderate exercise.

"*The doctor of the future will no longer treat the human frame with drugs, but rather will cure and prevent disease with nutrition.*"

—THOMAS EDISON

Chapter 23

CHIROPRACTIC AND THE FOUNTAIN OF YOUTH

real understanding of the relationship between health and disease cannot be achieved through knowledge of germs, inherited genes, medicines, surgery, or any of the many "diseases" that make people sick. Keeping up with these subjects is complex and doesn't really help people to take care of themselves. What we need right now are solutions for good health. The time is ripe to simplify. Understand what your cells need, how they work, and what causes them to malfunction. Your cells are what make your life possible.

When our cells begin to malfunction, the body will fight to get our health back on track. Sometimes when the malfunction is large and the cells are overwhelmed with toxins and are deficient of the nutrients necessary to rebuild the cells, they are no longer able to maintain homeostasis (balance) by regulating and repairing itself. This is the essence of disease, no matter what you call it or how it happens. Because we now know that only one disease exists, all we need to do is prevent the causes of that one disease—deficiency and toxicity.

As a chiropractor, we are taught the wonders of the body. However, when nerve supply is blocked, the organs that the nerves are supplying will become deficient and the cells will be vulnerable to malfunction. The body knows how to take care of itself, provided it has what it needs to do so.

I am proud to say my son, Dr. Jason Kaplan, and his fiancée, Dr. Stephanie Lyons, will be carrying on our family tradition in Wellington, Florida. These two young doctors are dedicating their lives to health and wellness. Nothing could make Mrs. Kaplan and I prouder than our children not only living our lifestyle, but embracing it. Stephanie will also be specializing in treating horses, as Wellington is horse country and animals need chiropractic as well. Healing is a family affair for the Kaplans.

One cure

The power that creates the body has the power to heal the body.

Chiropractic focuses on the relationship between the spine and the nervous system. When your nervous system is functioning properly, your body knows how to heal, regulate, and adapt appropriately to the many stressors of everyday life, while allowing you to live your life to the fullest. It is important to understand why everyone who wishes to be truly healthy needs to be checked by a chiropractor regularly to ensure optimal nerve function.

Chiropractors correct subluxation allowing for proper nerve supply once again. Freely flowing information across your nerve system is an essential element for health. While medicine is treating the disease of a sick person, the patients of chiropractors are focused on getting well and staying that way.

The need to simplify

What if we could all understand what causes disease? Wouldn't we be empowered to prevent disease? Can we actually do that? Can we distill simple truth from this complex mystery? Throughout man's history, great advancements in science have often come from people who were able to take extraordinarily complex subjects and simplify them. In this chapter we are trying to simplify the concepts of health and disease.

Consider this: Rather than thousands of diseases, there is only one disease. Does this sound simple or does it sound complex? We have been conditioned to think that there are many different diseases, rather than recognizing what is common to all disease. The most difficult aspect of this theory is that it requires you to look at health and disease in a completely different way. Using the concept of one disease dramatically simplifies how we perceive disease in general.

Everything living, every plant and animal on earth, is made of cells—the smallest units of life. Likewise, each human being started as one cell—a single cell encoded with all of the information needed to develop into the vastly complex, multi-trillion-celled organisms that we are today. But what if that pathway of information between your brain, your nervous system, and the organ or organs it was trying to communicate with got blocked? Like the reception on your television, it would not be functioning at 100%. This is why I love chiropractic, and it is the fastest growing natural healing system in the world. Any nerve deficiency makes make the cells susceptible to malfunction.

The role of a healthy spine is to protect the nerve system from stress, allowing it to transmit information. These messages travel at 325 mph through 45 miles of nerves. When each vertebra is in a healthy position and allowed to move properly, there is no stress on the nerve system. At its core, literally inside your spine, your spinal cord and nerve roots transmit information, connecting your brain to every organ in your body.

In a 24-hour span, this communication will result in:

- Your heart will beat 103,680 times
- You will breathe 23,040 times
- 2,100 gallons of blood will pump through nearly 62,000 miles of blood vessels

- 69 trillion red blood cells will be produced
- You will exercise about 7 million brain cells

A chiropractor's purpose is ensuring that the flow of vital information from your brain to your body occurs without interference. If not properly cared for, trauma or repetitive stress to the spine will interfere with this flow of information. An unhealthy spine will create stress on the nerve system. This is why chiropractors have had such success with conditions as diverse as high blood pressure, headaches, asthma, fertility issues, and ear infections.

The changes associated with a fixated joint or subluxation cause a decrease in normal joint motion, which results in decreased information being sent to the brain. This happens via receptors called proprioceptors. Proprioceptors send positive body signals. A decrease in information being sent to the brain (proprioception) is interpreted as stress by the nerve system. Stress, whether emotional, chemical, or physical (in the form of misalignments of the spine or other trauma) is responsible for lifestyle disease which kills 75% of all Americans. Through chiropractic adjustments, chiropractors are able to correct subluxations, restoring function and increasing positive body signals, therefore decreasing stress.

References: *Life* magazine; "A Fantastic Voyage Through the Human Body" Feb 1997; pg. 33

My background in health care began in chiropractic where I graduated from New York Chiropractic College in 1978. My mentor and the greatest teacher I ever knew, Dr. Donald Gutstein, taught me about the importance of combining Eastern and Western medicine. A convergence of trends where egos were put aside and the patient's health is of primary concern. He was a great teacher and his influence is written in the words throughout this book.

When a nerve is impinged, it cuts back the nerve supply. What if this nerve feeds the heart, the lungs, the liver, and more? One of the major causes of deficiencies in our body is "**nerve deficiency**" and this is the essence of chiropractic care. We must protect our cells from any deficiency.

Chiropractic is now taking its rightful place in the mainstream of the healing arts. Today, this profession is accepted by the public, insurance companies, and most medical doctors.

Chiropractors are also aware of the importance of healthy lifestyle practices (rest, drinking enough water, exercise, proper nutrition, and stress reduction) that can also positively influence the nervous system and immune response. All of this affects our telomeres in a positive way. Deficiency, whether it be nutritional or nerve related, must be recognized and treated.

Chiropractors even help patient's battle illnesses such as the flu. During the 1917–18 influenza epidemic that brought death and fear to many Americans, it has been estimated that 20 million people died throughout the world, including about 500,000 Americans. It was chiropractic's success in caring for flu victims that led to the profession's licensure in many states. My Uncle Al Brenner graduated from chiropractic school in 1920. When we were sick or allergy season was upon us, we went to see Uncle Al. Who knew then that my time with him would affect my life forever?

"These results are not so surprising given what we now know about the interaction between the nervous system and the immune system," stated Matthew McCoy DC, MPH. "Through research we know that chiropractic has beneficial effects on immunoglobulins, white blood cells, pulmonary function, and other immune system processes."

Chiropractic influence on oxidative stress and DNA repair

There is a growing body of evidence that wellness care provided by doctors of chiropractic reduces healthcare costs, improves health behaviors, and enhances a patient's quality of life. Until recently, however, little was known about how chiropractic adjustments affected the chemistry of biological processes on a cellular level. Now it is known and should be a part of your health regime. In a landmark study published in the *Journal of Vertebral Subluxation Research*, chiropractors collaborating with researchers at the University of Lund found that chiropractic care could influence basic physiological processes affecting oxidative stress and DNA repair. These findings offer a scientific explanation for the positive health benefits reported by patients receiving chiropractic care.

The researchers measured the levels of primary antioxidants (serum thiol) in patients under chiropractic care and compared those to patients in a non-chiropractic control group. Long-term chiropractic care of two or more years was shown to reestablish a normal physiological state independent of age, sex, or nutritional supplements. The test provides a surrogate estimate of DNA repair enzyme activity, which correlates with lifespan and aging.

One article, written by a friend and colleague of mine and also one of the researchers, Dr. Christopher Kent, explained, "Going through life, we experience physical, chemical, and emotional stress. These stresses affect the function of the nervous system. We hypothesized that these disturbances in nerve function could affect oxidative stress and DNA repair on a cellular level.

"Oxidative stress, metabolically generating free radicals, is now a broadly accepted theory of how we age and develop disease," Kent continued. "Oxidative stress results in DNA damage, and inhibits DNA repair. DNA repair is the mechanism which fixes the damage caused by environmental impact.

"Chiropractors apply spinal adjustments to correct disturbances of nerve function. Chiropractic care appears to improve the ability of the body to adapt to stress," continued Kent. "Further research is needed to gain additional insights that will ultimately lead to improved clinical outcomes."

Chiropractic is important to cellular health and cellular health is everything. According to some estimates, more than 10 million people a year visit chiropractors.

Researchers and scientists alike recognize that there is a critical link between the nervous system and the immune system. Physiologist Dr. Korr proposed that "spinal lesions" (similar to the vertebral subluxation complex) are associated with exaggerated sympathetic (a division of the nerve system) activity.

Sympathetic activity has been shown to release immune regulatory cells into the blood circulation, which alters immune function. The nervous system has a direct effect on the immune system due to the nerve supply to the important immune system organs.

One of the most important studies showing the positive effect chiropractic care can have on the immune system and general health was performed by Ronald Pero, PhD, chief of cancer prevention research at New York's Preventive Medicine Institute and professor of medicine at New York University. Dr. Pero measured the immune systems of people under chiropractic care as compared to those in the general population and those with cancer and other serious diseases. In his initial three-year study of 107 individuals who had been under chiropractic care for 5 years or more, the chiropractic patients were found to have a 200% greater immune competence than people who had not received chiropractic care and 400% greater immune competence than people with cancer and other serious diseases. The immune system superiority of those under chiropractic care did not diminish with age.

Another important study was performed at the Sid E. Williams Research Center of Life Chiropractic University, where my younger son, now Dr. Jason Kaplan, DC, received his bachelor's degree, before migrating to Parker University & Chiropractic College. He was lucky to work and get his training from two fine institutions. I am so proud of Jason who now teaches with me at Parker University.

In one recent study, researchers took a group of HIV-positive patients and adjusted them over a six-month period. What they found was that the "patients that were adjusted had an increase of 48% in the CD4 cells (an important immune system component)." The control group (the patients that were not adjusted) did not demonstrate this dramatic increase in immune function, but actually experienced a 7.96% decrease in CD4 cell counts over the same period.

When we read the results of that study we were shocked that we hadn't heard about it earlier. Why didn't it make the headline news and why wasn't it on the front page of every newspaper? Those are very impressive results with important implications.

Modern doctors of chiropractic work directly with the nerves because they understand that the nerves control and coordinate the functions, organs, and systems of the entire body. The system is vast and complex, it has been estimated that there are approximately 20 billion neurons throughout the nervous system and 10 billion neurons in the brain alone. Nerve impulses not only give us the ability to experience sensation, they make it possible to carry out movement. It is the nervous system that transmits all sensations to the brain that makes it possible for us to see, smell, taste, touch, and hear. It's our nerves that maintain the perfect balance of the body.

It's the nervous system that makes it possible for us to swallow and move our bowels. The nervous system controls the liver, lungs, spleen, pancreas, gall bladder, and kidneys. It also controls our ability to adjust to a wide range of temperatures. Perfect natural health is possible only when you have a complete, perfect, normally functioning nervous system.

Conversely, when there is interference with the nerve energy signals, a problem of some type will develop. An estimated 90% of all interference with nerves originates in the spinal area. Vertebrae slip out of position and pinch the nerves, thus diminishing or perhaps cutting off the vital force of the body. A misaligned bone will not necessarily cause pain at the time, but it will eventually give rise to symptoms. The symptoms will proliferate unless the bone is put into its proper place so that the nerve can be freed. And this is where chiropractic comes in.

Inflammatory based disease is influenced by both the nervous, endocrine, and immune systems. Nerve stimulation directly affects the growth and function of inflammatory cells. Researchers found that dysfunction in this pathway results in the development of various inflammatory syndromes such as rheumatoid arthritis and behavioral syndromes such as depression. Additionally, this dysfunctional neuro-endo-immune response plays a significant role in immune-compromised conditions such as chronic infections and cancer.

Chiropractors know that *the power that created the body has the power to heal the body.* The only difference between a live person and a dead body is the energy that flows through a living human being; we call this the life force. As a chiropractic student working on my first cadaver, I was awed by the profound difference between life and death. That corpse had every nerve, organ, and tissue I had. The only difference—and it was a huge one—was the energy flowing in my body. The true meaning of this was brought home to me the night of my mother's death. I went to the hospital and saw my mother lying there. Only three hours before, she was so full of life. Although she looked at peace, I could not help thinking of her as she was such a short time ago, when the life force was animating her.

When the life force is flowing as it should, the human body is perfect—a marvelous system working in complete harmony. The human body harbors an intelligence that is unmatched in power, capacity, and adaptability. A mother instinctively recognizes this; she has a personal understanding of the infinite wisdom of the miracle of life. She understands this without any special training or education. She has a special faith in her own body and the body of her child.

As a physician, one of my tasks is to recognize this perfection. It is the function of the chiropractor to help the body maintain its perfect balance, because if this balance is off even a fraction, the body will no longer be at ease.

Chiropractic has always been the people's doctor. Without the principles of chiropractic, this book would not exist; for I believe that chiropractic is as important to good health as proper diet, and exercise, and rest. If you have a health problem, it is highly probably that you also have a chiropractic problem. If your weight is a concern, it is possible that some form of nerve interference is making it impossible for your body to properly digest and utilize food.

It is important at this juncture of the book for me to remind you that doctors don't cure you and supplements don't cure you. *The power that created the body has the power to cure the body.*

Medical doctors recognize chiropractic benefits

The medical profession is beginning to share this view. Many medical doctors have conducted honest, open-minded investigations of chiropractic, and the response has been favorable. In my offices in Florida I employed many medical doctors. I had an orthopedic surgeon, a neurologist, as physiatrist, and an osteopath all on my payroll. I was one of the first fully integrated MD/DC clinics in the United States. I later took this knowledge to corporate America and worked diligently to get chiropractic benefits in the managed care arena. Modern chiropractic is changing our bodies one cell, one subluxation, at a time and the medical world is taking notice.

Chiropractic's position and status today with the American College of Surgeons is as follows: "There are no ethical or collective restraints to full professional cooperation between doctors of chiropractic and medical physicians. Such cooperation should include referrals, group practice, participation of all healthcare delivery systems, treatment and services in and through hospitals, participation in student exchange, programs between chiropractic and medical colleges in cooperation and research in continuing programs."

The American College of Radiology says, "There are and should be no ethical or collective impediments to inter-medical radiologists in any setting where such association may occur, such as a hospital, private practice, research, education, care of a patient, or other legal arrangement."

The American Hospital Association says, "The AHA has no objection to a hospital granting privileges to doctors of chiropractic for the purposes of administering chiropractic treatment furthering the clinical education and training of doctors of chiropractic or having X-rays, clinical laboratory tests and reports there are made for doctors of chiropractic and their patients and/or previously taken X-rays, clinical laboratory tests and reports made available to them upon patient authorization."

Individual physicians have also praised the results possible through chiropractic.

Ills traced to vertebrae

"It may never occur to them (his/her medical colleagues) that the headaches, stomach trouble, neuritis, or nervous irritability they are attempting to cure may be due to nothing more serious than a displaced vertebrae, which any competent chiropractor can restore in ten seconds."

—Rubin Herman, MD

Chiropractic Adjustment Works (referring to severe headaches during and after specific movements of the head)

"...a chiropractic adjustment will work on the cervical region. We find in the case of hypertension a drop from 25 to 30 mm Hg right after the adjustment is given."

—K. Gutzeit, MD

Performs miraculous cures

"From personal experience alone, I am of the opinion that many patients suffer from some type of dislocation on the vertebral structures. There is no doubt that the consciousness of the orthopedic surgeon was aroused originally by the success of bone-setters, the

early manipulators, and more recently the chiropractors. The latter group has undoubtedly performed their miraculous cures in individuals who have been misdiagnosed and mistreated by the practitioner of an internist."
—Harold T. Hyman, *American Journal of Medical Science.*

Patients find relief

"It is quite easy to replace the vertebrae with a moderate amount of manipulation, and...many patients find relief in the hands of chiropractors."
—James Brailsford, MD

Chiropractic First...Surgery Last

"It is better that the chiropractor treats these patients than to have them treated by a physician who thinks only in terms of surgery."
—H.B. Gotten, MD

Chiropractic succeeds where medicine fails

"Few medical practitioners could recommend manipulation because they were barred against it by their oath; however, it is indisputable that the exponents of chiropractic had brought relief to many patients in the past, after orthodox treatment had been tried and failed."
—John Mennel, MD

Results for medically "incurable"

"There was a time when I looked at chiropractic through a pair of bifocal lenses, the upper plus prejudice, the lower plus lack of investigation. But because medicine, with all its adjuncts, had failed to reach the complicated ailments of my invalid wife, I, like a drowning man, grasped for anything in sight.

"I learned of chiropractic through a friend of mine. I went at once to a school of chiropractic, and to my surprise, they were actually getting results on cases that were hopelessly incurable from the stand point of medicine. I soon saw that the theory they were working on was plausible and met the approval of common sense. All of this opened up a new field of thought to me which had never been presented through the study of medicine. The sooner the medical profession recognized the work of the chiropractor, the better! S/he is doing a work that medicine cannot do. S/he belongs exclusively to the specialists and should be recognized."

—M.E. King, MD

Misaligned spine affects organs

"It is possible that a slight irregularity in the disposition of the vertebrae by 'strangling' certain spinal nerves at their exit from the spine can have considerable organic effects, as the chiropractic school maintains."

—R.F. Allendy, MD

Medical doctors treated by chiropractors

"Most physicians are opposed to vertebral manipulation, yet they do not hesitate to correct other bony or articular displacements. This attitude causes them to have themselves taken care of by… chiropractors."

—James Cyria, MD

Often only cure

"The 600 cases that we have observed over a period of four years have taught us super abundantly that vertebrotherapy…often…constitutes the only means of curing and that in a manner which is at times spectacular…the manipulation extolled by chiropractors are multiple and varied, and do not concern back pain only."

—Charles Rocher, MD

Gaining favor among doctors

"An explanatory introduction to chiropractic is no longer necessary. The manipulation of the spine, or at least a strong interest in it, is gaining favor in a wide circle of doctors. Among patients it has almost become the fashion to let oneself be treated by chiropractic, be it by the few in Germany who have been trained professionally in the United States or by physicians who have familiarized themselves with the method of treatment."

—G. Zillinger, MD

Chiropractic enriches medical disciplines

"The great possibilities of chiropractic lie in the exactly purposeful removal of a blocking of the spinal dynamics. Chiropractic does not belong, therefore, in the realm of a medical specialty; rather does it cut across all medical disciplines, not superseding them, restraining them, but broadening, uniting, and enriching them."

—Albert Cramer, MD

Chiropractors make people better

We must now realize that the world is not full of cripples produced by chiropractors. Chiropractors do not make people worse, they make an awful lot of them better."

—W.J.S. Melvin, MD

Value not appreciated

"Subluxations of vertebrae occur in all parts of the spine and in all degrees. When the dislocation is so slight as not to affect the spinal cord, it will still produce disturbances in the spinal nerves, passing off through the spinal foramina (Channels). The value of (chiropractic) has not been fully appreciated."

— James P. Warbassee, MD

As you can see medical doctors no longer resist working with, referring to, or recognizing chiropractors. This is not just in our country but throughout the world.

Germany

"Chiropractic is scientifically well founded, is one of the most effective neurotherapeutic measures known, and belongs in the very center of medicine."
—Unknown

England

"Seventeen percent of my patients require manipulation and it is a tragic fact that the average physician learns of manipulation after his patient has been helped by someone outside the medical profession."
—Albert Cramer MD

Switzerland

"The attitude of clinical medicine toward chiropractic has radically changed...IN the mid-1930s, it was denounced...Today, however, many medical doctors are in favor of chiropractic and consider it to be an excellent therapeutic measure from certain diseases having their origin in changes within the spinal column."
—H. DeBrunner, MD

Australia

"There can be no disease which does not disturb the nerve cells concerned. If the cause of the disturbance of these conducting nerves can be ascertained or removed, the patient will be cured. If not, treatment merely diverts from the truth."
—R.J. Berry, MD

Canada

"The addition of chiropractic maneuvers to general management permits treatment of the cause rather than effect."
—R.A. Leeman, MD

Scotland

"Spinal manipulation is a method of treatment which has been long neglected by the medical profession. IN spite of the efforts of men...to demonstrate its value, there is still much prejudice against it and ignorance regarding the rational understanding of the treatment and methods for carrying it out."
—T. Millar, *The Clinical Journal*

Russia

"(In) many pathological processes...the nervous component remains from beginning to end the factor that determines their general state."
—A.D. Speransky

Great Britain

"It is regrettable that patients suffering from slight congestive spinal lesion should be advised to seek relief in a popular pain killer. No wonder that the manipulator who can, in a short time, often relieve intolerable backache and receives warm appreciation."
—*British Journal of Physical Medicine*

Denmark

"Manipulative treatment, which previously in this country, was given exclusively by chiropractors, has in later years been taken up by some physicians, among others, the writer, who has found that this therapy is of significant value...It must be emphasized that it requires great clinical experience and great technical skill to perform

these manipulations...If the physiotherapists want to use manipulative treatment, they ought to get an education just as thorough as that of chiropractors."
—Dr. Boje, Senior physician at Rigs Hospital, Copenhagen

France

"The 600 cases that we have observed over a period of 4 years have taught us super-abundantly that vertebra-therapy...often... constitutes the only means of curing, and that in a manner which is at times spectacular...the manipulations extolled by the chiropractors are multiple and varied, and do not concern back pains only."
—Charlies M. Rocher, MD

Argentina

"Chiropractic is a useful therapeutic method worthy of being introduced into the patrimony of medicine. We regard it as very fitting...to create a school of chiropractors, with the object of making known to physicians the existence of this therapeutic method and its accomplishments...and with the highly social objective of bringing the benefits of chirotherapy to even the humblest classes."
—Ministry of Public Health and Welfare

Germany

"Since the introduction of chiropractic methods in our polyclinic...it must undoubtedly be recognized that the percentage of success is great. . .No physical or psychic damage was done to the patients not successfully treated. Those not handled successfully were almost exclusively those who did not come regularly for treatment. This method is worth being brought to the attention of the widest possible medical circles."
—A.A. Hochfield

The Rand Study concluded, "Spinal manipulation is the most commonly used conservative treatment for low back pain in the United States. It is the treatment supported by the most research in its effectiveness in terms of early results and long-term benefits."

Study after study from the Rand Corporation to the *British Medical Journal* recognizes the benefits of chiropractic care. Chiropractic is the safe choice, the cost-effective choice, and the smart choice. It's not different to go to chiropractic anymore, it's just as smart.

If you have a health problem, it is highly probably that you also have a chiropractic problem. If your weight is a concern, it is possible that some form of nerve interference is making it impossible for your body to properly digest and utilize food.

In Ephesians 4:16, the Apostle Paul says, "All of the body, by being harmoniously joined together were being made to cooperate through every joint that gives what is needed, according to each respective member in due measure, makes for the growth of the body for building up itself." The human body has not changed since biblical times, and Paul's statement is as true now as it ever was.

According to WebMD, "About 22 million Americans visit chiropractors annually. Of these, 7.7 million, or 35%, are seeking relief from back pain from various causes, including accidents, sports injuries, and muscle strains. Other complaints include pain in the neck, arms, and legs, and headaches. Spinal manipulation and chiropractic care is generally considered a safe, effective treatment for acute low back pain, the type of sudden injury that results from moving furniture or getting tackled. Acute back pain, which is more common than chronic pain, lasts no more than six weeks and typically gets better on its own."

Tragically, more than three out of four Americans have medically significant cellular malfunction—a diagnosable disease of some kind. The overwhelming majority of us are somewhere between cellular malfunction and diagnosable disease. If this malfunction is due to a structural deficiency, research now clearly demonstrates that chiropractic will make a difference. Your cells cannot function at 100% if you have less than 100% nerve supply. This is the # 1 deficiency we are exposed to if not under chiropractic care. Is it any wonder why chiropractors always have a great attitude and live their lives the chiropractic way? They understand the importance of proper nerve supply, and now hopefully you do as well.

1. *Society desperately needs chiropractic care*
2. *Chiropractic care brings so much value to every human being and most of us have no idea how.*

Imagine for one minute that there existed a product that would help people revolutionize their cellular health, their personal health and well-being. Let's say this product or pill needed to be taken once a day for one week, then once per month from that point throughout their entire life. Now what if I told you, that evidence proved that this product helped reverse neuro-degeneration, increased immunity, stopped bone degeneration, increased telomere length (which decreases aging), reduced chronic disease physiology, and helped express good genes while suppressing bad genes. This all-natural product would take less than 10 minutes to administer and would begin producing an immediately healthy response. How much would people pay for such a product? How much would every community spend if Big Pharma held the lone patent?

The purpose of my hypothetical situation is obvious. The list in that analogy includes just a few of the many known and proven benefits of a chiropractic adjustment. Every Doctor of chiropractic holds the patent to the life-changing benefits stored in the power of an adjustment! Less than 100,000 doctors possess the knowledge, skill, and capability to deliver a precise adjustment that brings health to a society of millions of people badly in need of that very product.

Chiropractic is no longer a myth, it is a reality, and within the scope of chiropractic, miracles are taking place with every adjustment. Chiropractic has arrived and it is here to stay and should be part of your cellular health and telomere protection plan.

"Health is a relationship between you and your body."

—TERRI GUILLEMETS

Chapter 24

A NATURAL APPROACH
TO HEALTHCARE

As we begin to wind down on our journey, it is important we keep our eyes on the road and continue on our path to wellness—our quest to *Awaken the Wellness Within*.

You can see why I'm so excited about this. I just got done with my morning jog and my cells are happy, and my energy levels are better than ever before. Every day I work to age slower, healthier, and more gracefully.

To truly *Awaken the Wellness Within*, we must accept that there is only one disease—cytopathology. When cells are not at ease, they are at dis-ease. Once the cells are not at ease, they begin to weaken and malfunction and become diseased. When the cells are no longer in balance, the body is no longer able to maintain homeostasis by regulating and repairing itself; this is the essence of disease. Because only one disease exists, all we need to do is prevent the causes of that one disease. By doing this, we preserve fuel for our cells and lengthen our telomeres, which will hopefully extend our lives.

As we come to the end of this book, I have to remind you of where I began. It was one rainy afternoon in Atlanta at the Shepherd Center. My son had just wheeled me in my wheelchair to the garden. This was my first time outside in about two months. I remember sitting there and contemplating the meaning of life. Illness has a powerful way of providing perspective, and one of the most profound conclusions I have reached is that health is a choice and that often sickness and disease can be avoided. Each day we make choices and each day we must live with those choices.

Choose your future

With our choices, we get to choose our future. For every day we live, we prepare for our tomorrows. This starts with you and your current mindset. Our brains work like computers: Whether intended or unintended, they do what they have been programmed to do. A big part of using the psychological pathway to stay healthy is the ability to recognize your current programming and to learn new programs—new thoughts, attitudes, and behavior patterns.

Friends, let's face the facts: although perfect nutrition, perfect genes, a pure environment, and ideal behavior do not exist, these factors write the story of your life, including how many chapters you will finish. The interaction between inherited genes, nutritional intake, the environment, and our beliefs at any point in time are the triggers that determine our current state of health or disease, including how long we live.

By changing the conditions inside your body through nutrition, chiropractic, non-toxic living you can signal your cells to express in different ways. Our society tends to think that disease is the result of aging. Not true. Disease is a result of the rate at which we age, not the number of years we have inhabited the Earth. The rate is affected by "aging cells/telomeres," which we can choose to keep turned off.

Regardless of the recipe you start with, a dish is only as good as the ingredients put into it. The same goes for a cell. When a cell is provided with the proper nutrients, kept free from toxins, and placed in a supportive environment, health-supporting properties are activated, aging and disease-causing cells remain dormant, and

362

both your good cells and you are healthy. To move yourself in the right direction on the genetic pathway, create a healthy environment for your genes and protect them from damage.

There is only one disease: *Cytopathology*

When cells malfunction, the body is no longer able to maintain homeostasis (balance) by regulating and repairing itself. This is the essence of disease, no matter what you call it or how it happens. Because only one disease exists, all we need to do is prevent the causes of that one disease

There are only two causes of disease:

1. *Deficiency*
2. *Toxicity*

All you have to do for health is to give your cells what they need and protect them from what they don't need. Cells malfunction only if they suffer from a lack of nutrients (deficiency), toxic damage (toxicity), or a combination of both. Preventing these two causes of disease is made possible by our ability to choose how we live our lives.

We have learned throughout this book that health and disease are choices. We, as a society and as individuals, are the ones making those choices. Today, health is compromised at so many levels. If we want to improve our health, prevent or reverse disease, and extend life, we have to make special choices in order to compensate. We cannot rely on physicians to "fix" everything, especially if we have spent decades making ourselves sick by abusing our bodies and their cells.

The responsibility for health is yours, and you must embrace it and pay it forward. We must teach this to our children so they and their children can claim their birthright to lifelong good health. We must also ask our governments and society at large to make changes. Why do we allow soft drink and candy vending machines into our schools? Why is it that medical insurance covers failed traditional treatments but does not cover alternative treatments that are safer and more effective? Why do we allow our government to subsidize the dairy and sugar industries? Why do we allow genetically modified foods to be sold without labeling and without adequate testing for safety?

It amazes me that today throughout the country many schools still allow soft drink and candy vending machines into our schools. Why is it that medical insurance covers failed traditional treatments but does not cover alternative treatments that are safer and more effective? Shouldn't the care with the most risk be the alternative? We must change our countries paradigm from a symptom-based model to a model of prevention.

Yet ObamaCare will limit physician care and allow genetically modified foods to be sold without labeling and without adequate testing for safety? The key to the countries health care dilemma must focus on prevention. If elected, I promise to speak with President Trump, and as I know many of his beliefs on health care, I believe he will look for a better way.

We as Americans must speak up and no longer allow toxins like fluoride in our drinking water? How much money would the average American save if he trusted the water that came out of his tap? The water he pays taxes for.

Today, most of us, and almost all of our physicians, are living in a world of confusion and misunderstanding. The medical establishment has done a great job; in my eyes it is Big Pharma that is the major problem. They lobby for medical doctors to utilize and disperse their product, knowing of their many side effects. The current health paradigm of treating symptoms versus the cause is a distorted way of viewing health—treating symptoms alone is not solving our problems.

If we are continually taught and believe that thousands of diseases exist, then of course we must go to doctors for all our health problems; we are so overwhelmed and afraid that we must believe that only the doctor has the education to deal with all the different diseases and their treatments. The new perspective I offer you is that there is only one disease; health is then easier to understand, and the power to get healthy and to stay healthy lies within yourself. Aside from medical emergencies, which are indeed matters for trained professionals, maintaining your health is a matter of preventing deficiency and toxicity and requires little or no outside assistance.

The largest misconception in America is that most of us are healthy. In reality, most of us are on our way to getting sick and not reaching our health potential. We are living proof that it is entirely possible to achieve normal growth rates and have a healthy appearance while being undernourished and in a state of compromised health. Our unprecedented epidemic of chronic and degenerative disease is clearly the result of eating a diet consisting of adulterated and devitalized foods; exposure to the lethal effects of polluted air, water and food; and exposure to man-made electromagnetic radiation. Yet, as a society, we have failed to come to grips with this reality, partially because we are still stuck in the obsolete medical paradigm of the "germs and genes theory" of disease, and partially because powerful economic incentives exist to maintain the status quo.

Americans cannot continue to eat nutritionally deficient diets—diets rich in make-believe foods made from sugar, white flour, and processed oils; diets that will not even sustain healthy life in animals—and still be healthy?

I ask you now to consider your lifestyle and identify the areas that you must change. To be effective, please take a close look at your overall perspective on health and disease. Health is something we all want, yet so few of us give it serious thought until we get sick. That paradigm simply does not work. The practical new system for choosing health presented in this book is different from typical approaches. This new way to "see" health and disease is so simple it empowers the individual to take charge. That empowerment can help to end our current epidemic of chronic and degenerative disease, dramatically improving the health of our people.

Let me thank you for allowing me to share my theory of health and disease, one that is so simple and powerful that it gives you the ability to think about the really important things in life.

At my lowest point, while paralyzed, I asked myself whether or not I wanted to continue living. I was ashamed of my thoughts. I loved my wife, I loved my sons, but I was so weak, so sick, so disabled, and I was told there was no cure for botulism. It was one night while looking into my son's eyes, my son who still looked at me like I was his hero, that I made my decision. I decided that I did not want to die—I wanted to live. However, I chose not to accept my present disabled state or the prognosis of a life of disability that all the doctors envisioned. My only option was to find a way to become healthy again.

Once I made my decision, my healing began. I read everything and anything. Everywhere I went, everywhere I turned, led me to the cell.

This book is about health, healing, and *Awakening the Wellness Within*.

Only one cure

The greatest healer of all lies inside of you. *The power that created the body heals the body.* We must stop putting all our hope and faith into pills and potions and accept the power of the human body.

Every second that we're alive, the cells in our bodies are endlessly working to bring us back to a natural state of homeostasis or equilibrium. When we turn to medicines or physical manipulations of our body's systems to heal us, we are really only facilitating our body's natural ability to heal from within.

Each cell is a dynamic, living unit that is constantly monitoring and adjusting its own processes, ongoingly working to restore itself according to the original DNA code it was created with, and to maintain balance within the body.

More and more, people in the United States are getting wise to the fact that many diseases are avoidable, and preventing them is within our control. Whether it's the common cold or something more onerous such as heart disease or cancer, we have to work at keeping those illnesses away.

We must give thanks and acknowledge the great engineering feats of the body, the marvelous innate powers that protects its own vital interests. When we consider the wonderful mechanism of the human body, the certainty with which all organs perform their allotted work, the marvelous ingenuity with which the body meets our daily needs not to mention emergencies, its almost limitless powers of repair and recuperation, we develop a large respect and admiration for the healing powers of the body and learn to view with contempt and disgust the means that people employ in unintelligent efforts to "cure."

The greatest power in the universe is your own body, and its innate life force! The energy that keeps you alive also powers every bit of your healing! It must be your goal from here on in to use it to your full advantage or ignore and squander it, erroneously assuming your healing power is to be found elsewhere.

Your body is constantly working as best it can to preserve and improve its vital domain: repairing its parts when needed, regenerating, rebalancing, and optimizing all of its functions. This healing force is vigorous and thorough, under favorable conditions.

With rare exceptions, your cells contain the perfect instructions for all manner of self-healing; it happens automatically. All that is needed is that we intelligently cooperate with the body's calls for rest so that it can accomplish its tasks without interference. This means stepping out of the way and conserving energy so that our fullest energy potential is available for the healing work.

Our innate body intelligence knows best—it trumps the meddling mind and our futile tinkerings every time! Trust your body's wisdom—let it do its work and your "healing miracle" will take place in its own time. Healing can be fast or slow—we must be patient and accept that the body is always doing its best.

We hopefully have learned throughout this book that when we are sick or injured, the body's actions are unerring as it goes about its business of restoring health. Yes, occasionally, we may need some form of emergency care medical care and chiropractic manipulation to facilitate the natural healing of the entire organism. If we cooperate with the body, providing the optimum conditions for health, the healing job will be accomplished in minimal time.

Squandering our cells' innate self-healing power by bombarding our bodies with toxins and not being responsible for its deficiencies is a tragic mistake made too often by too many. We only delay healing and prolong suffering when we attempt to "fix" or "treat" the body with modalities. The body heals not because of, but in spite of such interventions! Allowing our innate power to do its work, while we patiently ride out the health restoration process, is a beautiful experience; it is always the most prudent approach. Best of all, it's free!

Healing can be as easy as lying down, closing your eyes and letting the God within take over.

Leading healthy lifestyles and consuming healthful (as opposed to toxic) diets will go a very long way in keeping us healthy, whether we are young or older.

This book is not about growing old, but growing your telomeres. The key to a long healthy life is your lifestyle.

As you consider your lifestyle and identify the areas that must change, take a close look at your overall perspective on health and disease. Health is something we all want, yet so few of us give it serious thought until we get sick. That approach simply does not work.

The practical new system for choosing health presented in this book is unique compared to many of the current approaches. This new paradigm to health is to see health and disease in such a simple form you can understand the process of health and aging. Doing this empowers you to take charge of your health, your life, and your cells. Your empowerment can help end our current epidemic of chronic and degenerative disease, dramatically improving your health and the health of your family and friends.

We live in a world where symptoms and disease dominate. Our current model of medicine is not about healthcare; it is about disease care. This model of medicine waits for disease to happen—instead of catching dis-ease at in its initial decline. We do this by ignoring the whole patient, including their diet and lifestyle. It ignores the effects of nutrition, toxins, and behavior and gives little or no recognition to the body's self-healing abilities.

The new perspective on health that I shared with you in this book is based not on waiting for disease to happen, but actively working to prevent disease. If disease does occur, then we must look for the true cause and restore health by removing the cause. This alternative approach recognizes, understands, and respects that the body is a self-regulating and self-healing organism. This approach incorporates all we have learned about the effects of nutrition, toxicity, and behavior. The underlying inspiration is that health is a choice and that almost all disease is preventable.

The key to health and wellness is cellular health. To maintain cellular health and longer telomeres, we must focus on the natural ways in which we can heal and nourish our cells, lengthen our telomeres, and lengthen our lives. People can take the easier road by trying to mask their symptoms and taking medication while ignoring their bad lifestyle habits—or they can take the purer, more natural approach that often takes longer for the effects to show but becomes a long-term solution.

Ultimately, we'll find that the extra time and energy needed for the more natural path is the road worth traveling.

Where do you go from here? How do you stay young, live young, and enjoy life? Begin with the basics: Cleanse and nourish the cell.

The secret to healthy cells and a long life of ageless aging is simple, but it does require daily discipline. The good news is it doesn't need to cost you a lot of money to stay healthy and to age gracefully.

This book is about healing yourself. To heal yourself you must have faith in your body's ability to heal itself. When your cells are functioning as they should, you have ample adaptive capacity to thrive in our constantly changing environment without ill effects. With properly functioning cells, you have strong resilience to various kinds of stress—physical, chemical, biological, and emotional. Your body has the innate ability to make daily repairs to your cells, the ability to build healthy new ones, and the ability to efficiently remove pathogenic microorganisms and toxins from your body.

Your body has an innate desire to self-heal because it wants to be in good health and remain healthy. However, on your road to health, don't panic if it takes more time than you thought; self-healing takes time. Your body is improving itself, bit by bit, moment by moment, and day by day. You need to be patient and have some degree of commitment and diligence to protecting your cells.

Most disease sufferers, knowingly or unknowingly, have made poor choices leading to their illness. This includes what they choose to eat and drink and also the choice to not lead an active life. Your lifestyle choices brought you to your current condition.

This book is about going back to the basics to remind us of the power of the human body, the greatest healer in the world. We've learned there is only *one disease, two causes, and one cure.*

All you have to do for health is to give your cells what they need and protect them from what they don't need. Cells weaken and die prematurely only if they are toxic and do not have the strength to fight off the toxins. If our cells suffer from a lack of nutrients (deficiency), toxic damage (toxicity), or a combination of both, they will weaken and disease will proliferate in our bodies. By making smart choices and preventing these two causes of disease we can literally age younger. It is our ability to choose how we live our lives, and this will determine the rate at which we age. Health depends on the choices we make daily. The right choices will lead us to the cure and prevention of disease. I wrote this book to help you make better choices. My brother Steve would want it this way.

Let each of us make an affirmation that from this day forward; we'll find that the extra time and energy needed for the more natural path will be well worth it. This is the road worth traveling. Here are some of the many benefits from a natural, preventative attitude to health and happiness:

- We need to treat the root causes of health problems instead of temporarily stopping symptoms.
- We need less medication, and possibly even eliminate medication (with your doctor's guidance), which will save you money and reduce suffering from side effects.
- We will work to develop a better attitude, achieve a better body weight, sleep better, feel more energetic...
- We will work to feel happier and healthier.

We must plan to live to an older age, while enjoying life as we age gracefully. This book is about healing yourself. To heal yourself, you must have faith in your body. Remember, when your cells are functioning as they should, you have ample adaptive capacity to thrive in our constantly changing environment without ill effects. With properly functioning cells, you have strong resilience to various kinds of stress—physical, chemical, biological and emotional. Your body has the innate ability to make daily repairs to your cells, the ability to build healthy new ones, and the ability to efficiently remove pathogenic microorganisms and toxins from your body.

Remember, the body is perfect in every way; we just have to treat it accordingly. Once we become one with our bodies, or in balance with our bodies and nature, we reach a mental and physical homeostasis. We must aspire to achieving good cellular health.

Hopefully you have learned that healthy people do not get sick, only sick people become sick. Once you start to compromise your cells you compromise your telomeres and your health. This happens through a series of events, your cells' experience. It starts with one cell. Once one cell becomes weakened, you're vulnerable for a number of cells to begin to malfunction. Once the body is no longer at ease, dis-ease enters and our immune system goes to war as our vulnerability to infections increase and dis-ease becomes disease.

Although we hate to face the facts, most disease sufferers invariably, if unknowingly, have made poor choices leading to illness. This includes their diet and their exercise regime (or lack of such a regime). In essence, their lifestyle choices. In the case of sick children, often the parents unknowingly have made poor choices on their behalf. Obesity and diabetes are on the rise in children. Is this a coincidence, or did they simply wear down the cells with toxins, sugars, processed foods, and carbohydrates?

We must accept responsibility for our health. Once we do this, we'll change our statistics in regard to healthcare. We need to be proactive, not reactive. The overall health of our cells determines the overall length of our telomeres, and thus our level of health.

There is only one disease: cytopathology. There are two causes: deficiency and toxicity. These are the only causes of disease. And there is only one cure: healing the cell and allowing the body to heal itself. If our cells are going to be replaced on a daily basis, doesn't it make sense to replace the poor cells with new, healthy cells?

A radical shift in paradigm

As you consider your new lifestyle and identify the areas that you must change, take a close look at your overall perspective on health and disease. Health is something we all want, yet so few of us give it serious thought until we get sick. We have learned chapter after chapter that approach simply does not work. Our practical new system for choosing health presented in this book is different from typical approaches. My goal as a doctor, author, husband, father, and friend was for this new paradigm I shared with you to make health and disease so easy to understand that it empowers you to take charge of your health. This new-found empowerment can help to end our current epidemic of chronic and degenerative disease, dramatically improving the health of our people.

When you change your lifestyle to possess healthy habits and to create healthy cells, you will attain longer telomeres and better health. There are no shortcuts to ageless aging.

Once we are able to embrace health and avoid illness by educating ourselves and our families on how to make healthy choices, we'll take a proactive position in regards to our health. Once we are able to lower our levels of deficiency by providing the body with the supplements we need to protect the cells and removing the toxins that alter our cells, we can promote cellular health, the key to ageless aging.

Fortunately, you can accept responsibility for your health at any time and make lifestyle choices that will bring good health and a long life. You need to be proactive, not reactive. The overall health of your cells determines the overall length of your telomeres, your level of health, and length of life.

When you change your lifestyle to possess healthy habits, to create healthy cells, you will preserve both your telomeres and your health.

Once we embrace health and avoid illness by educating ourselves and our families on how to make healthful choices, the right choices, we will take a proactive position on our health. By removing toxins and deficiencies, we can protect and heal the cells and promote cellular health, the key to *Awakening the Wellness Within.*

One Disease—Two Causes—One Cure

THE BEGINNING.

Epilogue

LIFE EXIST—LIFEXIST = THE FUTURE

Throughout time man has searched for the mythical *Fountain of Youth*: Drinking from it was supposed to stop aging and restore youthfulness. Legend has it that Ponce de León went searching for it in the early 1500s and discovered Florida in the process. In current times, the once vision of the cure-all fountain has been replaced by the wish for medications that can stop or reverse aspects of the aging process. We learned health and wellness do not come in a bottle, that it begins at a cellular level. We have learned that the symptoms of aging, memory loss, and dementia concerns are particularly frightening yet with diet and lifestyle change may be avoided. As a doctor, I have remained on that quest every day of my life. This book has taken on many roads, many pathways, and my search will continue till the day I die. I now know by understanding the cell, understanding cellular health, that there is a way; there are clinics that look to restore the bodies innate healing powers.

Life is for the living. Our Founding Fathers were right about the pursuit of happiness being as critical as life and liberty. Happiness boosts the immune system and helps tamp down stress. Involvement with activities, people, and experiences that bring joy and contentment also boost optimism and positive attitude, both of which are linked to longevity. Our attitude affects our cells, which maintains our telomeres. Happy person, happy cells. Life is for living, loving, laughing, and learning, not just whining, worrying, and working. Fact is, pursuing reasonable pleasures helps one live more fully in the moment, rather than dwelling on the past or suffering until some future happiness comes along in the form of a vacation because you are overworked and not meeting your health potential.

Throughout this book we have learned so much about health. But what do we do now? Where do we go? Throughout my travels, I have looked for that One-Stop shop to anti-aging and wellness. Well good news my friends, I may have found it. The name of this new brand this upcoming franchise is LifeXist. I met with Dr. Eric Nepute and franchise king Todd Beckman, with over 15 years of franchise experience. Meeting Todd was fun, his office is like a Disneyland for adults, filled with cars and racing memorabilia. He is a man of 50 with the stamina of a 25-year-old. His energy was boundless, and his enthusiasm for life was contagious. Meeting him and Dr. Nepute got me very excited as they explained to myself and Dr. Bard their concept. Dr. Nepute is one of the leading alternative practitioners in the United States. His focus and health model is a brain-based cellular management program. It's true healing from the inside out. Diligently he works to combine the best of Eastern and Western Medicine. Imagine one place where the best medicine and chiropractic work together, providing balance of your cells and removing toxins and deficiencies, the two causes of the one disease—cytopathology.

LifeXist, is their new model, which they plan on being a "one-stop shop" for anti-aging. They utilize a proprietary approach to aging, health, and wellness that is both accessible and affordable. Their model focuses on the importance of the cell and cellular health. Once we discussed my One Disease Paradigm, Todd and Eric went wild. "This is it," Todd, said. "This is our concept." Aging naturally, healthfully, gracefully. A franchise committed to making you feel younger and healthier at an affordable rate. Imagine one location working with you, helping you be the best you that you can be.

Aging, a steady decline:

Let's face the facts: Every day we age; we get a day older. Yet, why do so many celebrities look good beyond their years. Yes, you can say plastic surgery, but look deeper and you will notice their muscle tone, their energy. What do they know that you don't? The history of the world is filled with stories of individuals trying to find eternal youth—wealthy people going to private centers for magic elixirs, many individuals taking mega doses of certain vitamins, drinking green tea, using coenzyme Q10, etc. hoping to find the "fountain of youth." Let's take a closer look and see what happens to our bodies as we age.

Earlier in the book we discussed the two T's of anti-aging. Telomeres and Turmeric. To the many traditional cultures around the world that have long utilized the spice in cooking and medicine, turmeric's amazing anti-inflammatory, antioxidant, and anti-cancer benefits are no secret. But modern, Western cultures are only just now beginning to learn of the incredible healing powers of turmeric, which in more recent days have earned it the appropriate title of "king of all spices." And as more scientific evidence continues to emerge, turmeric is quickly becoming recognized as a fountain of youth "superspice" with near-miraculous potential in modern medicine. This spice also aids in protecting our telomeres.

Scientific studies published in recent years have shown that taking turmeric on a regular basis can actually lengthen lifespan and improve overall quality of life. A study conducted on roundworms, for instance, found that small amounts of curcumin, the primary active ingredient in turmeric, increased average lifespan by about 39%. A similar study involving fruit flies revealed a 25% lifespan increase as a result of curcumin intake. Yet, this great product is rarely recommended by conventional doctors today.

In the first study mentioned above, researchers found that turmeric helped reduce the number of reactive oxygen species in roundworms, as well as reduce the amount of cellular damage that normally occurs during aging. Curcumin was also observed to improve roundworms' resistance to heat stress compared to those not taking the spice. And in fruit flies, curcumin appeared to trigger increased levels of superoxide dismutase (SOD), an antioxidant compound that protects cells against oxidative damage.

Dr. Nepute, Dr. Bard and I, like many doctors, understand nature's healing herbs. The problem is so few doctors recommend these products. Which brings us back to the values to aiding the cells proficiency.

Even with all the data showing that it can help boost energy levels, cleanse the blood, heal digestive disorders, dissolve gallstones, treat infections, and prevent cancer, some health experts have been reluctant to recommend taking turmeric in medicinal doses until human clinical trials have been conducted. But unlike pharmaceutical drugs, taking turmeric is not dangerous, and civilizations have been consuming large amounts of it for centuries as part of their normal diets.

According to consumption data collected back in the 1980s and 1990s, the average Asian person consumes up to 1,000 milligrams of turmeric a day, or as much as 440 grams per year, which equates to roughly 90 milligrams of active curcuminoids per day at the higher end of the concentration spectrum. And these figures, of course, primarily cover just the amount of turmeric consumed as food in curries and other traditional dishes, which means supplements with similar concentrations are perfectly safe and effective.

Time alone is not the enemy

Growth hormone declines steadily at the age of 31 and at the rate of 14% per decade. Along with aging, we become vulnerable to diseases. Our ability to fight illness declines, the body's ability to metabolize sugar, handle cholesterol, and clear the kidneys of toxins becomes more and more difficult. Ultimately, the slow deadly disease of aging creeps in.

As a person ages, hormone levels fall. Decreasing levels of certain hormones shows symptoms such as:

- Gray hair
- Wrinkly skin
- Reduced skin thickness
- Forgetfulness
- Low sex drive
- Weight gain
- Bone or joint problems
- Immune system weakens
- Decreased muscle strength

These symptoms can be the possible result of reduced human growth hormone. Until age 21, human growth hormone is abundant in the body, being solely responsible for muscle building, bone growth, skin elasticity, increased energy, lean body mass, and sexual vigor.

Graying hair

One of the first signs of aging is graying hair. What causes this and can it be reversed? Graying hair is caused by the slowing production of melanin over time within the hair follicles. When this happens, the hair follicles produce less and less melanin, and the result is a loss of hair, color and strength.

The skin

The next telltale sign of aging is the skin. Fact is, the hormonal breakdown and free radicals is the major contributor of skin aging because of the reduction of the body's hormone production or lack of. Hormones such as human growth hormone and testosterone are only produced in noticeable quantities up to the age of 20. These hormones are responsible for physical fitness, regeneration, and the immune system. Due to a declining hormone level, the breakdown of organs, tissues, and cells begins.

Another factor are free radicals. These are parts of molecules that are found in the human body. As a result of external factors such as ultraviolet light (too much sun), smoking or unhealthy eating habits, under these circumstances free radicals are inclined to react. Meaning that they are in search of other chemical substances to bond themselves with. Ultimately, the breakdown of the skin begins. The body protects itself against these aggressors with naturally occurring antioxidants. Until you reach the age of 20 and onwards, this natural defense mechanism slowly declines, until eventually the skin can no longer defend itself.

What can be done about aging?

Well, about your actual age—nothing, but could a healthier lifestyle, proper diet, or maybe vitamin and supplement intake help turn back the aging clock? Is there something out there that could:

- Alleviate menopausal and premenstrual symptoms
- Reduce body fat
- Restore gray hair
- Increase energy
- Increase sex drive enhancement in both men and women
- Restore the function of organs and glands
- Improve memory

- Improve vision
- Enhance one's spirits
- Stabilize blood pressure
- Enhance the immune system

My answer is yes to all of the above. Within the genius of Dr. Nepute and the business acumen of Todd Beckman comes a new type of clinic that has me excited. A one-stop shop for anti-aging in an affordable manner. A concept that provides ongoing treatment to improve one's health that is not solely for the rich and famous. With LifeXist, membership truly has its privileges.

LifeXist
"Helping you break through health and aging barriers."

The facts are simple: Health care is complicated. To travel life without a map is wellness suicide. Their program is committed to knowing where you are healthwise and exactly where you are meant to be! Specializing in customized solutions to assist with physical, emotional, and mental problems.

Through education and empowerment, LifeXist will guide you on your very own, unique road to wellness! What makes it even better is it's not simply fee-for-service. It is membership based. I have never seen such an exclusive product so affordable. This paradigm will revolutionize wellness as McDonald's did hamburgers.

Do you currently have an injury or illness that prevents you from enjoying life?

Want to increase the calm in your mind throughout your busy, jam-packed week?

What if we could change that? LifeXist's goal is to help its members make it to 100—but let's face it, some people age a lot more gracefully than others. What's the difference between someone who looks and feels vibrant in midlife and beyond—and someone who's sick, sad, and already *old*?

Scientists are turning up some surprising key factors: approaches to attitude and lifestyle that not only add years to your life but add a better quality of life to your years.

"Studies on successful aging have shown that only one third of what predicts how well we age is controlled by genetics. About two thirds is based on our personal lifestyle choices—and is therefore under our control," says psychiatrist Gary Small, director of the UCLA Center.

LifeXist shares a great Mission Statement: "To give every man and woman the opportunity to achieve their God-given maximum potential in life. To empower their members not only to live life, but to thrive and LifeXist.

Here are some longevity factors you can do something about:

Health—The key to happiness

Without health you have nothing. Daily, everyone's bodies lose essential vitamins and hormones as they age. This leads for weakened cells and thus causes our cells to malfunction. With One Disease and Two Causes, deficiency plays a primary role to cellular optimization to total wellness. LifeXist and their team of doctors are revolutionizing wellness. Their doctors work closely with each patient to identify the deficiencies of their client and their guide cells while working to develop a program to restore cellular optimization.

Most people aren't good at knowing what makes them happy, what makes them healthy. No one wants to get or feel old. Daily we need to pay extra-close attention to not only our diet but our mood for a few days. Jot down what's happening during times when you feel particularly happy, as well as what circumstances drain you or trigger anxiety. Who are you with? What are you doing? What are you thinking about? How do you feel physically and why? How can you get more of those good feelings and minimize the less-good ones? Aging attacks us in so many ways. Deficiency will manifest itself in the form of depression. Depression is more than just a mental condition; sometimes our bodies are depressed because they are nutrient deficient.

Time for something new

If you do the same thing the same way, you can only expect the same result. Life is about change. The brain loves novelty; it excites the energy maker, the "mitochondria" of the cells. Although different types of mental skills change with age—for example, mental computations slow—the brain never loses the ability to grow. And trying or learning new things builds new neural connections all through life. We learned throughout this book that *the power that creates the body heals the body*; however, a car, the best car, can't go far without gasoline. LifeXist offers a unique program where weekly you engage in cellular optimization. They identify the deficiencies of each client and develop a program designed specifically for them.

We need to daily maximize cell and brain fitness and the body's health will follow in kind. Staying receptive to new ideas also fuels curiosity, open-mindedness, and creativity—traits linked to healthier aging.

Unfortunately, habits also ossify with age, which can make us prone to dismiss new things or feel intimidated by them. Cellular health, the preservation of our telomeres, is the key to aging gracefully.

Be your own best friend

People often fall into the trap of being kinder, more loving, and more forgiving to those around them than to themselves. We beat ourselves up about an imperfect diet or a missed opportunity. We hate our looks (waist, hair, nose—there's always something). We neglect self-care. In general, we fail to be our own number-one cheerleader. Lacking compassion and a sense of worth about your-self leads to making unfortunate choices that can damage health and well-being.

"Stress occurs when the mind perceives you're not enough or don't have enough," says Eva Selhub, the senior staff physician at the Benson/Henry Institute for Mind/Body Medicine at Massachusetts General Hospital and author of *The Love Response* (Ballantine).

Liking one's self, on the other hand, infuses everything you do with a more positive outlook. You make better choices—about what to eat, whether to smoke or drink, what you deserve in relationships. And you build greater stores of resiliency that can help you bounce back from outside stressors.

LifeXist goes through the body mind connection, connecting your sympathetic and parasympathetic nervous system. This is the Yin and Yang of Health care. Their doctors will work to pinpoint cravings or addictions you might be using to fill yourself up in the absence of self-love: food, drugs, excessive Internet use, unsafe sex, and cigarettes. **Smoke Arrest** is the system they will be using, of which they have reported up to a 90% success rate, and it is the only laser doctor-supervised system in our country recognized by leading doctors today.

According to a growing body of research, people who are socially connected live longer, maintain better cognitive health, and have overall better mental and physical well-being. Humans are meant to be social animals. "The 'American disease' is isolation," Sel-hub says. "We live longer and better when we feel important, valid, and valued, and when we feel that we'll be remembered. Living within a community helps us feel that we exist and that we did exist for a reason."

Imagine a community dedicated to:

- Age-Management
- Nutrition Infusion

- Oral Nutrition
- Metabolic Boosting
- Hormone Management
- Weight Loss
- Stress management
- Brain Body Work
- Wellness Care
- Smoking Cessation

Doctors throughout history have also pursued the Fountain of Youth, and the LifeXist model is the most complete model that offers a comprehensive, affordable solution. Increasing snowdrifts of studies point to the same conclusion: Among all other lifestyle factors, cellular health is the linchpin to good health.

The study of anti-aging as we learned throughout this book is based on solid medical research. Anti-aging began to develop as a separate area of research in the mid-1980s. In 1997, Harvard University established the first medical board examination for anti-aging practitioners in such futuristic fields as cryogenics, regeneration, gene mapping, genetic engineering, and cloning. Each of these fields promises biomedical breakthroughs as efforts to enhance health and prolong life continue to advance.

Diet, nutrition, supplementation are germane. Eliminating toxins and deficiencies are the road to health. People who eat right, avoid toxins, and exercise regularly have a lower risk of developing cardiovascular diseases, dementia, diabetes, depression, and osteoarthritis. They're also more likely to maintain a stable, healthy weight and less likely to be obese, which is itself a risk factor for those diseases.

Now a series of compelling independent studies published in an early 2010 issue of the *Archives of Internal Medicine* underscores the message that exercise can stave off many diseases. An analysis from the large Nurses Health Study, for example, found that women who jogged three hours a week or walked briskly for five hours a week were

76% more likely to age successfully, with less chronic disease or mental impairment, an effect that's held among all ages and weights. So what is holding you back? This book has offered you a road and a destination to being the best you that you can be.

Rethink your idea of "health" and focus on cellular protection and support of all kinds. Aim for a three-way mix of body, mind, and spirit, a health regime, a formula to prevent toxins and deficiencies.

Life with a purpose

What drives the human desire for longer life that these scientists are feverishly working to secure? Prolonging physical life has been a preoccupation of people in all ages. Have you wondered why there are "immortal longings," as William Shakespeare put it, in people's hearts? Some might say it originates in the fear of death, or in a longing for better opportunities, or just to see grandchildren and great-grandchildren. Certainly we would all welcome a better quality of life for those who suffer from inherited diseases that shorten life or compromise its quality.

We would also probably agree that length of life alone is not enough. What we truly seek is fulfilling, exciting, and rewarding lives replete with opportunities for vigorous pursuits and continuing achievements. Although length of life is largely genetically programmed, our achievements in life are personally determined by opportunity, means, and a sense of purpose.

Humankind's potential for eternal life is the central theme of the Hebrew scriptures and apostolic writings—the Bible. That book says that God does have a purpose for humanity, and that He offers immortality to all, not just to those who are wealthy enough to pay for it.

Hopefully this book has taken you on a journey, and maybe LifeXist is in your future—it is mine.

Here's one last story I want to share with you.

A young woman went to her grandmother and told her about her life and how things were so hard for her—her husband had cheated on her and she was devastated. She did not know how she was going to make it and wanted to give up. She was tired of fighting and struggling. It seemed as soon as one problem was solved, a new one arose.

Her grandmother took her to the kitchen. She filled three pots with water and placed each on a high fire. Soon the pots came to boil. In the first she placed carrots, in the second she placed eggs, and in the last she placed ground coffee beans. She let them sit and boil, without saying a word.

In about twenty minutes she turned off the burners. She fished the carrots out and placed them in a bowl. She pulled the eggs out and placed them in a bowl. Then she ladled the coffee out and placed it in a bowl.

Turning to her granddaughter, she asked, "Tell me what you see."

"Carrots, eggs, and coffee," she replied.

Her grandmother brought her closer and asked her to feel the carrots. She did and noted that they were soft. The grand-mother then asked the granddaughter to take an egg and break it. After pulling off the shell, she observed the hard-boiled egg.

Finally, the grandmother asked the granddaughter to sip the coffee. The granddaughter smiled as she tasted its rich aroma. The granddaughter then asked, "What does it mean, grandmother?"

Her grandmother explained that each of these objects had faced the same adversity: boiling water. Each reacted differently. The carrot went in strong, hard, and unrelenting. However, after being subjected to the boiling water, it softened and became weak. The egg had been fragile. Its thin outer shell had protected its liquid interior, but after sitting through the boiling water, its inside became hardened. The ground coffee beans were unique, however. After they were in the boiling water, they had changed the water.

"Which are you?" she asked her granddaughter. "When adversity knocks on your door, how do you respond? Are you a carrot, an egg, or a coffee bean?

Think of this: Which am I? Am I the carrot that seems strong, but with pain and adversity? Do I wilt and become soft and lose my strength?

Am I the egg that starts with a malleable heart, but changes with the heat? Did I have a fluid spirit, but after a death, a breakup, a financial hardship, or some other trial, have I become hardened and stiff? Does my shell look the same, but on the inside am I bitter and tough with a stiff spirit and hardened heart?

Or am I like the coffee bean? The bean actually changes the hot water, the very circumstance that brings the pain. When the water gets hot, it releases the fragrance and flavor. If you are like the bean, when things are at their worst, you get better and change the situation around you. When the hour is the darkest and trials are their greatest, do you elevate yourself to another level?

How do you handle adversity? Are you a carrot, an egg, or a coffee bean?

May you have enough happiness to make you sweet, enough trials to make you strong, enough sorrow to keep you human, and enough hope to make you happy.

The happiest of people don't necessarily have the best of everything; they just make the most of everything that comes along their way. The brightest future will always be based on a forgotten past; you can't go forward in life until you let go of your past failures and heartaches.

When you were born, you were crying and everyone around you was smiling. Live your life so at the end, you're the one who is smiling and everyone around you is crying. May we all be like the coffee bean.

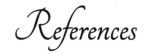

References

A Natural Product Telomerase Activator As Part of a Health Maintenance Program.

ABC News-Cox

Aben A, Danckaerts M. Omega-3 and omega-6 fatty acids in the treatment of children and adolescents with ADHD. Tijdschr Psychiatr. 2010;52(2):89-97.

Adam O, Beringer C, Kless T, et al. Anti-inflammatory effects of a low arachidonic acid diet and fish oil in patients with rheumatoid arthritis. Rheumatol Int. 2003 Jan;23(1):27-36.

Adirim TA, Cheng TL. Overview of injuries in the young athlete. Sports Med. 2003;33(1):75-81.

Allendy, R.F., MD. Orientation Des Idees Medicales.

Alternative Medicine, the Burton Goldberg Group, Future Medicine Publishing, Inc.

Alternative Medicine: The Definitive Guide, The Burton Goldberg Group, Future Medicine Publishing, Inc.

Andrews WH, Boerma CL, Rawson JRY.

Andrews WH, Funk WD, West MD

Andrews WH, Rawson JRY.

Andrews, W. H. and J. R. Y. Rawson

Andrews, W. H. and J. R. Y. Rawson

Angerer P, von Schacky C. n-3 polyunsaturated fatty acids and the cardiovascular system. Curr Opin Lipidol. 2000;11(1):57-63.

Antiproliferative small molecule inhibitors of transcription factor LSF reveal oncogene addiction to LSF in hepatocellular carcinoma

Aoki H, Hisada T, Ishizuka T, et al. Protective effect of resolvin E1 on the development of asthmatic airway inflammation. Biochem Biophys Res Commun. 2010 Sep 10;400(1):128-33.

Appleton, Nancy. Lick the Sugar Habit. (Garden City Park, NY: Avery Publishing Group), 1996.

Aronson WJ, Glaspy JA, Reddy ST, Reese D, Heber D, Bagga D. Modulation of omega-3/omega-6 polyunsaturated ratios with dietary fish oils in men with prostate cancer. Urology. 2001;58(2):283-288.

Aronson WJ, Kobayashi N, Barnard RJ, et al. Phase II prospective randomized trial of a low-fat diet with fish oil supplementation in men undergoing radical prostatectomy. Cancer Prev Res (Phila). 2011 Dec;4(12):2062-71.

Ascensão A, Ferreira R, Magalhaes J. Exercise-induced cardioprotection—biochemical, morphological and functional evidence in whole tissue and isolated mitochondria Int J Cardiol 2007;117:16-30.[CrossRef][Web of Science][Medline]

B.P. Alter et al., "Very short telomere length by flow fluorescence in situ hybridization identifies patients with dyskeratosis congenita," Blood, 110:1439-47, 2007.

B.P. Alter, et al, "Cancer in dyskeratosis congenital," Blood, 113:6549-57, 2009.

Baeurle SA, et al. Effect of the counterion behavior on the frictional-compressive properties of chondroitin sulfate solutions. Polymer 2009;50(7):1805–1813.

Bahadori B, Uitz E, Thonhofer R, et al. omega-3 Fatty acids infusions as adjuvant therapy in rheumatoid arthritis. JPEN J Parenter Enteral Nutr. 2010;34(2):151-5.

Balfour, E.B. The Living Soil. (New York: Universe Books), 1976.

Balk EM, Lichtenstein AH, Chung M et al. Effects of omega-3 fatty acids on serum markers of cardiovascular disease risk: A systematic review. Atherosclerosis. 2006 Nov;189(1):19-30.

Barrett B. Viral upper respiratory infection. In: Rakel DP, ed. Integrative Medicine

Bays HE. Safety considerations with omega-3 Fatty Acid therapy. Am J Cardiol. 2007;99(6A):S35-43.

Bazan NG, Musto AE, Knott EJ. Endogenous signaling by omega-3 docosahexaenoic acid-derived mediators sustains homeostatic synaptic and circuitry integrity. Mol Neurobiol. 2011 Oct;44(2):216-22.

Bazan NG. Neuroprotectin D1-mediated anti-inflammatory and survival signaling in stroke, retinal degenerations, and Alzheimer's disease. J Lipid Res. 2009 Apr;50 Suppl:S400-5. Epub 2008 Nov 18.

Beasley, J. D., and Swift, J. J. The Kellogg Report. (Annandale-on-Hudson, NY: The Institute of Health Policy and Practice/Bard College Center), 1989.

Becker, R. O. The Body Electric. (New York: Quill/William Morrow), 1985.

Becker, S.L., Will milk make them grow? An episode in the discovery of the vitamins. In Chemistry and Modern Society (J. Parascandela, editor) pp. 61-83, American Chemical Society, Washington, D.C. (1983).

Bellenger J, Bellenger S, Bataille A, et al. High pancreatic n-3 fatty acids prevent STZ-induced diabetes in fat-1 mice: inflammatory pathway inhibition. Diabetes. 2011 Apr;60(4):1090-9.

Bello AE, Oesser S. Collagen hydrolysate for the treatment of osteoarthritis and other joint disorders: a review of the literature. Curr Med Res Opin 2006 Nov;22(11):2221-2232.

Belluzzi A, Boschi S, Brignola C, Munarini A, Cariani C, Miglio F. Polyunsaturated fatty acids and inflammatory bowel disease. Am J Clin Nutr. 2000;71(suppl):339S-342S.

Bendix L et al. Leukocyte telomere length and physical ability among Danish Twins age 70+. Mech Aging Dev. 2011 Oct 12. doi: 10.1016/j.mad.2011.10.003

Bendyk A, Marino V, Zilm PS, Howe P, Bartold PM. Effect of dietary omega-3 polyunsaturated fatty acids on experimental periodontitis in the mouse. J Periodontal Res. 2009 Apr;44(2):211-6.

Berbert AA, Kondo CR, Almendra CL et al. Supplementation of fish oil and olive oil in patients with rheumatoid arthritis. Nutrition. 2005;21:131-6.

Berbert AA, Kondo CR, Almendra CL, Matsuo T, Dichi I. Supplementation of fish oil and olive oil in patients with rheumatoid arthritis. Nutrition. 2005 Feb;21(2):131-6.

Berson EL, Rosner B, Sandberg MA, et al. Clinical trial of docosahexaenoic acid in patients with retinitis pigmentosa receiving vitamin A treatment. Arch Ophthalmol. 2004;122(9):1297-1305.

Bilal S, Haworth O, Wu L, Weylandt KH, Levy BD, Kang JX. Fat-1 transgenic mice with elevated omega-3 fatty acids are protected from allergic airway responses. Biochim Biophys Acta. 2011 Sep;1812(9):1164-9.

Biltagi MA, Baset AA, Bassiouny M, Kasrawi MA, Attia M. Omega-3 fatty acids, vitamin C and Zn supplementation in asthmatic children: a randomized self-controlled study. Acta Paediatr. 2009 Apr;98(4):737-42.

Biochemistry 20, 2639-2644. (1981)

Biochemistry 31, 11595-11599 (1992)

Black C et al. The clinical effectiveness of glucosamine and chondroitin supplements in slowing or arresting progression of osteoarthritis of the knee: a systematic review and economic evaluation. Health Technol Assess 2009 Nov;13(52):1-148.

Blasbalg TL, Hibbeln JR, Ramsden CE, Majchrzak SF, Rawlings RR. Changes in consumption of omega-3 and omega-6 fatty acids in the United States during the 20th century. Am J Clin Nutr. 2011;93(5):950-62.

Blasco MA. Telomeres and human disease: aging, cancer and beyond Nat Rev Genet 2005;6:611-622. [CrossRef][Web of Science][Medline]

Boelsma E, Hendriks HF. Roza L. Nutritional skin care: health effects of micronutrients and fatty acids. Am J Clin Nutr. 2001;73(5):853-864.

Boskou, D. Olive oil. World Rev Nutr Diet. 2000;87:56-77.

Bradbury J, Myers SP, Oliver C et al. An adaptogenic role for omega-3 fatty acids in stress; a randomised placebo controlled double blind intervention study (pilot)ISRCTN22569553. Nutr J. 2004 Nov 28;3:20.

Brailsford, James, M. Journal of Surgery.

Brekhman, I. I. and Nesterenko, I. F. Brown Sugar and Health. (New York: The Pergamon Press), 1983.

Brostow DP, Odegaard AO, Koh WP, et al. Omega-3 fatty acids and incident type 2 diabetes: the Singapore Chinese Health Study. Am J Clin Nutr. 2011;94(2):520-6.

Brothers VM, Kuhn I, Paul LS, Gabe JD, Andrews WH, Sias SR, McCaman MT, Dragon EA, Files JG.

Bruyere O, et al. Evaluation of symptomatic slow-acting drugs in osteoarthritis using the GRADE system. BMC Musculoskelet Disord 2008 Dec 16;9:165.

Buckley MS, Goff AD, Knapp WE, et al. Fish oil interaction with warfarin. Ann Pharmacother. 2004;38:50-2.

Buitrago-Lopez et al. Chocolate consumption and cardiometabolic disorders: systematic review and meta-analysis. British Medical Journal 2011;343:d4488. doi: 10.1136/bmj.d4488

Burgess J, Stevens L, Zhang W, Peck L. Long-chain polyunsaturated fatty acids in children with attention-deficit hyperactivity disorder. Am J Clin Nutr. 2000;71(suppl):327S-330S.

Burr ML, Dunstan FD, George CH et al. Is fish oil good or bad for heart disease? Two trials with apparently conflicting results. J Membr Biol. 2006;206:155-63.

Calo L, Bianconi L, Colivicchi F et al. N-3 Fatty acids for the prevention of atrial fibrillation after coronary artery bypass surgery: a randomized, controlled trial. J Am Coll Cardiol. 2005;45:1723-8.

Cangemi FE. TOZAL Study: an open case control study of an oral antioxidant and omega-3 supplement for dry AMD. BMC Ophthalmol. 2007;7:3.

Carlo T, Levy BD. Chemical mediators and the resolution of airway inflammation. Allergol Int. 2008 Dec;57(4):299-305.

Carneiro, T., Khair, L., Reis, C.C., Borges, V., Moser, B.A., Nakamura, T.M. and Ferreira, M.G. (2010)

Caron MF, White CM. Evaluation of the antihyperlipidemic properties of dietary supplements. Pharmacotherapy. 2001;21(4):481-487.

Carpenter, K.J., Beriberi, White Rice and Vitamin B, University of California Press, Berkeley (2000).

Carpenter, K.J., The History of Scurvy and Vitamin C, Cambridge University Press, New York (1986).

Carper, Jean, Miracle Cures, Harper Collins.

Casdorph, Richard and Walker, Morton. Toxic Metal Syndrome. (Garden City Park, NY: Avery Publishing Group), 1995.

Cataloging Altered Gene Expression in Young and Senescent Cells using Enhanced Differential Display.

Cawthon RM, Smith KR, O'Brien E, Sivatchenko A, Kerber RA. Association between telomere length in blood and mortality in people aged 60 years or older Lancet 2003;361:393-395.[CrossRef][Web of Science][Medline]

Cell Biology 79, 320A.

Cell Biology 83, 357A.

Cell-Line and Site-Specific Attachment of Chondroitin Sulfate to Recombinant Human Thrombomodulin.

Chan EJ, Cho L. What can we expect from omega-3 fatty acids? Cleve Clin J Med. 2009 Apr;76(4):245-51. Review.

Chapter 10

Characterization of a Surface Antigen of Eimeria-Tenella Sporozoites and Synthesis from a Cloned Complementary DNA in Escherichia-Coli.

Chattipakorn N, Settakorn J, Petsophonsakul P, et al. Cardiac mortality is associated with low levels of omega-3 and omega-6 fatty acids in the heart of cadavers with a history of coronary heart disease.Nutr Res. 2009;29(10):696-704.

Cheraskin, E., Ringsdorf, W. M., Jr., and Sisley, E. L. The Vitamin C Connection. (New York: Bantam Books), 1983.

Chiropractic Acclaimed Worldwide, Parker College.

Cho E, Hung S, Willet WC, Spiegelman D, Rimm EB, Seddon JM, et al. Prospective study of dietary fat and the risk of age-related macular degeneration. Am J Clin Nutr. 2001;73(2):209-218.

Chopra, Deepak. Ageless Body, Timeless Mind. (New York: Harmony Books), 1993.

Chopra, Deepak. Creating Health. (Boston, MA: Houghton Mifflin), 1987.

Chopra, Deepak. Quantum Healing. (New York: Bantam Books), 1989.

Christensen B, et al. Effect of anti-inflammatory medication on the running-induced rise in patella tendon collagen synthesis in humans. J Appl Physiol. 2011 Jan;110(1):137-41.

Christensen JH, Skou HA, Fog L, Hansen V, Vesterlund T, Dyerberg J, Toft E, Schmidt EB. Marine n-3 fatty acids, wine intake, and heart rate variability in patients referred for coronary angiography. Circulation. 2001;103:623-625.

Clarke JH, Light DR, Blasko E, Parkinson JF, Nagashima M, McLean K, Vilander L, Andrews WH, Morser J, Glaser CB.

Cleland LG, Caughey GE, James MJ, Proudman SM. Reduction of cardiovascular risk factors with longterm fish oil treatment in early rheumatoid arthritis. J Rheumatol. 2006 Oct;33(10):1973-9.

Clin Res 40, 352A (1992)

Cloning of a cDNA Encoding a Receptor Related to the Formyl Peptide Receptor of Human Neutrophils.

Cloning of a Human Formyl Peptide Receptor Gene.

Cloning of Chloroplast DNA in Bacterial Plasmid Vectors

Cloning of the Gene Coding for a Human Receptor for Formyl Peptides Characterization of a Promoter Region and Evidence for Polymorphic Expression.

Cohen, A. M.; Bavly, S.; Poznanski, R. "Change of Diet of Yemenite Jews in Relation to Diabetes and Ischaemic Heart Disease." The Lancet (1961) 2:1399-1401.

Cohen, Robert. Milk: The Deadly Poison. (Englewood Cliffs, NJ: Argus Publishing), 1997.

Cole GM, Frautschy SA. DHA may prevent age-related dementia. J Nutr. 2010 Apr;140(4):869-74. 70. Jicha GA, Markesbery WR. Omega-3 fatty acids: potential role in the management of early Alzheimer's disease. Clin Interv Aging. 2010;5:45-61.

Cole GM. Omega-3 fatty acids and dementia. Prostaglandins Leukot Essent Fatty Acids. 2009;81(2-3):213-21.

Colgan M. Beat Arthritis. Vancouver: Apple Publishing, 2000.

Complementary and Alternative Medicine for the Treatment of Depressive Disorders in Women. Psychiatric Clinics of North America. 2010;33(2).

Coulter, Harris. Vaccination, Social Violence, and Criminality: The Medical Assault on the American Brain. (Berkely, CA: North Atlanta Books), 1990.

Courtney ED, Matthews S, Finlayson C, et al. Eicosapentaenoic acid (EPA) reduces crypt cell proliferation and increases apoptosis in normal colonic mucosa in subjects with a history of colorectal adenomas. Int J Colorectal Dis. 2007 Jul;22(7):765-76.

Coussens M, Davy P, Brown L, Foster C, Andrews WH, Nagata M, Allsopp R.

Cramer, Albert, MD. Hippocrates.

Cyria, James, MD, Médecine et Hygiène.

da Silva TM, Munhoz RP, Alvarez C, et al. Depression in Parkinson's disease: a double-blind, randomized, placebo-controlled pilot study of omega-3 fatty-acid supplementation. J Affect Disord. 2008 Dec;111(2-3):351-9.

Dangardt F, Osika W, Chen Y, et al. Omega-3 fatty acid supplementation improves vascular function and reduces inflammation in obese adolescents. Atherosclerosis. 2010 Oct;212(2):580-5.

Daniel CR, McCullough ML, Patel RC, Jacobs EJ, Flanders WD, Thun MJ, Calle EE. Dietary intake of omega-6 and omega-3 fatty acids and risk of colorectal cancer in a prospective cohort of U.S. men and women. Cancer Epidemiol Biomarkers Prev. 2009 Feb;18(2):516-25.

Das UN. Do polyunsaturated fatty acids behave like an endogenous "polypill"? Med Hypotheses. 2008;70(2):430-4. Epub 2007 Jul 10.

Das UN. Essential fatty acids and their metabolites could function as endogenous HMG-CoA reductase and ACE enzyme inhibitors, anti-arrhythmic, anti-hypertensive, anti-atherosclerotic, anti-inflammatory, cytoprotective, and cardioprotective molecules. Lipids Health Dis. 2008;7:37.

Davidson MH. Omega-3 fatty acids: new insights into the pharmacology and biology of docosahexaenoic acid, docosapentaenoic acid, and eicosapentaenoic acid. Curr Opin Lipidol. 2013;24(6):467-74.

De Silva V et al. Evidence for the efficacy of complementary and alternative medicines in the management of osteoarthritis: a systematic review. Rheumatology (Oxford) 2010 Dec 17. (Epub ahead of print)

Dewailly E, Blanchet C, Lemieux S, et al. n-3 fatty acids and cardiovascular disease risk factors among the Inuit of Nunavik. Am J Clin Nutr. 2001;74(4):464-473.

Diamond, Harvey and Marilyn. Fit for Life.

Dichi I, Frenhane P, Dichi JB, Correa CR, Angeleli AY, Bicudo MH, et al. Comparison of omega-3 fatty acids and sulfasalazine in ulcerative colitis. Nutrition. 2000;16:87-90.

Differential arrival of leading and lagging strand DNA polymerases at fission yeast telomeres.

Dona M, Fredman G, Schwab JM, et al. Resolvin E1, an EPA-derived mediator in whole blood, selectively counterregulates leukocytes and platelets. Blood. 2008 Aug 1;112(3):848-55.

Dopheide JA, Pliszka SR. Attention-deficit-hyperactivity disorder: an update. Pharmacotherapy. 2009 Jun;29(6):656-79. (Epub ahead of print)

Dr. Mercola's article of 4/19/2011: http://articles.mercola.com/sites/articles/archive/2011/04/18/is-this-the-key-to-living-longer-than-150-years-old.aspx

Dunstan JA, Mori TA, Barden A, et al. Fish oil supplementation in pregnancy modifies neonatal allergen-specific immune responses and clinical outcomes in infants at high risk of atopy: a randomized, controlled trial. J Allergy Clin Immunol. 2003 Dec;112(6):1178-84.

E.H. Blackburn et al., "Telomeres and telomerase: the path from maize, Tetrahymena and yeast to human cancer and aging," Nat Med, 12:1133-38, 2006.

El-Sharkawy H, Aboelsaad N, Eliwa M, et al. Adjunctive treatment of chronic periodontitis with daily dietary supplementation with omega-3 Fatty acids and low-dose aspirin. J Periodontol. 2010 Nov;81(11):1635-43.

Enstrom, J.E. et al, Vitamin C. Intake and Mortality Among A Sample Of U.S. Population. Epedimiol 3. (3)pp. 194-202, 1994

Enzymatic Properties of Bovine Prochymosin Synthesized in Escherichia coli.

Expression Efficiency of the Human Thrombomodulin-Encoding Gene in Various Vector and Host Systems.

Expression of Cloned Chloroplast DNA from Euglena gracilis in an In Vitro DNA-Dependent Transcription-Translation System Prepared from E. coli.

Expression of Cloned Chloroplast DNA in E. coli Minicells

Fakhrzadeh H, Ghaderpanahi M, Sharifi F, et al. The effects of low dose n-3 fatty acids on serum lipid profiles and insulin resistance of the elderly: a randomized controlled clinical trial. Int J Vitam Nutr Res. 2010 Apr;80(2):107-16.

Farooqui AA, Ong WY, Horrocks LA, Chen P, Farooqui T. Comparison of biochemical effects of statins and fish oil in brain: the battle of the titans. Brain Res Rev. 2007 Dec;56(2):443-71.

Farzaneh-Far, R., et al, "Association of Marine Omega-3 Fatty Acid Levels With Telomeric Aging in Patients With Coronary Heart Disease," JAMA. 2010;303(3):250-257.

Fatty fish consumption and ischemic heart disease mortality in older adults: The cardiovascular heart study. Presented at the American Heart Association's 41st annual conference on cardiovascular disease epidemiology and prevention. AHA. 2001.

Feng J, Funk WD, Wang S-S, Weinrich SL, Avilion AA, Chiu C-P, Adams RA, Chang E, Allsopp, RC, Yu J, Le S, West MD, Harley CB, Andrews WH, Greider CW, Villeponteau B.

Feng, J., W. D. Funk, et al. (1995). The RNA component of human telomerase. Science 269(5228): 1236-1241.

Fenton WS, Dicerson F, Boronow J, et al. A placebo controlled trial of omega-3 fatty acid (ethyl eicosapentaenoic acid) supplementation for residual symptoms and cognitive impairment in schizophrenia. Am J Psychiatry. 2001;158(12):2071-2074.

Fibrinolysis 4, 109 (1990)

Field DT et al. Consumption of cocoa flavanols results in an acute improvement in visual and cognitive functions. Physiology & Behavior 103 (3-4): 255-60. doi: 10.1016/j.physbeh.2011.02.013

Fiorucci S, Wallace JL, Mencarelli A, et al. A beta-oxidation-resistant lipoxin A4 analog treats hapten-induced colitis by attenuating inflammation and immune dysfunction. Proc Natl Acad Sci U S A. 2004 Nov 2;101(44):15736-41.

Firestein. Kelley's Textbook of Rheumatology. 8th ed. St. Louis, MO: Elsevier Saunders; 2008.

Fission yeast Tel1ATM and Rad3ATR promote telomere protection and telomerase recruitment.

Flachs P, Ruhl R, Hensler M, et al. Synergistic induction of lipid catabolism and anti-inflammatory lipids in white fat of dietary obese mice in response to calorie restriction and n-3 fatty acids. Diabetologia. 2011 Oct;54(10):2626-38.

Follow us: @UMMC on Twitter | MedCenter on Facebook

Formyl Peptide Receptor Chimeras Define Domains Involved in Ligand Binding.

Fotuhi M, Mohassel P, Yaffe K. Fish consumption, long-chain omega-3 fatty acids and risk of cognitive decline or Alzheimer disease: a complex association. Nat Clin Pract Neurol. 2009 Mar;5(3):140-52. Review.

Frangou S, Lewis M, McCrone P et al. Efficacy of ethyl-eicosapentaenoic acid in bipolar depression: randomised double-blind placebo-controlled study. Br J Psychiatry. 2006;188:46-50

Fredman G, Serhan CN. Specialized proresolving mediator targets for RvE1 and RvD1 in peripheral blood and mechanisms of resolution. Biochem J. 2011 Jul 15;437(2):185-97.

Fredman G, Van Dyke TE, Serhan CN. Resolvin E1 regulates adenosine diphosphate activation of human platelets. Arterioscler Thromb Vasc Biol. 2010 Oct;30(10):2005-13.

Freeman VL, Meydani M, Yong S, Pyle J, Flanigan RC, Waters WB, Wojcik EM. Prostatic levels of fatty acids and the histopathology of localized prostate cancer. J Urol. 2000;164(6):2168-2172.

Freund-Levi Y, Eriksdotter-Jonhagen M, Cederholm T, et al. Omega-3 fatty acid treatment in 174 patients with mild to moderate Alzheimer disease:

Omegad study: a randomized double-blind trial. Arch Neurol. 2006 Oct;63(10):1402-8.

Freund-Levi Y, Hjorth E, Lindberg C, Cederholm T, Faxen-Irving G, Vedin I, Palmblad J, Wahlund LO, Schultzberg M, Basun H, Eriksdotter Jönhagen M. Effects of omega-3 fatty acids on inflammatory markers in cerebrospinal fluid and plasma in Alzheimer's disease: the OmegAD study. Dement Geriatr Cogn Disord. 2009;27(5):481-90.

Freund-Levi YF, Eriksdotter-Jonhagen M, Cederholm T, et al. Omega-3 fatty acid treatment in 174 patients with mild to moderate Alzheimer disease: OmegAD Study. Arch Neurol. 2006;63:1402-8.

Fritsch D, Allen TA, Dodd CE, et al. Dose-titration effects of fish oil in osteoarthritic dogs. J Vet Intern Med. 2010 Sep-Oct;24(5):1020-6.

Furumoto, K., et al, "Age-dependent telomere shortening is slowed down by enrichment of intracellular vitamin C via suppression of oxidative stress," Life Sci. 1998;63(11):935-48.

Fuster JJ, Andres V. Telomere biology and cardiovascular disease Circ Res 2006;99:1167-1180.[Abstract/Free Full Text]

Gabbe. Obstetrics: Normal and Problem Pregnancies. 6th ed. Philadelphia, PA: Elsevier Saunders; 2012.

Gabe JD, Chang R-J, Slomiany R, Andrews WH, McCaman MT.

Galli C, Risé P. Fish consumption, omega-3 fatty acids and cardiovascular disease. The science and the clinical trials. Nutr Health. 2009;20(1):11-20. Review.

Gangemi S, Pescara L, D'Urbano E, et al. Aging is characterized by a profound reduction in anti-inflammatory lipoxin A4 levels. Exp Gerontol. 2005 Jul;40(7):612-4.

Geelen A, Brouwer IA, Schouten EG et al. Effects of n-3 fatty acids from fish on premature ventricular complexes and heart rate in humans. Am J Clin Nutr. 2005;81:416-20.

Geerling BJ, Badart-Smook A, van Deursen C, et al. Nutritional supplementation with N-3 fatty acids and antioxidants in patients iwth Crohn's disease in remission: effects on antioxidant status and fatty acid profile. Inflamm Bowel Dis. 2000;6(2):77-84.

Gene 118, 303-304 (1992)

Gene 147, 287-292 (1994)

Ginty AT, Conklin SM. Preliminary evidence that acute long-chain omega-3 supplementation reduces cardiovascular reactivity to mental stress: a randomized and placebo controlled trial. Biol Psychol. 2012 Jan;89(1):269-72.

Glaser CB; Morser J; Clarke JH; Blasko E; McLean K; Kuhn I; Chang RJ; Lin JH; Vilander L; Andrews WH.

Goldberg RJ, Katz J. A meta-analysis of the analgesic effects of omega-3 polyunsaturated fatty acid supplementation for inflammatory joint pain. Pain. 2007 Feb 28; [Epub ahead of print].

Gonzalez-Periz A, Claria J. Resolution of adipose tissue inflammation. ScientificWorldJournal. 2010;10:832-56.

Gonzalez-Periz A, Horrillo R, Ferre N, et al. Obesity-induced insulin resistance and hepatic steatosis are alleviated by omega-3 fatty acids: a role for resolvins and protectins. FASEB J. 2009 Jun;23(6):1946-57.

Gotten, H.B., MD. Journal of Tennessee Medical Association.

Gow RV, Sumich A, Vallee-Tourangeau F, et al. Omega-3 fatty acids are related to abnormal emotion processing in adolescent boys with attention deficit hyperactivity disorder. Prostaglandins Leukot Essent Fatty Acids. 2013;88(6):419-29.

Grant TJ, Bishop JA, Christadore LM, Barot G, Chin HG, Woodson S, Kavouris J, Siddiq A, Gredler R, Shen X, Sherman J, Meehan T, Fitzgerald KJ, Pradhan S, Briggs LA, Andrews WH, Sarkar D, Schaus SE, Hansen U.

Greene ER, Huang S, Serhan CN, Panigrahy D. Regulation of inflammation in cancer by eicosanoids. Prostaglandins Other Lipid Mediat. 2011 Nov;96(1-4):27-36.

Greider CW, Autexier C, Buchkovich K, Collins K, Blasco M, Avilion A, Mantell L, Prowse K, Harley C, Funk W, Andrews W, Feng J, Villeponteau B.

Greider CW, Blackburn EH. (1985) Identification of a specific telomere terminal transferase activity in Tetrahymena extracts. Cell 43: 405-413.

Grosso G, Pajak A, Marventano S, et al. Role of omega-3 fatty acids in the treatment of depressive disorders: a comprehensive meta-analysis of randomized clinical trials. PLoS One. 2014;9(4):e96905.

Gruenwald J, Petzold E, Busch R, Petzold HP, Graubaum HJ. Effect of glucosamine sulfate with or without omega-3 fatty acids in patients with osteoarthritis. Adv Ther. 2009 Sep;26(9):858-71.

Gutzeit, K., MD. The Spine as Causative Factor Disease.

HAATI survivors replace canonical telomeres with blocks of generic heterochromatin.

Hagen KB, Byfuglien MG, Falzon L, Olsen SU, Smedslund G. Dietary interventions for rheumatoid arthritis. Cochrane Database Syst Rev. 2009 Jan 21;(1):CD006400. Review.

Hakim AA, Petrovich H, Burchfiel CM, et al. Effects of walking on mortality among nonsmoking retired men N Engl J Med 1998;338:94-99.[CrossRef] [Web of Science][Medline]

Hall MN, Campos H, Li H, Sesso HD, Stampfer MJ, Willett WC, Ma J. Blood levels of long-chain polyunsaturated fatty acids, aspirin, and the risk of colorectal cancer. Cancer Epidemiol Biomarkers Prev. 2007;16(2):314-21.

Halpern GM. Anti-inflammatory effects of a stabilized lipid extract of Perna canaliculus (Lyprinol). Allerg Immunol (Paris). 2000 Sep;32(7):272-278.

Hambrecht R, Fiehn E, Weigl C, et al. Regular physical exercise corrects endothelial dysfunction and improves exercise capacity in patients with chronic heart failure Circulation 1998;98:2709-2715. [Abstract/Free Full Text]

Hambrecht R, Wolf A, Gielen S, et al. Effect of exercise on coronary endothelial function in patients with coronary artery disease N Engl J Med 2000;342:454-460.[CrossRef][Web of Science][Medline]

Harley CB, Andrews W, Chiu C-P, Feng J, Funk W, Gaeta F, Hirsch K, Kin NW, Kozlowski M, Wang S-S, Weinrich SL, West MD, Avilion A, Le S, Grieder CW, Villeponteau B

Harley CB, Liu W, Blasco M, Vera E, Andrews WH, Briggs LA, Raffaele JM.

Hartweg J, Farmer AJ, Holman RR, Neil A. Potential impact of omega-3 treatment on cardiovascular disease in type 2 diabetes. Curr Opin Lipidol. 2009 Feb;20(1):30-8.

Haworth O, Levy BD. Endogenous lipid mediators in the resolution of airway inflammation. Eur Respir J. 2007 Nov;30(5):980-92.

Hayflick, L. (1965). The limited in vitro lifetime of human diploid cell strains. Exp. Cell Res. 37 (3): 614-636.

Hayflick, L. (1965). The limited in vitro lifetime of human diploid cell strains. Exp. Cell Res. 37 (3): 614-636.

Health Alert, Volume Three, no. 1.

Hellmann J, Tang Y, Kosuri M, Bhatnagar A, Spite M. Resolvin D1 decreases adipose tissue macrophage accumulation and improves insulin sensitivity in obese-diabetic mice. FASEB J. 2011 Jul;25(7):2399-407.

Hewitt MJ. Writing an exercise prescription. In: Rakel DP, ed. Integrative Medicine

HIF1alpha as critical for telomerase function in murine embryonic stem cells.

Hisada T, Ishizuka T, Aoki H, Mori M. Resolvin E1 as a novel agent for the treatment of asthma. Expert Opin Ther Targets. 2009 May;13(5):513-22.

Ho KJ, Spite M, Owens CD, et al. Aspirin-triggered lipoxin and resolvin E1 modulate vascular smooth muscle phenotype and correlate with peripheral atherosclerosis. Am J Pathol. 2010 Oct;177(4):2116-23.

Hooper L, Thompson R, Harrison R et al. Omega-3 fatty acids for prevention and treatment of cardiovascular disease. Cochrane Database Syst Rev. 2004;CD003177.

Hornig B, Maier V, Drexler H. Physical training improves endothelial function in patients with chronic heart failure Circulation 1996;93:210-214. [Abstract/Free Full Text]

Human Formyl Peptide Receptor Ligand Binding Domain(s) - Studies Using an Improved Mutagenesis/Expression Vector Reveal a Novel Mechanism for the Regulation of Receptor Occupancy.

Human Telomerase Inhibition and Cancer.

Hyman, Harold T. American Journal of Medical Science.

I, Briggs L, Wheeler J, Sampathkumar J, Gonzalez R, Larocca D, Murai J, Snyder E,

In Methods in Chloroplast Molecular Biology. ed. M. Edelman, R. B. Hallick, and N. H. Chua. Elsevier/North Holland. 493-506 (1982)

In Methods in Chloroplast Molecular Biology. ed. M. Edelman, R. B. Hallick, and N. H. Chua. Elsevier/North Holland. 565-571 (1982)

In-vivo and In-vitro Expression of Recombinant DNA Molecules Carrying Euglena-Gracilis Chloroplast Restriction Endo Nuclease DNA Fragments. Infection and Immunity 63, 142-148 (1994)

Irving GF, Freund-Levi Y, Eriksdotter-Jonhagen M, et al. Omega-3 fatty acid supplementation effects on weight and appetite in patients with Alzheimer's disease: the omega-3 Alzheimer's disease study. J Am Geriatr Soc. 2009 Jan;57(1):11-7.

Iso H, Rexrode KM, Stampfer MJ, Manson JE, Colditz GA, Speizer FE et al. Intake of fish and omega-3 fatty acids and risk of stroke in women. JAMA. 2001;285(3):304-312.

Isolation of Extracytoplasmic Proteins from Serpulina hyodysenteriae B204 and Molecular Cloning of the flaB1 Gene Encoding a 38-Kilodalton Flagellar Protein.

Itomura M, Hamazaki K, Sawazaki S et al. The effect of fish oil on physical aggression in schoolchildren - a randomized, double-blind, placebo-controlled trial. J Nutr Biochem. 2005;16:163-71.

Ivker RS. Chronic sinusitis. In: Rakel DP, ed. Integrative Medicine

J Biol Chem 268, 2292-2295 (1993)

J Biol Chem 268, 6309-6315 (1993)

J Biol Chem 269, 22485-22487 (1994)

J Biol Chem 269, 25021-25030 (1994)

J Cell Biol 87, 186A (1980)

J Clin Invest 90, 2565-73 (1992)

J. Biol. Chem. 285(8): 5327-5337. (doi:10.1074/jbc.M109.078840)

J. Biotechnology 2, 177-190 (1985)

J.M. Houben et al., "Telomere length and mortality in elderly men: the Zutphen Elderly Study," J Gerontol A Biol Sci Med Sci, 66:38-44, 2011.

Jain, D., Hebden, A.K., Nakamura, T.M., Miller, K.M. and Cooper, J.P. (2010)

James MJ, Gibson RA, Cleland LG. Dietary polyunsaturated fatty acids and inflammatory mediator production. Am J Clin Nutr. 2000 Jan;71(1 Suppl):343S-8S.

Janakiram NB, Mohammed A, Rao CV. Role of lipoxins, resolvins, and other bioactive lipids in colon and pancreatic cancer. Cancer Metastasis Rev. 2011 Dec;30(3-4):507-23.

Janakiram NB, Rao CV. Role of lipoxins and resolvins as anti-inflammatory and proresolving mediators in colon cancer. Curr Mol Med. 2009 Jun;9(5):565-79.

Jeschke MG, Herndon DN, Ebener C, Barrow RE, Jauch KW. Nutritional intervention high in vitamins, protein, amino acids, and omega-3 fatty acids improves protein metabolism during the hypermetabolic state after thermal injury. Arch Surg. 2001;136:1301-1306.

Jiang W, Oken H, Fiuzat M, et al. Plasma omega-3 polyunsaturated fatty acids and survival in patients with chronic heart failure and major depressive disorder. J Cardiovasc Transl Res. 2012 Feb;5(1):92-9.

Jimenez-Gomez Y, Marin C, Peerez-Martinez P, et al. A low-fat, high-complex carbohydrate diet supplemented with long-chain (n-3) fatty acids alters the postprandial lipoprotein profile in patients with metabolic syndrome. J Nutr. 2010 Sep;140(9):1595-601.

Jing K, Wu T, Lim K. Omega-3 polyunsaturated fatty acids and cancer. Anti-cancer Agents Med Chem. 2013;13(8):1162-77.

Johansson AS, Noren-Nystrom U, Larefalk A, Holmberg D, Lindskog M. Fish oil delays lymphoma progression in the TLL mouse. Leuk Lymphoma. 2010 Nov;51(11):2092-7.

Johnson EJ, Chung HY, Caldarella SM, Snodderly DM. The influence of supplemental lutein and docosahexaenoic acid on serum, lipoproteins, and macular pigmentation. Am J Clin Nutr. 2008 May;87(5):1521-9.

Johnson EJ, McDonald K, Caldarella SM, Chung HY, Troen AM, Snodderly DM. Cognitive findings of an exploratory trial of docosahexaenoic acid and lutein supplementation in older women. Nutr Neurosci. 2008 Apr;11(2):75-83.

Johnson R, Knopp W. Nonorthopaedic conditions. In: DeLee JC, Drez D Jr, Miller MD, eds. DeLee and Drez's Orthopaedic Sports Medicine.

Jordan KM. Arden NK. An evidence based approach to the management of knee osteoarthritis: Report of a Task Force of the Standing Committee for International Clinical Studies Including Therapeutic Trials (ESCISIT)". Ann Rheum Dis 2003;62 (12): 1145–1155.

Jordan KM. Arden NK. An evidence based approach to the management of knee osteoarthritis: Report of a Task Force of the Standing Committee for International Clinical Studies Including Therapeutic Trials (ESCISIT)". Ann Rheum Dis 2003;62 (12): 1145–1155.

Joy CB, Mumby-Croft R, Joy LA. Polyunsaturated fatty acid supplementation for schizophrenia. Cochrane Database Syst Rev. 2006 Jul 19;3:CD001257. Review.

K. G. Hairston, M. Z. Vitolins, J. M. Norris, A. M. Anderson, A. J. Hanley, and L. E. Wagenknecht. Lifestyle Factors and 5-Year Abdominal Fat Accumulation in a Minority Cohort: The IRAS Family Study. Obesity.(Silver. Spring), 2011. doi: 10.1001/archinternmed.2011.18.

Kalman DS, et al. Effect of a natural extract of chicken combs with a high content of hyaluronic acid (Hyal-Joint) on pain relief and quality of life in subjects with knee osteoarthritis: a pilot randomized double-blind placebo-controlled trial. Nutr J 2008;Jan 21(7):3.

Kar S. Omacor and omega-3 fatty acids for treatment of coronary artery disease and the pleiotropic effects. Am J Ther . 2014;21(1):56-66.

Karlstrom BE, Jarvi AE, Byberg L, Berglund LG, Vessby BO. Fatty fish in the diet of patients with type 2 diabetes: comparison of the metabolic effects of foods rich in n-3 and n-6 fatty acids. Am J Clin Nutr. 2011;94(1):26-33.

Kelley DS, Siegel D, Fedor DM, Adkins Y, Mackey BE. DHA supplementation decreases serum C-reactive protein and other markers of inflammation in hypertriglyceridemic men. J Nutr. 2009 Mar;139(3):495-501.

Kent et al. Toxicol in Vitro 2003 Feb;17(1):27-33. doi:10.1016/S0887-2333(02) 00119-4

Kesavalu L, Bakthavatchalu V, Rahman MM, et al. Omega-3 fatty acid regulates inflammatory cytokine/mediator messenger RNA expression in Porphyromonas gingivalis-induced experimental periodontal disease. Oral Microbiol Immunol. 2007 Aug;22(4):232-9.

Keyes KT, Ye Y, Lin Y, et al. Resolvin E1 protects the rat heart against reperfusion injury. Am J Physiol Heart Circ Physiol. 2010 Jul;299(1):H153-64.

Khair, L., Subramanian, L., Moser, B.A. and Nakamura, T.M. (2010)

King, M.E., MD. Therapeutic Review.

Koh KK, Quon MJ, Shin KC, et al. Significant differential effects of omega-3 fatty acids and fenofibrate in patients with hypertriglyceridemia. Atherosclerosis. 2012 Feb;220(2):537-44.

Kopecky J, Rossmeisl M, Flachs P, et al. n-3 PUFA: bioavailability and modulation of adipose tissue function. Proc Nutr Soc. 2009 Nov;68(4):361-9. Epub 2009 Aug 24.

Kotani S, Sakaguchi E, Warashina S, et al. Dietary supple-mentation of arachidonic and docosahexaenoic acids improves cognitive dysfunction. Neurosci Res. 2006 Oct;56(2):159-64.

Krauss RM, Eckel RH, Howard B, et al. AHA Scientific Statement: AHA Dietary guidelines Revision 2000: A statement for healthcare professionals from the nutrition committee of the American Heart Association. Circulation. 2000;102(18):2284-2299.

Kremer JM. N-3 fatty acid supplements in rheumatoid arthritis. Am J Clin Nutr. 2000;(suppl 1):349S-351S.

Kris-Etherton P, Eckel RH, Howard BV, St. Jeor S, Bazzare TL. AHA Science Advisory: Lyon Diet Heart Study. Benefits of a Mediterranean-style, National Cholesterol Education Program/American Heart Association Step I Dietary Pattern on Cardiovascular Disease. Circulation. 2001;103:1823.

Kromhout D, Geleijnse JM, de Goede J, et al. n-3 fatty acids, ventricular arrhythmia-related events, and fatal myocardial infarction in post-myocardial infarction patients with diabetes. Diabetes Care. 2011 Dec;34(12):2515-20.

Kruse LG, Ogletree RL. Omega-3 fatty acids and cardiovascular risk. J Miss State Med Assoc. 2013;54(6):156-7.

Kumar S, Sutherland F, Teh AW, et al. Effects of chronic omega-3 polyunsaturated fatty acid supplementation on human pulmonary vein and left atrial electrophysiology in paroxysmal atrial fibrillation. Am J Cardiol. 2011 Aug 15;108(4):531-5.

Kurz et al. Chronic oxidative stress compromises telomere integrity and accelerates the onset of senescence in human endothelial cells. J Cell Sci 2004. doi: 10.1242/jcs.01097.

Kwak SM, Myung SK, Lee YJ, Seo HG. Efficacy of omega-3 fatty acid supplements (eicosapentanoic acid and docosahexaenoic acid) in the secondary prevention of cariovascular disease: a meta-analysis of randomized, double-blind, placebo-controlled trials. Arch Intern Med. 2012;172(9):686-94.

Leach, Robert, DC. The Chiropractic Theories: A Synopsis of Scientific Research.

Lee JH, O'Keefe JH, Lavie CJ; Harris WS. Omega-3 fatty acids: cardiovascular benefits, sources and sustainability. Nat Rev Cardiol. 2009;6(12):753-8.

Leeb BF, et al. A meta-analysis of chondroitin sulfate in the treatment of osteoarthritis. J Rheumatol 2000 Jan;27(1):205-11.

Leemans J, Cambier C, Chandler T, et al. Prophylactic effects of omega-3 polyunsaturated fatty acids and luteolin on airway hyperresponsiveness and inflammation in cats with experimentally induced asthma. Vet J. 2010 Apr;184(1):111-4.

Leffler CT, et al. Glucosamine, chondroitin, and manganese ascorbate for degenerative joint disease of the knee or low back: a randomized, double-blind, placebo-controlled pilot study. Military Med 1999;164(2):85-91.

Levy BD, Bonnans C, Silverman ES, Palmer LJ, Marigowda G, Israel E. Diminished lipoxin biosynthesis in severe asthma. Am J Respir Crit Care Med. 2005 Oct 1;172(7):824-30.

Levy BD, De Sanctis GT, Devchand PR, et al. Multi-pronged inhibition of airway hyper-responsiveness and inflammation by lipoxin A(4). Nat Med. 2002 Sep;8(9):1018-23.

Levy BD, Kohli P, Gotlinger K, et al. Protectin D1 is generated in asthma and dampens airway inflammation and hyperresponsiveness. J Immunol. 2007 Jan 1;178(1):496-502.

Lewontin, Richard. Human Diversity. (New York: W. H. Freeman & Co.), 1982.

Lin J-H, Light D, McLean K, Andrews W, Young T, Morser J.

Lin J-H, Wang M, Andrews WH, Wydro R, Morser J.

Lin JH, McLean K, Morser J, Young TA, Wydro RM, Andrews WH, Light DR.

Lin PY, Chiu CC, Huang SY, Su KP. A meta-analytic review of polyunsaturated fatty acid compositions in dementia. J Clin Psychiatry. 2012;73(9):1245-54.

Linskens MH, Feng J, Andrews WH, Enlow BE, Saati SM, Tonkin LA, Funk WD, Villeponteau B.

Lipski, Elizabeth. Digestive Wellness. (New Canaan, CT: Keats Publishing), 1996.

Liu, Q., et al, "Effects of sodium selenite on telomerase activity and telomere length," Sheng Wu Hua Xue Yu Sheng Wu Wu Li Xue Bao (Shanghai) Dec Dec. 2003;35(12):1117-22.

Lopez-Alarcon M, Martinez-Coronado A, Velarde-Castro O, Rendon-Macias E, Fernandez J. Supplementation of n3 long-chain polyunsaturated fatty acid synergistically decreases insulin resistance with weight loss of obese prepubertal and pubertal children. Arch Med Res. 2011 Aug;42(6):502-8.

Lopez, D. A., Williams, R. M., and Miehlke, K. Enzymes: The Fountain of Life. (Charleston, SC: The Neville Press), 1994.

Lorente-Cebrian S, Costa AG, Navas-Carretero S, Zabala M, Martinez JA, Moreno-Aliaga MJ. Role of omega-3 fatty acids in obesity, metabolic syndrome, and cardiovascular diseases: a review of the evidence. J Physiol Biochem. 2013;69(3):633-51.

Lukiw WJ, Cui JG, Marcheselli VL, et al. A role for docosahexaenoic acid-derived neuroprotectin D1 in neural cell survival and Alzheimer disease. J Clin Invest. 2005 Oct;115(10):2774-83.

Macsai MS. The role of omega-3 dietary supplementation in blepharitis and meibomian gland dysfunction (an AOS thesis). Trans Am Ophthalmol Soc. 2008;106:336-56.

Mangano KM, Walsh SJ, Insogna KL, Kenny AM, Kerstetter JE. Calcium Intake in the United States from Dietary and Supplemental Sources across Adult Age Groups: New Estimates from the National Health and Nutrition Examination Survey 2003-2006. J Am Diet Assoc 2011;111:687-95.

Manson JE, Greenland P, LaCroix AZ, et al. Walking compared with vigorous exercise for the prevention of cardiovascular events in women N Engl J Med 2002;347:716-725.[CrossRef][Web of Science][Medline]

Matsuyama W, Mitsuyama H, Watanabe M, et al. Effects of omega-3 poly-unsaturated fatty acids on inflammatory markers in COPD. Chest. 2005 Dec;128(6):3817-27.

Mattar M, Obeid O. Fish oil and the management of hypertriglyceridemia. Nutr Health. 2009;20(1):41-9. Review.

McCaman, M. T., W. H. Andrews, and J. G. Files

McGee, C. T. How to Survive Modern Technology. (New Canaan, CT: Keats Publishers), 1979.

McTaggart, Lynne. What Doctor's Don't Tell You. (San Francisco, CA: Thorsons/Harper Collins), 1996.

Mead, Nathaniel. "Don't Drink Your Milk," Natural Health, July/August, 1994, 70.

Melvin, W.J.S., MD. President of Ontario Medical Association.

Mendelsohn, R. S. Confessions of a Medical Heretic. (Chicago, IL: Contempoary Books), 1979.

Mennell, John, MD. "The Science and Art of Joint Manipulation."

Merched AJ, Ko K, Gotlinger KH, Serhan CN, Chan L. Atherosclerosis: evidence for impairment of resolution of vascular inflammation governed by specific lipid mediators. FASEB J. 2008 Oct;22(10):3595-606.

Micke P et al. Eur J Clin Invest 2001 Feb;32(2):171-8. doi: 10.1046/j.1365-2362.2001.00781

Mickleborough TD, Lindley MR, Ionescu AA, Fly AD. Protective effect of fish oil supplementation on exercise-induced bronchoconstriction in asthma. Chest. 2006 Jan;129(1):39-49.

Mickleborough TD, Murray RL, Ionescu AA, Lindley MR. Fish oil supplementation reduces severity of exercise-induced bronchoconstriction in elite athletes. Am J Respir Crit Care Med. 2003 Nov 15;168(10):1181-9.

Mitchell EA, Aman MG, Turbott SH, Manku M. Clinical characteristics and serum essential fatty acid levels in hyperactive children. Clin Pediatr (Phila). 1987;26:406-411.

Modulation of Glycosaminoglycan Addition in Naturally Expressed and Recombinant Human Thrombomodulin.

Moertl D, Hammer A, Steiner S, Hutuleac R, Vonbank K, Berger R. Dose-dependent effects of omega-3-polyunsaturated fatty acids on systolic left ventricular function, endothelial function, and markers of inflammation in chronic heart failure of nonischemic origin: a double-blind, placebo-controlled, 3-arm study. Am Heart J. 2011 May;161(5):915 e1-9.

Mol Biochem Parasitol 28, 235-248 (1988)

Mol Biol Cell 3, 66A (1992)

Molecules with Both Fibrinolytic and Antithrombotic Activities.

Montori V, Farmer A, Wollan PC, Dinneen SF. Fish oil supplementation in type 2 diabetes: a quantitative systematic review. Diabetes Care. 2000;23:1407-1415.

Mori TA. Omega-3 fatty acids and blood pressure. Cell Mol Biol (Nosiy-legrand). 2010;56(1):83-92.

Morreale P, et al. Comparison of the anti-inflammatory efficacy of chondroitin sulfate and diclofenac sodium in patients with knee osteoarthritis. J Rheumatol 1996;23:1385-91.

Morser J, Aguilera M, Andrews WH, Blasko E, Clarke J, Kuhn I, Light D, McLean K, Vilander L.

Moser, B.A., Chang, Y.-T., Kosti, J. and Nakamura, T.M. (2011)

Moser, B.A., Subramanian, L., Chang, Y.-T., Noguchi, C., Noguchi, E. and Nakamura, T.M. (2009)

Moser, B.A., Subramanian, L., Khair, L., Chang, Y.-T. and Nakamura, T.M. (2009)

Mozaffarian D et al. Changes in Diet and Lifestyle and Long-Term Weight Gain in Women and Men. N Engl J Med 2011; 364(25): 2392-404.

Mozaffarian D, Geelen A, Brouwer IA et al. Effect of Fish Oil on Heart Rate in Humans. A Meta-Analysis of Randomized Controlled Trials. Circulation. 2005;112(13):1945-52.

Mozaffarian D, Lemaitre RN, King IB, et al. Circulating long-chain omega-3 fatty acids and incidence of congestive heart failure in older adults: the cardiovascular health study: a cohort study. Ann Intern Med. 2011 Aug 2;155(3):160-70.

Mozzaffarian D, Marchioli R, Macchia A, et al. Fish oil postoperative atrial fibrillation: the Omega-3 Fatty Acids for Prevention of Post-operative Atrial Fibrillation (OPERA) randomized trial. JAMA. 2012;308(19):2001-11.

Mozzaffarian D, Wu JH. Omega-3 fatty acids and cardiovascular disease: effects on risk factors, molecular pathways, and clinical events. J Am Coll Cardiol. 2011;58(20):2047-67.

Muir, Maya, Antibiotics Resistance, Alternative Complimentary Therapies, vol.2, no. 3, May/June 1996, p. 141.

Müller HJ. (1938) The remaking of chromosomes. Collecting Net 13: 181-198.

McClintock B. (1941) The stability of broken ends of chromosomes in Zea mays. Genetics 26: 234-282.

Mumcuoglu, Madeleine, Sambucus, Black Elderberry Extract, RSS Publishing, Inc.

Murphy RA, Mourtzakis M, Chu QS, Baracos VE, Reiman T, Mazurak VC. Nutritional intervention with fish oil provides a benefit over standard of care for weight and skeletal muscle mass in patients with nonsmall cell lung cancer receiving chemotherapy. Cancer. 2011 Apr 15;117(8):1775-82.

Murphy RA, Mourtzakis M, Chu QS, Baracos VE, Reiman T, Mazurak VC. Supplementation with fish oil increases first-line chemotherapy efficacy in patients with advanced nonsmall cell lung cancer. Cancer. 2011 Aug 15;117(16):3774-80.

Murphy, Suzanne et al. "Demographic and economic factors associated with dietary quality for adults in the 1987–88 Nationwide Food Consumption Survey." Journal of the American Dietetic Association, Vol. 92, No. 11, November 1992.

N.S. Heiss et al., "X-linked dyskeratosis congenita is caused by mutations in a highly conserved gene with putative nucleolar functions," Nat Genet, 19:32-38, 1998.

Nagakura T, Matsuda S, Shichijyo K, Sugimoto H, Hata K. Dietary supplementation with fish oil rich in omega-3 polyunsaturated fatty acids in children with bronchial asthma. Eur Resp J. 2000;16(5):861-865.

Nakamura TM, Morin GB, Chapman KB, Weinrich SL, Andrews WH, Lingner J, Harley CB, Cech TR.

Naqvi AZ, Buettner C, Phillips RS, Davis RB, Mukamal KJ. n-3 fatty acids and periodontitis in US adults. J Am Diet Assoc. 2010 Nov;110(11):1669-75.

Nat. Struct. Mol. Biol. 18: 1408-1413. (doi:10.1038/nsmb.2187)

Nature 467(7312): 223-227. (doi:10.1038/nature09374)

Nature 467(7312): 228-232. (doi:10.1038/nature09353)

Nature Genetics 17, 498-502 (1997)

Nelson, William. The Real Truth About Health.

Neu, H.C., Science, 1992, p. 257, 1064-1073

New England Journal of Medicine, "Iatrogenic Illness on a General Medical Service at a University Hospital" (304–11) Mar. 12, 1981: 638-642.

Newcomer LM, King IB, Wicklund KG, Stanford JL. The association of fatty acids with prostate cancer risk. Prostate. 2001;47(4):262-268.

Nodari S, Triggiani M, Campia U, et al. n-3 polyunsaturated fatty acids in the prevention of atrial fibrillation recurrences after electrical cardioversion: a prospective, randomized study. Circulation. 2011 Sep 6;124(10):1100-6.

Noori N, Dukkipati R, Kovesday CP, et al. Dietary omega-3 fatty acid, ratio of omega-6 to omega-3 intake, inflammation, and survival in long-term hemodialysis patients. Am J Kidney Dis. 2011;58(2):248-56.

Norris PC, Dennis EA. Omega-3 fatty acids cause dramatic changes in TLR4 and purinergic eicosanoid signaling. Proc Natl Acad Sci U S A. 2012 May 29;109(22):8517-22.

Nucleic Acids Research 23, 3244-3251 (1995).

Null, Gary. Get Healthy Now. (New York: Seven Stories Press), 1999.

O.T. Njajou et al., "Association between telomere length, specific causes of death, and years of healthy life in health, aging, and body composition, a population-based cohort study," J Gerontol A Biol Sci Med Sci, 64:860-64, 2009.

O'Brien. 2011. "Exercise May Prevent Impact of Stress on Telomeres, A Measure of Cell Health." University of California, San Francisco (UCSF). April 4, 2011.

Oh H, Taffet GE, Youker KA, et al. Telomerase reverse transcriptase promotes cardiac muscle cell proliferation, hypertrophy, and survival Proc Natl Acad Sci U S A 2001;98:10308-10313.[Abstract/Free Full Text]

Okamoto M, Misunobu F, Ashida K, et al. Effects of dietary supplementation with n-3 fatty acids compared with n-6 fatty acids on bronchial asthma. Int Med. 2000;39(2):107-111.

Olovnikov AM. (1971) Principle of marginotomy in template synthesis of polynucleotides. Doklady Akademii nauk SSSR. 201(6):1946-9. Watson, J. D. (1972) Origin of concatemeric T7 DNA. Nat New Biol. 239(94): 197-201.

Olsen SF, Osterdal ML, Salvig JD, et al. Fish oil intake compared with olive oil intake in late pregnancy and asthma in the offspring: 16 y of registry-based follow-up from a randomized controlled trial. Am J Clin Nutr. 2008 Jul;88(1):167-75.

Olsen SF, Secher NJ. Low consumption of seafood in early pregnancy as a risk factor for preterm delivery: prospective cohort study. BMJ. 2002;324(7335):447-451.

Ornstein, Robert and Sobel, David. The Healing Brain. (New York: Simon & Schuster), 1987.

Orr SK, Bazinet RP. The emerging role of docosahexaenoic acid in neuroinflammation. Curr Opin Investig Drugs. 2008 Jul;9(7):735-43.

Oski, Frank. Don't Drink Your Milk. (Brushton, NY: TEACH Services), 1983.

Ott, John. Health and Light. (Columbus, OH: Ariel Press), 1976[...]"

Oxidation of a specific methionine in thrombomodulin by activated neutrophil products blocks cofactor activity. A potential rapid mechanism for modulation of coagulation.

P. Scheinberg et al., "Association of telomere length of peripheral blood leukocytes with hematopoietic relapse, malignant transformation, and survival in severe aplastic anemia," JAMA, 304:1358-64, 2010.

Palacios-Pelaez R, Lukiw WJ, Bazan NG. Omega-3 essential fatty acids modulate initiation and progression of neurodegenerative disease. Mol Neurobiol. 2010 Jun;41(2-3):367-74.

Paniagua JA, Perez-Martinez P, Gjelstad IM, et al. A low-fat high-carbohydrate diet supplemented with long-chain n-3 PUFA reduces the risk of the metabolic syndrome. Atherosclerosis. 2011 Oct;218(2):443-50.

Parcell S. Sulfur in human nutrition and applications in medicine. Altern Med Rev 2002 Feb;7(1):22-44. Davies JR, Chang YM, Snowden H et al. The determinants of serum vitamin D levels in participants in a melanoma case-control study living in a temperate climate. Cancer Causes Control 2011;22(10):1471-82. doi: 10.1007/s10552-011-9827-3

Park Y,Subar AF, Hollenbeck A, Schatzkin A. Dietary Fiber Intake and Mortality in the NIH-AARP Diet and Health Study. Arch Intern Med. 2011 Jun 27;171(12):1061-8. Epub 2011 Feb 14. doi: 10.1001/archinternmed.2011.18.

Parker HM, Johnson NA, Burdon CA, Cohn JS, O'Connor HT, George J. Omega-3 supplementation and non-alcoholic fatty liver disease: a systematic review and meta-analysis. J Hepatol. 2012 Apr;56(4):944-51.

Patterson RE, Flatt SW, Newman VA, et al. Marine fatty acid intake is associated with breast cancer prognosis. J Nutr. 2011 Feb;141(2):201-6.

Paul, L., et al, "Telomere Length in Peripheral Blood Mononuclear Cells Is Associated with Folate Status in Men," J. Nutr. July 2009:139(7);1273-1278.

Pauwels EK, Kostkiewicz M. Fatty acid facts, Part III: Cardiovascular disease, or, a fish diet is not fishy. Drug News Perspect. 2008 Dec;21(10):552-61.

Peat JK, Mihrshahi S, Kemp AS, et al. Three-year outcomes of dietary fatty acid modification and house dust mite reduction in the Childhood Asthma Prevention Study. J Allergy Clin Immunol. 2004 Oct;114(4):807-13.

Pedersen MH, Molgaard C, Hellgren LI, Lauritzen L. Effects of fish oil supplementation on markers of the metabolic syndrome. J Pediatr. 2010 Sep;157(3):395-400.

Perez DH, Vilander L, Andrews WH, Holmes R.

Perez HD, Holmes R, Kelly E, McClary J, Andrews WH.

Perez HD, Holmes R, Kelly E, McClary J, Andrews WH.

Perez HD, Holmes R, Kelly E, McClary J, Chou Q, Andrews WH.

Perez HD, Holmes R, Vilander LR, Adams RR, Manzana W, Jolley D, Andrews WH. Plasmid 8, 148-163 (1982)

PLoS Genet. 5(8): e1000622. (doi:10.1371/journal.pgen.1000622)

Proc Natl Acad Sci U S A. (submitted for publication 12/30/2011, accepted 2/2/2012).

Proc Natl Acad Sci USA. 107(31):13842-7 (2010).

Proceedings of the American Association for Cancer Research 36, 672 (1995).

Proceedings of the American Association for Cancer Research 36, 671-672. (1995)

R.M. Cawthon et al., "Association between telomere length in blood and mortality in people aged 60 years or older," Lancet, 361:393-95, 2003.